EAT THIS NOT THAT!® 2010

The No-Diet Weight Loss Solution
Completely Updated and Expanded

BY DAVID ZINCZENKO
WITH MATT GOULDING

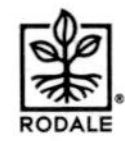

Notice

This book is intended as a reference volume only, not as a medical manual.
The information given here is designed to help you make informed decisions about your health.
It is not intended as a substitute for any treatment that may have been prescribed by your doctor.
If you suspect that you have a medical problem, we urge you to seek competent medical help.

Mention of specific companies, organizations, or authorities in this book does not imply endorsement by the author or publisher, nor does mention of specific companies, organizations, or authorities imply that they endorse this book, its author, or the publisher.

Internet addresses and telephone numbers given in this book were accurate at the time it went to press.

Rodale books may be purchased for business or promotional use or for special sales. For information, please write to: Special Markets Department, Rodale Inc., 733 Third Avenue, New York, NY 10017

Printed in the United States of America

Rodale Inc. makes every effort to use acid-free ♾, recycled paper ♻

Book design by George Karabotsos

Cover photographs by Jeff Harris.
Food styling by Ed Gabriels for Halley Resources. Hand model: Ashly Covington

All interior photos by Mitch Mandel and Thomas MacDonald/Rodale Images with the exception of the following: pages 47, 48, 275–280 ©Jeff Harris; pages 80, 81, 116, 117 ©Michael LoBiondo; pages 92–95, 120–125 ©Orly Catz; pages 170, 171 ©Shawn Taylor
Rodale Images food styling by Melissa Reiss with the exception of pages 301, 306, 318 by Diane Simone Vezza

Library of Congress Cataloging-in-Publication Data is on file with the publisher

ISBN-10: 1-60529-538-8 paperback

ISBN-13: 978-1-60529-538-1 paperback

Distributed to the trade by Macmillan

2 4 6 8 10 9 7 5 3 1 paperback

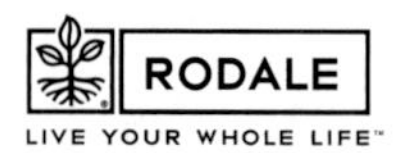

We inspire and enable people to improve their lives and the world around them

For more of our products visit **rodalestore.com** or call 800-848-4735

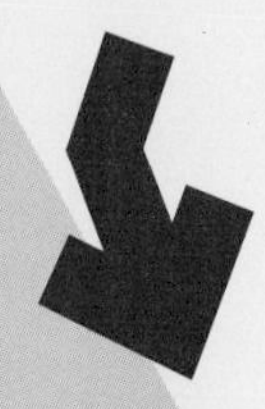

EAT THIS NOT THAT! 2010

DEDICATION

To the five million men and women who have made ***EAT THIS, NOT THAT!*** a publishing phenomenon and who have spread the word to friends and relatives about the importance of knowing what's really in our food. Because of your passionate efforts, food manufacturers and restaurant chains have woken up to the fact that more and more of us demand good, solid information about our food and healthy choices that will let us drop pounds and stay lean for life.

And to the men and women working in America's fields, farms, and supermarkets, waiting tables, and toiling in kitchens everywhere: It is because of your hard work that Americans have so many options. This book is designed to help us choose the best of what you've created.

—Dave and Matt

ACKNOWLEDGMENTS

This book is the product of thousands of meals, hundreds of conversations with nutritionists and industry experts, and the collective smarts, dedication, and raw talent of dozens of individuals. Our undying thanks to all of you who have inspired this project in any way. In particular:

To Steve Murphy and the Rodale family, whose dedication to improving the lives of their readers is apparent in every book and magazine they put their name on.

To George Karabotsos and his crew of immensely talented designers, including Laura White, Mark Michaelson, Emily Kehe, Elizabeth Neal, John Gilman, and Rob Campos. You're the reason why each book looks better than the last.

To our crack team of researchers, including Clint Carter, Carolyn Kylstra, Anna Maltby, and Sophie Fitzgerald: Your relentless pursuit of the truth about our food is what makes these books vital.

To Tara Long, who spends more time in the drive-thru and the supermarket aisles than anyone on the planet, all in the name of making us look good.

To the Rodale book team: Steve Perrine, Karen Rinaldi, Chris Krogermeier, Debbie McHugh, Nancy Bailey, Sara Cox, Mitch Mandel, Tom MacDonald, Troy Schnyder, Melissa Reiss, Nikki Weber, Jennifer Giandomenico, Wendy Gable, Keith Biery, Liz Krenos, Brooke Myers, Marc Sirinsky, Sean Sabo, and Caroline McCall. You continue to do whatever it takes to get these books done. We appreciate your heroic efforts.

Special thanks to Allison Falkenberry and Brett LeVecchio, whose talent and dedication help millions of Americans learn how to eat better.

—Dave and Matt

Check out the other informative books in the ***EAT THIS, NOT THAT!***® series:

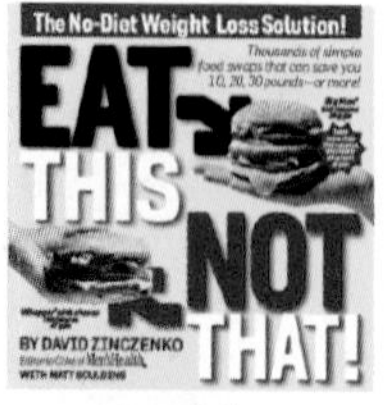

***Eat This, Not That!* (2007)**

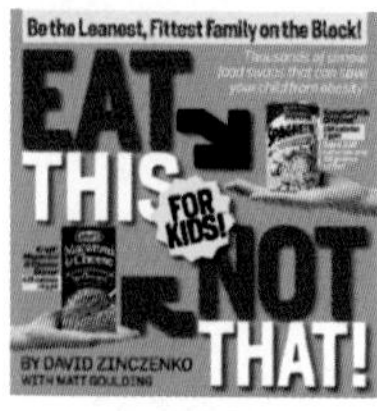

***Eat This, Not That! for Kids!* (2008)**

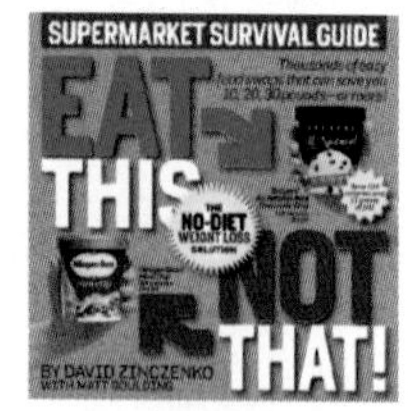

***Eat This, Not That! Supermarket Survival Guide* (2009)**

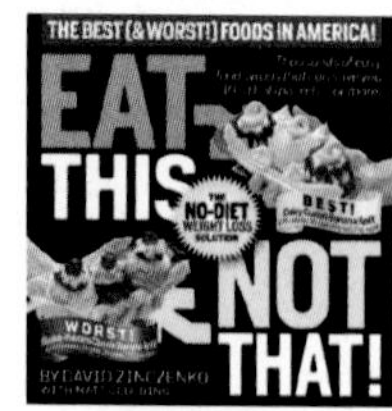

***Eat This, Not That! The Best (& Worst!) Foods in America!* (2009)**

CONTENTS

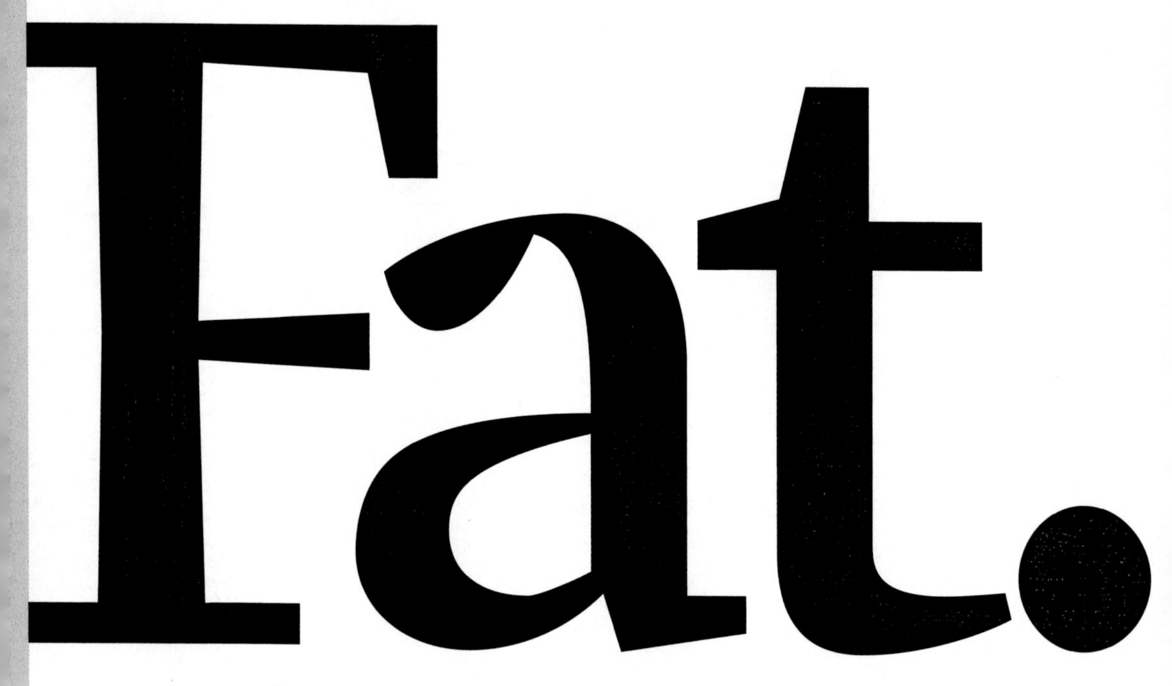

It's all around us.

Fat cells? They encase our internal organs, form a ring around our gut, spin through our circulatory system, and follow our butt wherever we go. Our bodily fat surrounds us, no matter how hard we try to wriggle free.

Fat people? Every trip to the market or the mall is a Close Encounter of the Wider Kind. Sixty-six percent of adult Americans are overweight or obese, and by 2030 that number is expected to approach 87 percent!

Fat food? Every aisle of the grocery store, even the ones that used to be healthy like the produce and dairy sections, has become loaded with new products that hide extra calories within, like little dietary suicide bombers that explode your gut when you eat them.

And yet even if you lost every bit of fat in your body (something you wouldn't want to do, by the way, since 70 percent of the protective coating in your brain is fat); even if you never left your house; even if you ate nothing but lentils and couscous for the rest of your life, you still couldn't escape the fat. Because, eventually, you'd probably turn on the TV.

And that's where fat is born.

The top 44 food and beverage marketers spent an estimated $1.6 billion in 2006, just promoting food and drink products to kids and adolescents under the age of 17. (And when was the last time a kids' program carried an ad for apples, spinach, or blueberries?) Add on top of that the pitches for your local fast-food joint, the pizza come-ons, the never-ending advertising assault criticizing you for not drinking the right sports beverage or eating at the right chain restaurant and you've got an electronic fat-delivery system, shooting straight into your eyeballs, trying to lure you into investing your hard-earned cash in what?

More fat.

We are so overwhelmed with teases, temptations, and twisted truths that it's hard to know what to eat anymore.

And that's why we created *EAT THIS, NOT THAT!*

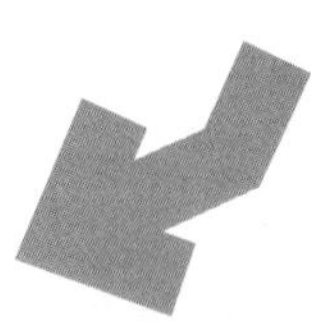

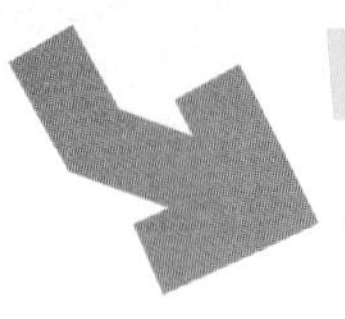

A Weight-Loss Coach in Your Pocket

EAT THIS, NOT THAT! isn't a typical book.

Sure, it's packed with intensely researched, passionately written, life-altering advice. It's filled with great images that convey massive amounts of useful information. And it's dense with hidden extras about your body and the foods that help it—and harm it. But a typical book is to be read, absorbed, and placed on your bookshelf for possible future reference. And that's not what **EAT THIS, NOT THAT!** is designed for. Sure, I want you to read this book. But more important, I want you to *use* it!

See, this book is designed to go with you, on whatever food adventure you might be headed on—and let's face it, in America today every day is a food adventure. Whether you're doing the mall, hitting the supermarket, or just driving around in your car, food advertising messages are everywhere, and so are the products they tout. And the last thing you want to do is deny yourself when you're craving a bite or feel like you have to go hungry rather than give in to temptation.

In fact, **EAT THIS, NOT THAT!** is a practical guidebook to giving in to temptation. We'll just show you how to do it smartly, no matter where you are. For example:

> ***Let's say you're shopping at the mall.*** You pass by the food court, the aromatic allure of hot, cinnamon-dusted baked goods in the air. On one side, Auntie Anne's is selling those delicious Cinnamon Sugar Pretzels. On the other, Cinnabon's Caramel Pecanbon beckons. Which way do you head? The amazing truth: If you pick the Cinnabon over the Auntie Anne's, you'll nosh down an additional 630 calories—almost a third of your whole day's allotment! (Make that wrong choice just twice a month and you'll pack on almost 5 pounds of body fat in a year!)

> ***Or maybe you stop at the gas station*** to fill up your car's tank and you notice your own tank is feeling a little empty. You could grab a 100 Grand bar

to fix your nutty chocolate jones or pick the old standby Snickers. But pick the wrong one and you'll be choking down almost an extra 100 calories and nearly twice the fat! (Hint: The right choice is grand, and the wrong choice might make people snicker at you.)

> ***Or perhaps it's up to you to do the family shopping this week.*** Frozen dinners are always convenient, so you wipe the fog from the glass and stare in at two similar dishes—Marie Callender's Oven Baked Chicken meal and Stouffer's White Meat Chicken Pot Pie. Would you believe the right choice will save you 840 calories and an entire day's worth of saturated fat? And by making it just once a week for a year, you'll save you and your family members more than 12 pounds of body fat. (They don't call it a "pot" belly for nothing!)

> ***Or maybe you're just driving around town*** and the kids are getting antsy in the backseat. To quell the clamor and calm your nerves, you decide to pull into Mickey D's for a snack. Child A orders the Vanilla Reduced-Fat Ice Cream Cone, and Child B wants the Chocolate Triple Thick Milkshake. Pretty similar, right? Well, you've just fed Child B 1,000 calories more than Child A—plus 150 extra grams of sugar. (To put that in context, a teaspoon of sugar is 4.2 grams. So Child B just got an extra 35½ teaspoons of sugar—as much as you'd find in 21 Cinnamon Twist dougnuts from Krispy Kreme! Makes you wonder how the next dentist appointment is going to go, huh?)

You make these kinds of decisions day in and day out, and you probably don't even realize it. Every time you choose one restaurant meal or bag of chips or fast-food hamburger over another, you're making a decision that will have a ripple effect—quite literally—on your body. And whether that body stays lean and healthy or begins to droop and drag depends on making more informed choices.

That's where this book comes in.

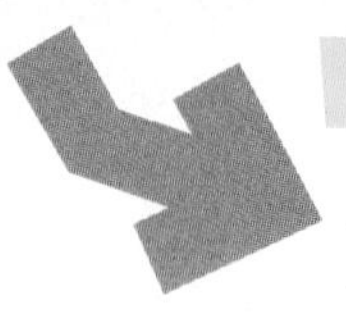

Smart Choices, Proven Results

As the editor-in-chief of *Men's Health* and the editorial director of *Women's Health*—along with my esteemed coauthor Matt—it's my job to scour the studies, interview the experts, test out the trends, and compile the newest, smartest, most authoritative information on weight loss available.

But even the most up-to-date diet advice only works when you have control over what, how, and when you're eating. And as you well know, most of the time you don't have that control.

Sure, you can cook your own dinner. You can brown-bag your own lunch. You can have a cup of yogurt in the morning and eat a healthy snack before bedtime. But you can't control what's being offered at the office cafeteria (unless you own the company) or what's being served at Mom's house for Thanksgiving (unless you're Mom). And you can't stand in the kitchen at Olive Garden or Burger King and tell the cook to go easier on the vegetable oil, either.

Yet there are few places to turn to for information. A handful of local municipalities—New York City, Seattle, and Portland, Oregon—have implemented legislation forcing restaurants to tell consumers what's in the food they're serving. But eat anywhere between the two coasts and you're entirely on your own. That's how T.G.I. Friday's can get away with serving potato skins that pack 2,270 calories; how Baskin-Robbins can serve a Chocolate Chip Cookie Dough Shake—a drink!—with a whopping 1,690 calories (that's three Big Macs!); and how P.F. Chang's can sell a bowl of Egg Drop Soup (as an appetizer) that contains nearly a full day's worth of sodium.

And it's not any better in the supermarket. Even though we're supposedly protected by labeling laws that force manufacturers to reveal calories and ingredients, what goes on the front of the box can be more than a little deceptive; that's how Quaker can make its Natural Granola, Oats & Honey & Raisins look healthy even though it has twice as much sugar as a bowl of Cocoa Pebbles!

But the tide has begun to turn, thanks to you: The popularity of the ***EAT THIS, NOT THAT!*** series has forced big food companies to stand up and take notice. In fact, since publishing ***EAT THIS, NOT THAT!***; ***EAT THIS, NOT THAT! FOR KIDS!***; and ***EAT THIS, NOT THAT! SUPERMARKET SURVIVAL GUIDE***, we've seen food industry giants snap to attention.

* After **CHILI'S AWESOME BLOSSOM** took the runner-up spot on our annual "Worst Foods in America" list, Chili's removed the calorie bomb from their menu entirely.

* **PEPPERIDGE FARM** followed suit after being placed on the Worst Foods list and discontinued their **ROASTED CHICKEN POT PIE**.

* When we released our list of the Worst Kids' Meals in America, **MACARONI GRILL** sprang into action and cut the calorie count of their **DOUBLE MACARONI 'N' CHEESE** dish in half, from 1,210 calories to just 670.

* When we put the spotlight on **BASKIN-ROBBINS' HEATH BAR SHAKE** as one of the most egregious calorie offenders (2,310 calories!), the drink was abolished from their menu.

* And when **JAMBA JUICE** earned a citation on our Worst Drinks in America list, they stopped serving the largest size of their **CHOCOLATE MOO'D** smoothie and wrote to inform us of their goal to become one of the healthiest restaurant chains in the nation.

Overall, 10 of the 20 items on our Worst Foods list in the original ***EAT THIS, NOT THAT!*** book either improved dramatically or disappeared entirely. And restaurants that had historically declined to provide nutritional information began posting calorie counts for the first time, including nationwide favorites Quiznos, Red Lobster, and Olive Garden. (In fact, Red Lobster's Restaurant Report Card grade jumped from an F, for failure to disclose, to an A-, thanks to a ton of low-calorie, high-protein entrées and healthy sides.)

But that's not all. One of the most encouraging trends we've seen since the first **EAT THIS, NOT THAT!** book was published is states and municipalities beefing up their nutrition laws. I mean, mention the phrase "nutrition laws" 5 years ago and you'd get nothing but puzzled stares or exclamations of "That'll be the day!" But it's happening.

★ In New York, a law was put into effect in July 2009, that required food-service establishments (ones that are part of a chain of 15 or more restaurants nationally) to list calories for their menu items on menu boards and food item display tags. The type size was even regulated—it has to be as large as the font used for the name or price!

★ In July 2007, in Seattle, the King County Board of Health voted on a new law requiring nutrition disclosure for chain restaurants. The law went into full effect on January 1, 2009—it requires chain restaurants with 15 or more national locations and $1 million in annual sales to display nutrition information. But Seattle went a step further than even NYC: They're requiring calories *plus* saturated fat, sodium, and carbohydrates.

★ Then the Portland, Oregon, area got wind of what was going on and passed its own menu labeling measure. They'll start fining noncompliant restaurants in January 2010—chains with 15 or more national locations who don't post calories and provide saturated fat, trans fat, carbohydrate, and sodium info upon request.

★ Other states and counties aren't far behind. Those with passed laws that have recently been implemented or will be soon include the state of California; Davidson County, Tennessee; Philadelphia; San Francisco City and County; Santa Clara County, California; Suffolk County, New York; and Ulster County, New York.

★ And that doesn't even scratch the surface of local and state governments that have introduced similar bills—those include New York's Albany and

Rockland Counties, Oregon's Lane County, and the states of Arizona, Connecticut, Georgia, Hawaii, Illinois, Indiana, Iowa, Kentucky, Louisianna, Maine, Maryland, Massachusetts, Missouri, New Jersey, New York, Ohio, Oregon, South Carolina, Tennessee, Texas, Vermont, Washington, and West Virginia.

That's a *lot* of impact. But we feel like we're forgetting something. What's that other huge, incredibly encouraging change we've seen since getting the ***EAT THIS, NOT THAT!*** franchise off the ground? Those great stories we hear every day that remind us why we're still so passionate about all this stuff?

Oh, *that's* right! It's all the weight you've lost! We're lucky enough to get countless e-mails, letters, Facebook messages, and even Tweets every single day about the insane success you've had using ***EAT THIS, NOT THAT!*** to lose weight. Here's just a tiny sample.

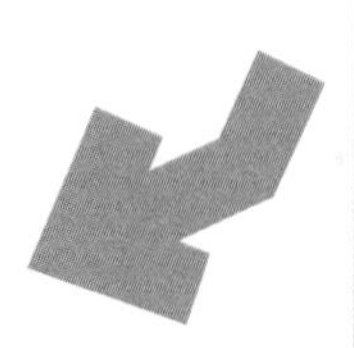

- **DARLENE COBURN** *lost 40 pounds* and dropped from a size 14 to a size 8 *in just 4 months*. "It's just so easy with these books," she says. "I now control my food instead of my food controlling me. I'm losing weight without even trying."

- **DUSTY ROBINSON AND HIS PARENTS** *lost a combined 70 pounds* in just 6 weeks—without ever feeling hungry. "We eat out all the time, and this is the fastest, cheapest, smartest plan I can imagine," he says. "It's really revitalized our family."

- **GINGER McNEELY FELICE** combined the books with exercise to *lose 70 pounds in just 8 months*. "*Eat This, Not That!* is written for lazy, lazy, lazy people like me!" she says. (We'll take issue with that a bit—after all, the busier you are, the more you need *Eat This, Not That!*) "It was so easy to understand. If it weren't for *ETNT*'s straightforward clarity about how food is made and packaged, I don't think my weight loss attempt would have worked."

▶ **KIRK ROBERTSON'S** health was at stake to the point where doctors told him he needed gastric bypass. "I knew the health risk involved, and I did not want to go through the surgery," he says. But once he started using *Eat This, Not That!* Kirk found hope and a healthy new body. "I weighed 330 pounds, and now I'm down to 181," he says. That's nearly ***150 pounds!***

But it's not all fireworks and confetti. While plenty of food companies have made the effort to make their foods a little healthier, many are still finding new ways to layer extra calories, fat, sodium, and other additives into our food. And new products are being introduced every day, on restaurant menus and grocery store shelves around the country. And if the mad food scientists aren't going to rest? Well, neither are we.

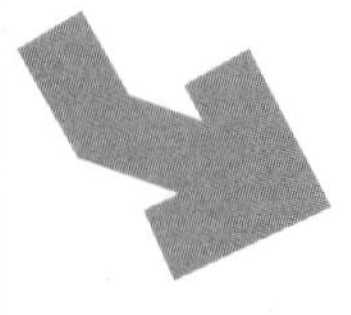

So here it is: a new volume with the most up-to-date information on the most current food offerings on the market. Whether you're shopping for the family dinner, swinging by the drive-thru for lunch, or taking the gang out to your favorite restaurant, **EAT THIS, NOT THAT!** is your secret weapon. Take it with you. Use it. And start reaping the benefits today!

For thousands of food comparisons and enough savvy, nutritional advice to help you lose 10, 20, or 30 pounds in two months, join the EAT THIS, NOT THAT! premium online service. Find out more at **EATTHIS.COM**

How to lose weight with this book

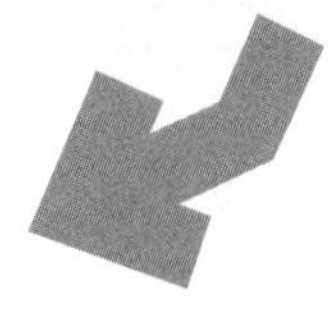

If you want to shed belly fat, there's only one formula you need to know, and luckily for you, it's easier than anything you encountered in ninth grade algebra.

The magic formula is this: Calories in – calories out = total weight loss or gain. This is the equation that determines whether your body will shape up to look more like a slender 1 or a paunchy 0, a flat-bellied yardstick or a pot-bellied protractor. That's why it's absolutely critical that you have some understanding of what sort of numbers you're plugging into this formula.

On the "calories out" side, we have your daily activities: cleaning house, standing in line at the post office, hauling in groceries, and so on. Oftentimes when people discover extra flab hanging around their midsections, they assume there's something wrong with this side of the equation. Maybe so, but more likely it's the front-end of the equation—the "calories in" side—that's tipping the scale. That side keeps track of all the cookies, fried chicken, and piles of pasta that you eat every day.

In order to maintain a healthy body weight, a moderately active female between the ages of 20 and 50 needs only 2,000 to 2,200 calories per day. A male fitting the same profile needs 2,400 to 2,600. Those numbers can fluctuate depending on whether you're taller or shorter than average or whether you spend more or less time exercising, but they represent reasonable estimations for most people. (For a more accurate assessment, use the calorie calculator at mayoclinic.com,)

Let's take a closer look at the numbers: It takes 3,500 calories to create a pound of body fat. So if you eat an extra 500 per day—the amount in one Dunkin' Donuts' Multigrain Bagel with Reduced Fat Cream Cheese—than you'll earn 1 new pound of body fat each week. Make that a habit—like so many of us do unwittingly—and you'll gain 52 pounds of flab per year!

That's where this book comes in. Within these pages are literally hundreds of simple food swaps that will save you from 10 to 1,000 calories or more apiece. The more often you choose "Eat This" foods over "Not That" options, the quicker you'll notice layers of fat melting away from your body. Check this out:

- A single cup of **CINNAMON TOAST CRUNCH** cereal has 173 calories. Switch to **CINNA-GRAHAM HONEY COMBS** five times per week and you'll drop 6 pounds this year.
- A **GRANDE JAVA CHIP FRAPPUCCINO** from Starbucks has 340 calories. Switch to an **ICED COFFEE WITH MOCHA SYRUP** three times per week and you'll shed 5 pounds in 6 months.
- **BANQUET'S FRIED CHICKEN FROZEN DINNER** has 380 calories. Make the switch to **SWANSON'S** version of the same meal three times per week and you'll drop an extra 1½ pounds every 3 months.
- A **CHICKEN FAJITA ROLLUP** from Applebee's packs in an astounding 1,450 calories. Instead order the **ITALIAN CHICKEN & PORTOBELLO SANDWICH** two times per week—or make a comparative swap at some other restaurant—and you'll blast away 5 pounds of body fat in just 2 months.

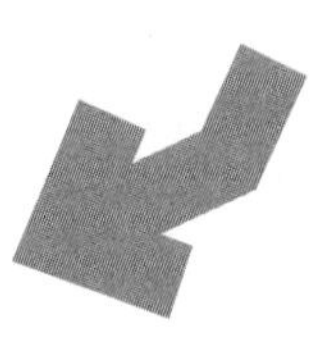

And here's best news of all: These swaps aren't isolated calorie savers. If you commit yourself to just the four on this list, the cumulative calorie-saving effect will stamp out one pound of body fat every week this year. Take that, multigrain bagel! Check out 12 more of our favorite calorie-squashing, fat-melting Top Swaps in the following pages.

Burgers

Save!
230 calories
and
19 g fat!

Eat This!
McDonald's Big Mac
540 calories
29 g fat
(10 g saturated, 1.5 g trans)
1,040 mg sodium

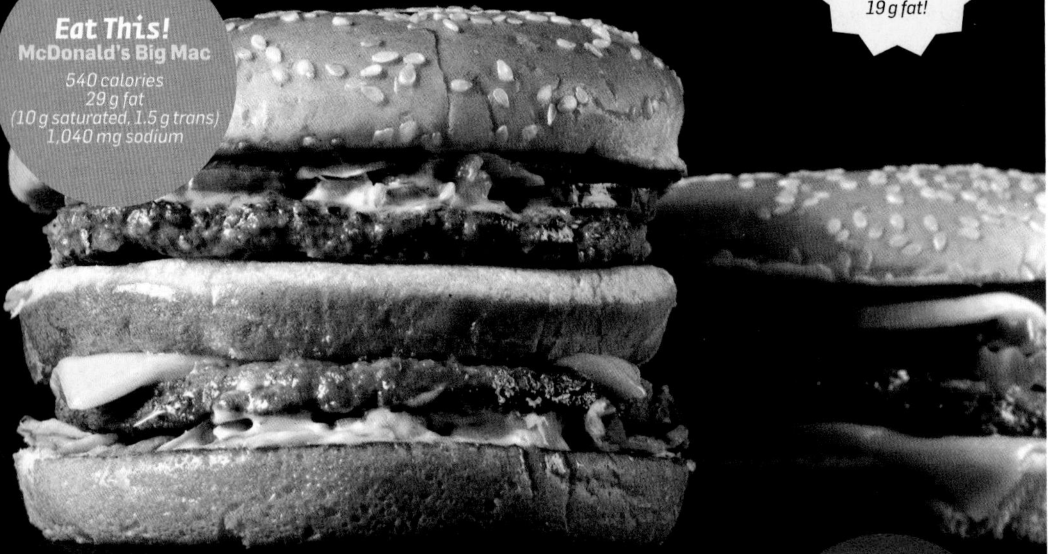

Not That!
Whopper with Cheese
770 calories
48 g fat
(16 g saturated, 1.5 g trans)
1,450 mg sodium

We love this iconic American showdown between the two biggest fast-food purveyors and their two most famous burgers. Despite the tri-bun and the special sauce, the Big Mac prevails by a respectable margin. Blame the Whopper's defeat on a massive bun and a 160-calorie sheen of mayo adorning the patty. (McDonald's may prevail, but both BK and Mickey D need to do something about the trans fat in their burgers...immediately.)

Sandwiches

Save!
620 calories and 56 g fat!

Eat This!
Subway 6" Double Roast Beef with Provolone Cheese
450 calories
11 g fat (4.5 g saturated)
1,535 mg sodium

Not That!
Quiznos Prime Rib Cheesesteak Sub (regular)
1,070 calories
67 g fat
(16.5 g saturated, 1.5 g trans)
1,835 mg sodium

Quiznos sandwiches all follow the same basic architectural formula: meat, heavy sauce, melted cheese. This bulky beef sandwich is no exception. In a mere 8", they manage to cram in a full day's worth of fat and 75 percent of your daily sodium allotment. Seek solace in Subway's 6" roast beef. Normally it doesn't have the heft to compare with Quiznos's regular-size sandwiches, but the double meat option is a genius way to up the protein for a tiny caloric cost. Plus, Subway has about a dozen different vegetables you can pile on your sandwich gratis. Take full advantage.

Iced Coffee

Drink This!
Dunkin' Donuts
Mocha Spice Iced Latte
(small; 16 oz)
220 calories
6 g fat (4 g saturated)
32 g sugars
Save!
250 calories
and
27 g sugars!
DUNKIN'
DONUTS
STARBUCKS
COFFEE
Not That!
Starbucks
Iced White Chocolate
Mocha with whip
(grande; 16 oz)
470 calories
18 g fat (12 g saturated)
59 g sugars

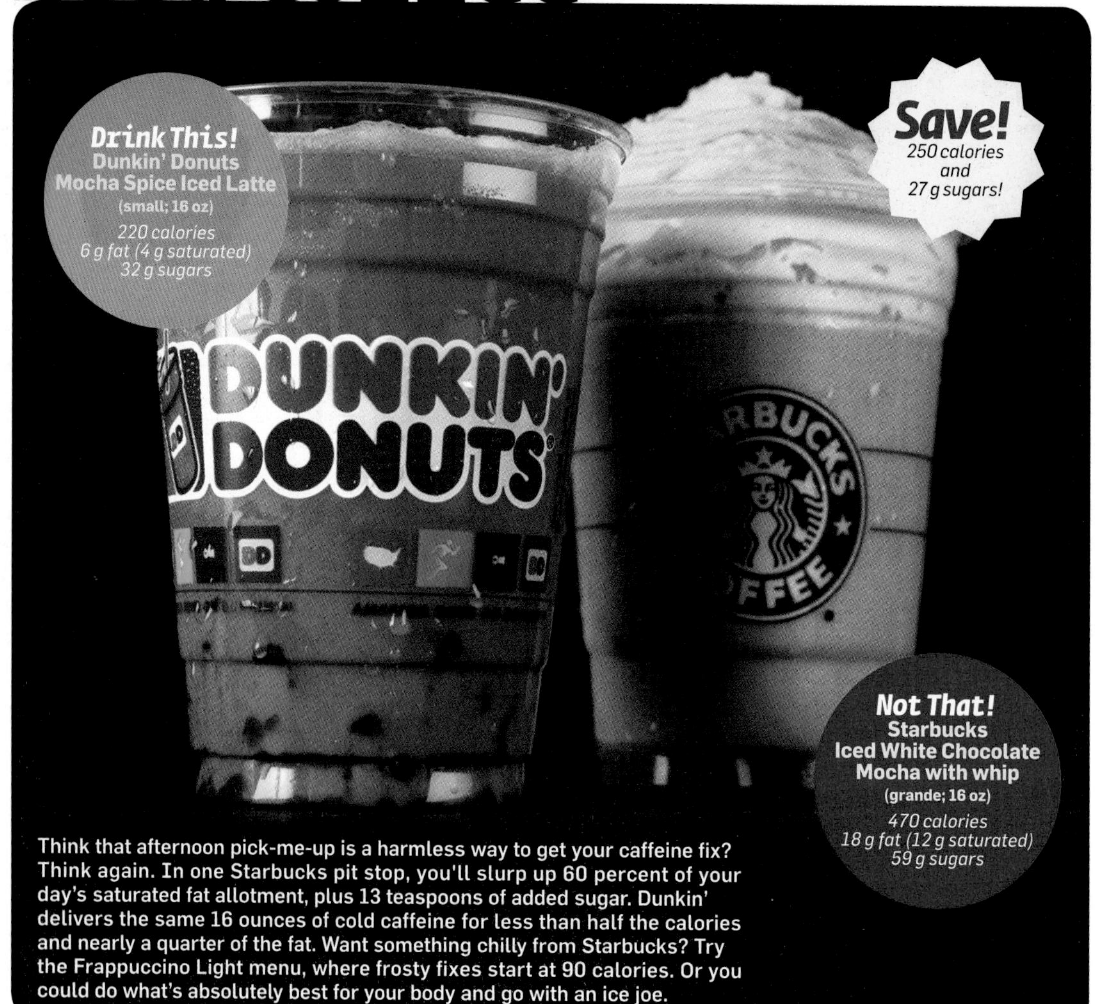

Think that afternoon pick-me-up is a harmless way to get your caffeine fix? Think again. In one Starbucks pit stop, you'll slurp up 60 percent of your day's saturated fat allotment, plus 13 teaspoons of added sugar. Dunkin' delivers the same 16 ounces of cold caffeine for less than half the calories and nearly a quarter of the fat. Want something chilly from Starbucks? Try the Frappuccino Light menu, where frosty fixes start at 90 calories. Or you could do what's absolutely best for your body and go with an ice joe.

Breakfast

Not That!
Panera Bacon, Egg & Cheese Grilled Breakfast Sandwich
510 calories
24 g fat
(10 g saturated, 0.5 g trans)
1,060 mg sodium

Eat This!
McDonald's Egg McMuffin
300 calories
12 g fat (5 g saturated)
820 mg sodium

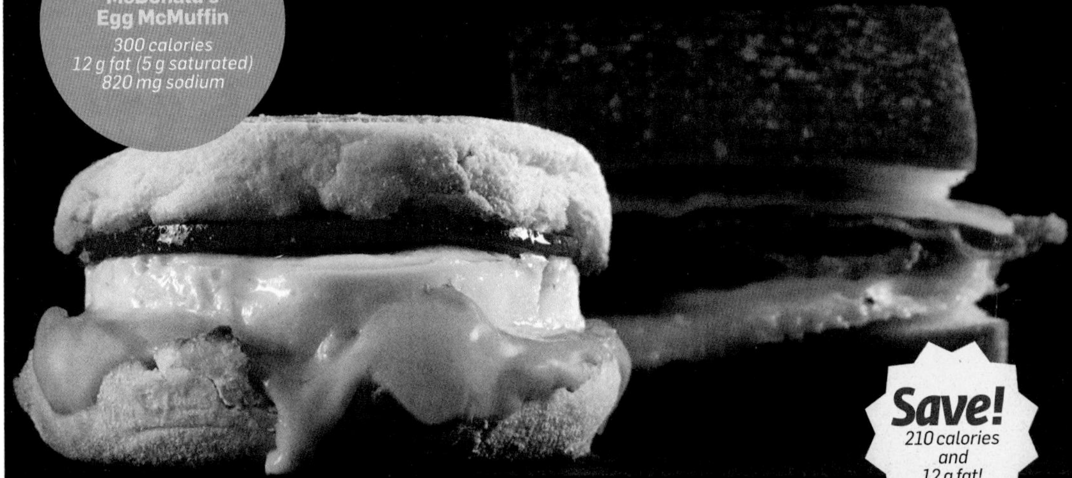

Save!
210 calories and 12 g fat!

What can we say, we have a soft spot for the Egg McMuffin. But our affection has been fully earned by this ubiquitous sandwich, which offers up 18 grams of protein—the nutritional equivalent of an alarm clock for your metabolism—for an impressively low caloric cost. Panera, on the other hand, serves up one lackluster piece of food after the next in the morning hours. The few dishes that aren't based on refined carbs, like this breakfast sandwich, are loaded down with excess fat and 4 digits' worth of sodium. Come back to Panera for lunch, but for breakfast head to the Golden Arches.

Frozen Dinner

Eat This!
Swanson Classics Boneless Fried Chicken with Mashed Potatoes and Carrots
240 calories
13 g fat (3 g saturated)
520 mg sodium

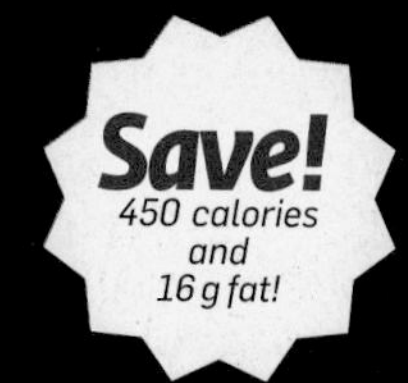

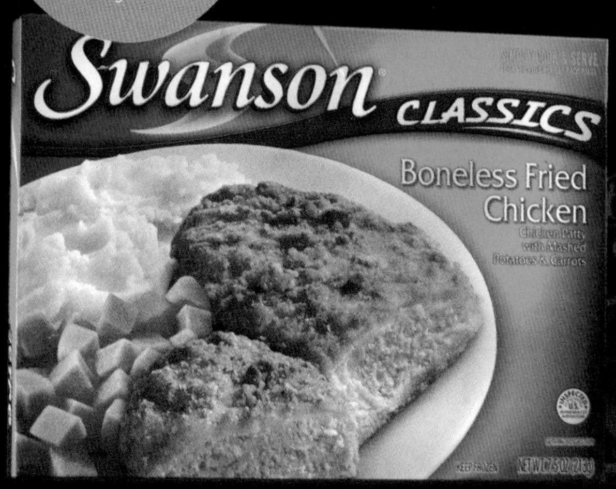

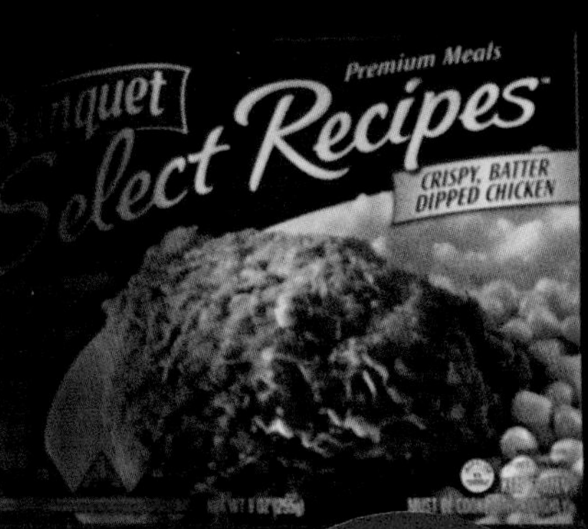

Not That!
Banquet Select Recipes Classic Fried Chicken Thigh with Mashed Potatoes and Corn
690 calories
29 g fat
(7 g saturated, 1.5 g trans)
950 mg sodium

Don't think that the supermarket is devoid of staggering mismatches. On the contrary, some of the easiest, most meaningful swaps you can make come in the most familiar aisles—especially in the freezer section. Here, fierce rivals Swanson and Banquet put out identical TV dinners with nutritional vitals that couldn't be less similar. Blame Banquet's slightly larger portion size, plus their reliance on a fattier cut of chicken. Beyond the caloric discrepancy, Banquet also brings nearly a full day of trans fat to the table by relying on partially hydrogenated oil to create this lackluster dish.

Italian Food

Save!
360 calories
and
51 g fat!
Not That!
Romano's
Macaroni Grill
Spaghetti and Meat
Sauce (dinner)
1,120 calories
69 g fat (33 g saturated)
2,290 mg sodium
Eat This!
Uno Chicago Grill
Penne Bolognese
760 calories
18 g fat (7 g saturated)
1,880 mg sodium

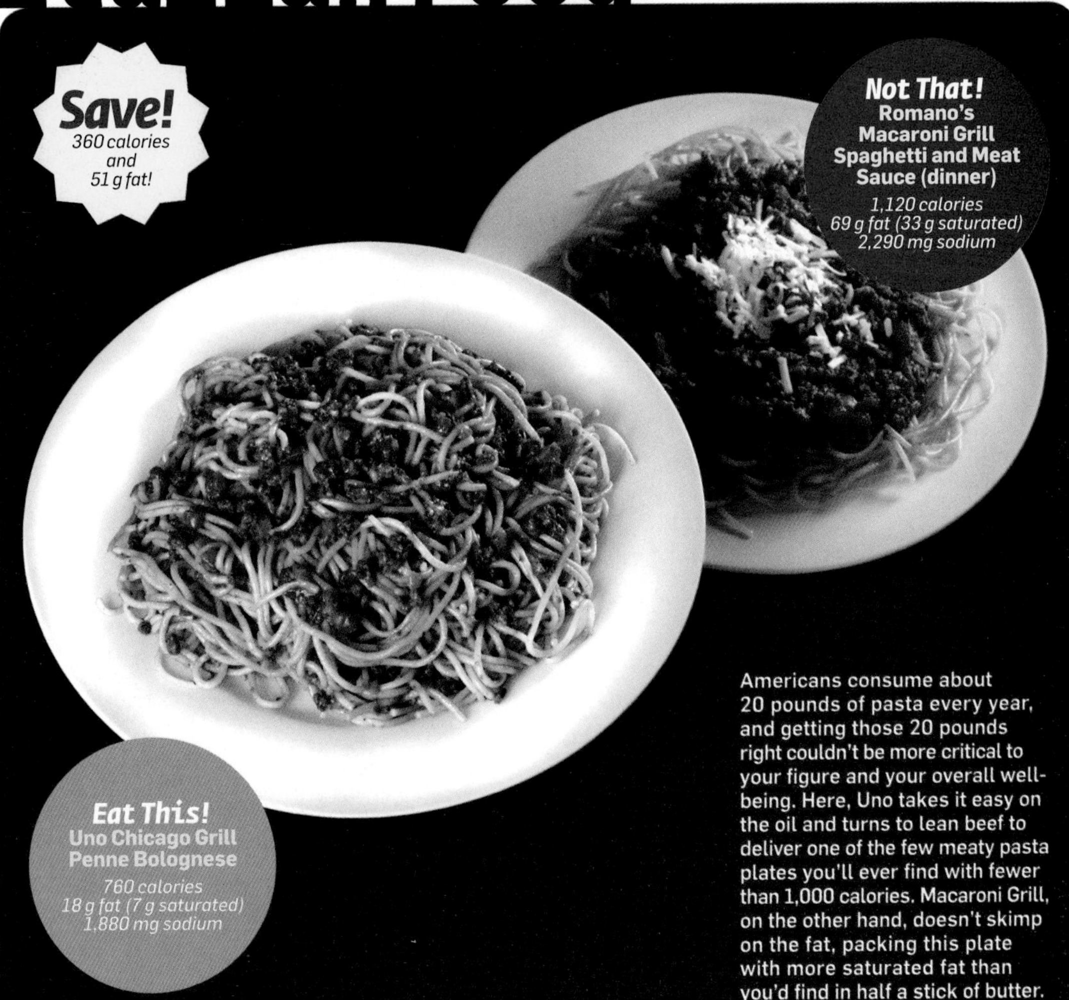

Americans consume about 20 pounds of pasta every year, and getting those 20 pounds right couldn't be more critical to your figure and your overall well-being. Here, Uno takes it easy on the oil and turns to lean beef to deliver one of the few meaty pasta plates you'll ever find with fewer than 1,000 calories. Macaroni Grill, on the other hand, doesn't skimp on the fat, packing this plate with more saturated fat than you'd find in half a stick of butter.

Mexican Food

Save!
1,660 calories
and
125 g fat!
Not That!
On the Border
Dos XX Fish Tacos
with Creamy
Red Chile Sauce (3)
2,350 calories
152 g fat (31 g saturated)
4,060 mg sodium
Eat This!
Baja Fresh
Grilled Mahi Mahi
Tacos (3)
690 calories
27 g fat (4.5 g saturated)
900 mg sodium

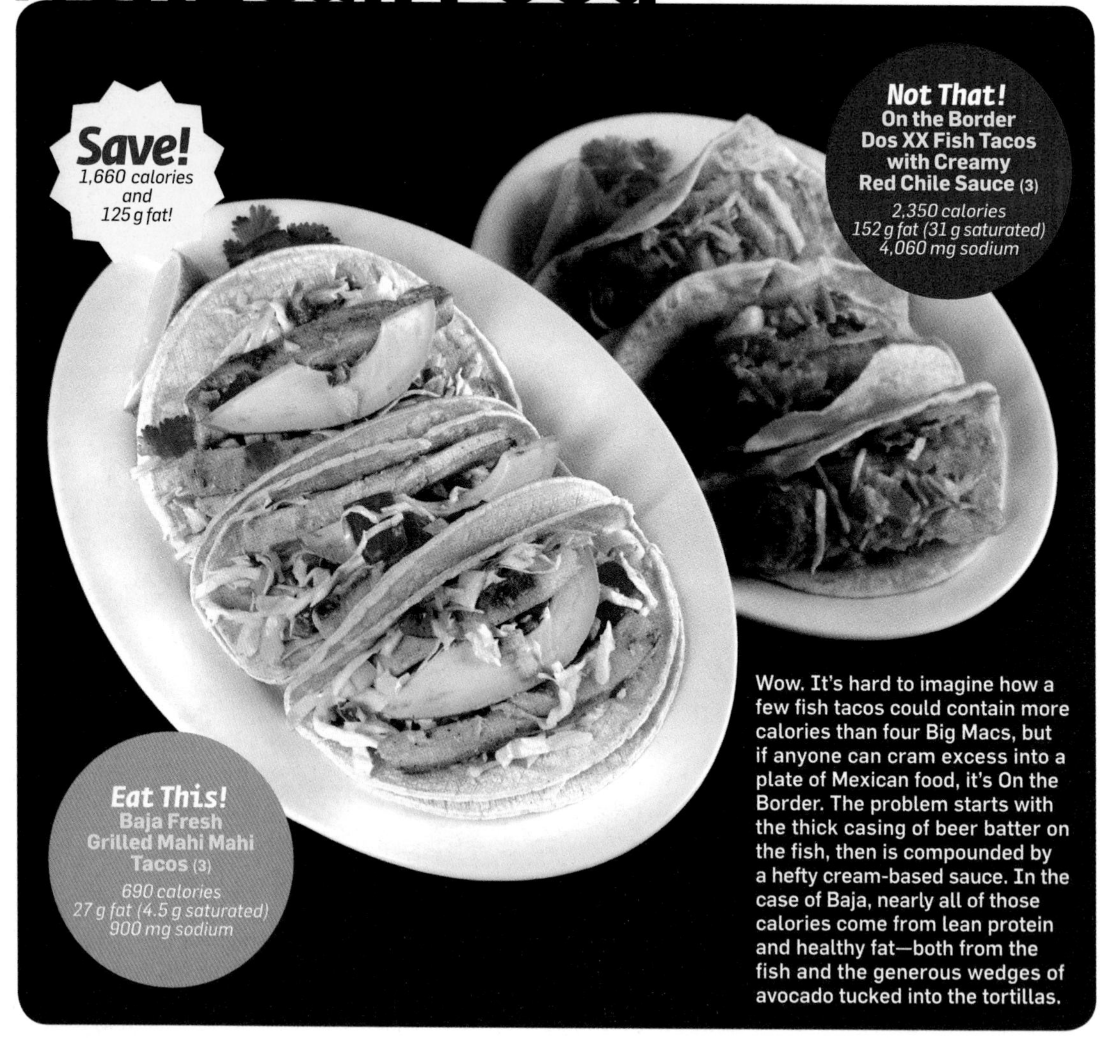

Wow. It's hard to imagine how a few fish tacos could contain more calories than four Big Macs, but if anyone can cram excess into a plate of Mexican food, it's On the Border. The problem starts with the thick casing of beer batter on the fish, then is compounded by a hefty cream-based sauce. In the case of Baja, nearly all of those calories come from lean protein and healthy fat—both from the fish and the generous wedges of avocado tucked into the tortillas.

Pizza

Save!
1,740 calories and 142 g fat!
Not That!
Uno Chicago Grill Chicago Classic Deep Dish Individual Pizza
2,310 calories
165 g fat (54 g saturated)
4,920 mg sodium
Eat This!
Pizza Hut All Natural Pepperoni and Mushroom Personal Pan Pizza
570 calories
23 g fat (9 g saturated)
1,260 mg sodium

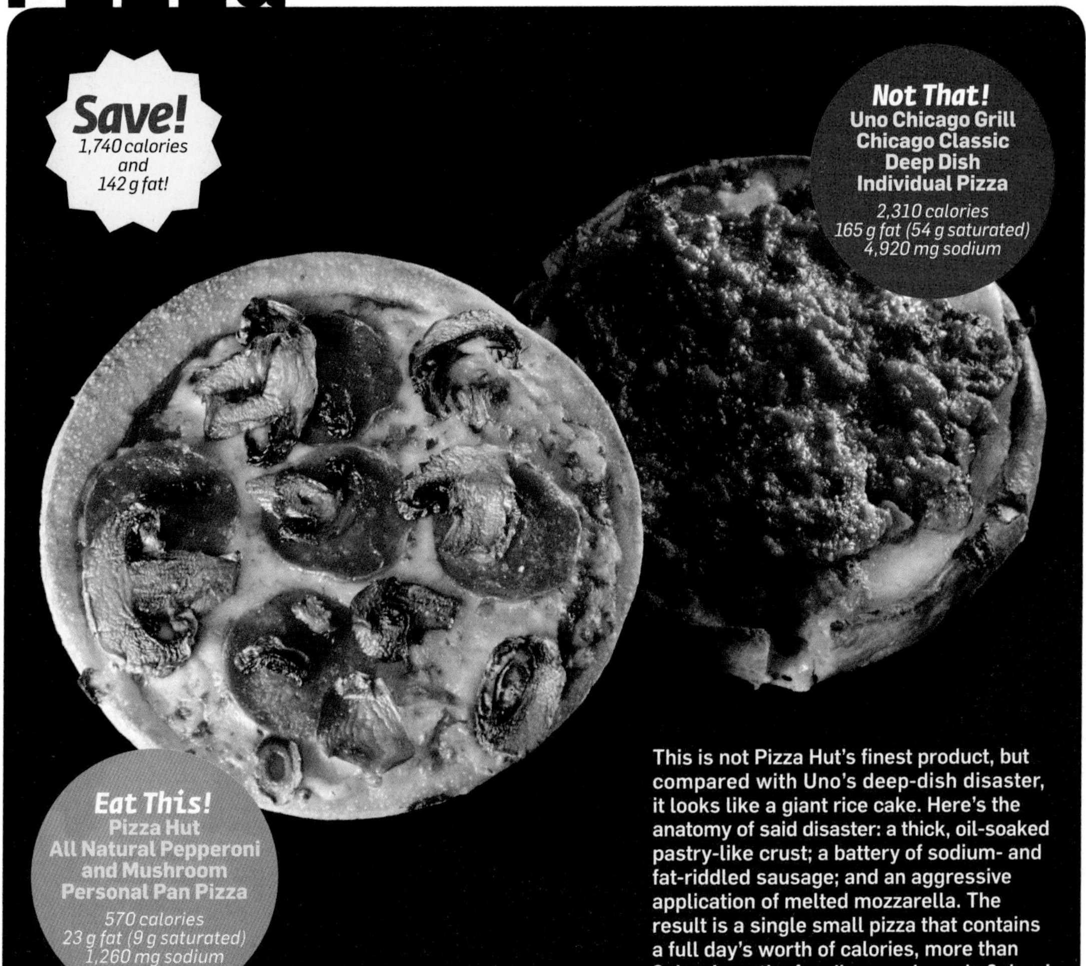

This is not Pizza Hut's finest product, but compared with Uno's deep-dish disaster, it looks like a giant rice cake. Here's the anatomy of said disaster: a thick, oil-soaked pastry-like crust; a battery of sodium- and fat-riddled sausage; and an aggressive application of melted mozzarella. The result is a single small pizza that contains a full day's worth of calories, more than 2 days' worth of sodium, and nearly 3 days' worth of fat.

Salads

Save!
1,110 calories and 96 g fat!

Not That!
On the Border Grande Taco Salad with Taco Beef and Smoked Chipotle Vinaigrette Dressing
1,620 calories
118 g fat (37 g saturated)
3,010 mg sodium

Eat This!
Chipotle Steak Salad with Black Beans, Guacamole, and Red Tomatillo Salsa
510 calories
22 g fat (4 g saturated)
1,275 mg sodium

Don't be thrown off by the word "salad" used to describe On the Border's monster bowl. Think of it instead as the world's largest taco, cradled by an oversize fried tortilla trough. A Chipotle salad can be dangerous, too, but only if you let them dress it with their 290-calorie vinaigrette. Instead, use one of their many salsas to dress the greens for as low as 15 calories, then reinvest those savings on a scoop of guac, which brings plenty of satisfying healthy fat to this exemplary salad.

Chinese Food

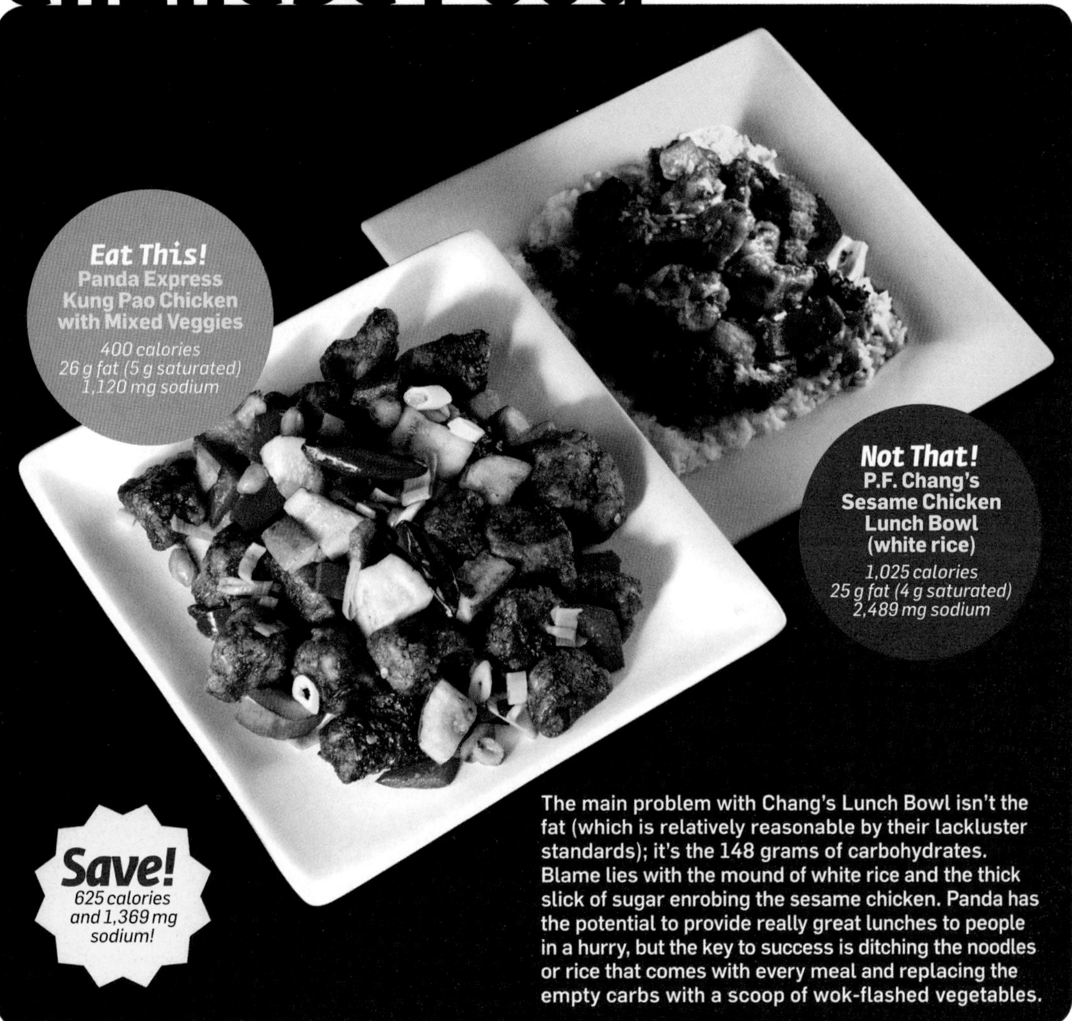

Eat This!
Panda Express Kung Pao Chicken with Mixed Veggies
400 calories
26 g fat (5 g saturated)
1,120 mg sodium

Not That!
P.F. Chang's Sesame Chicken Lunch Bowl (white rice)
1,025 calories
25 g fat (4 g saturated)
2,489 mg sodium

Save!
625 calories and 1,369 mg sodium!

The main problem with Chang's Lunch Bowl isn't the fat (which is relatively reasonable by their lackluster standards); it's the 148 grams of carbohydrates. Blame lies with the mound of white rice and the thick slick of sugar enrobing the sesame chicken. Panda has the potential to provide really great lunches to people in a hurry, but the key to success is ditching the noodles or rice that comes with every meal and replacing the empty carbs with a scoop of wok-flashed vegetables.

Seafood

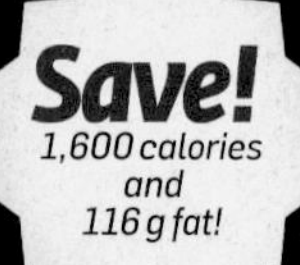

Not That!
Romano's Macaroni Grill Parmesan-Crusted Sole
2,190 calories
141 g fat (58 g saturated)
2,980 mg sodium

Eat This!
Olive Garden Parmesan-Crusted Tilapia
590 calories
25 g fat (10 g saturated)
910 mg sodium

The two dishes couldn't be more similar in name and appearance, so how does Macaroni Grill's end up with nearly four times the calories and more than five times the fat? Without access to the restaurants' recipes, it's tough to discern every drastic measure Mac Grill is taking to torture this poor sole, but in the end they produce one of the worst fish dishes we've ever seen—stricken with nearly 3 full days' worth of saturated fat. Like most restaurant blunders, a massive portion size and an abundance of cheap oil are most likely to blame here.

Banana Split

Save!
490 calories and 52 g sugars!
Not That!
Baskin-Robbins Classic Banana Split
1,010 calories
34 g fat (20 g saturated)
125 g sugars
Eat This!
Dairy Queen Banana Split
520 calories
13 g fat (10 g saturated)
73 g sugars

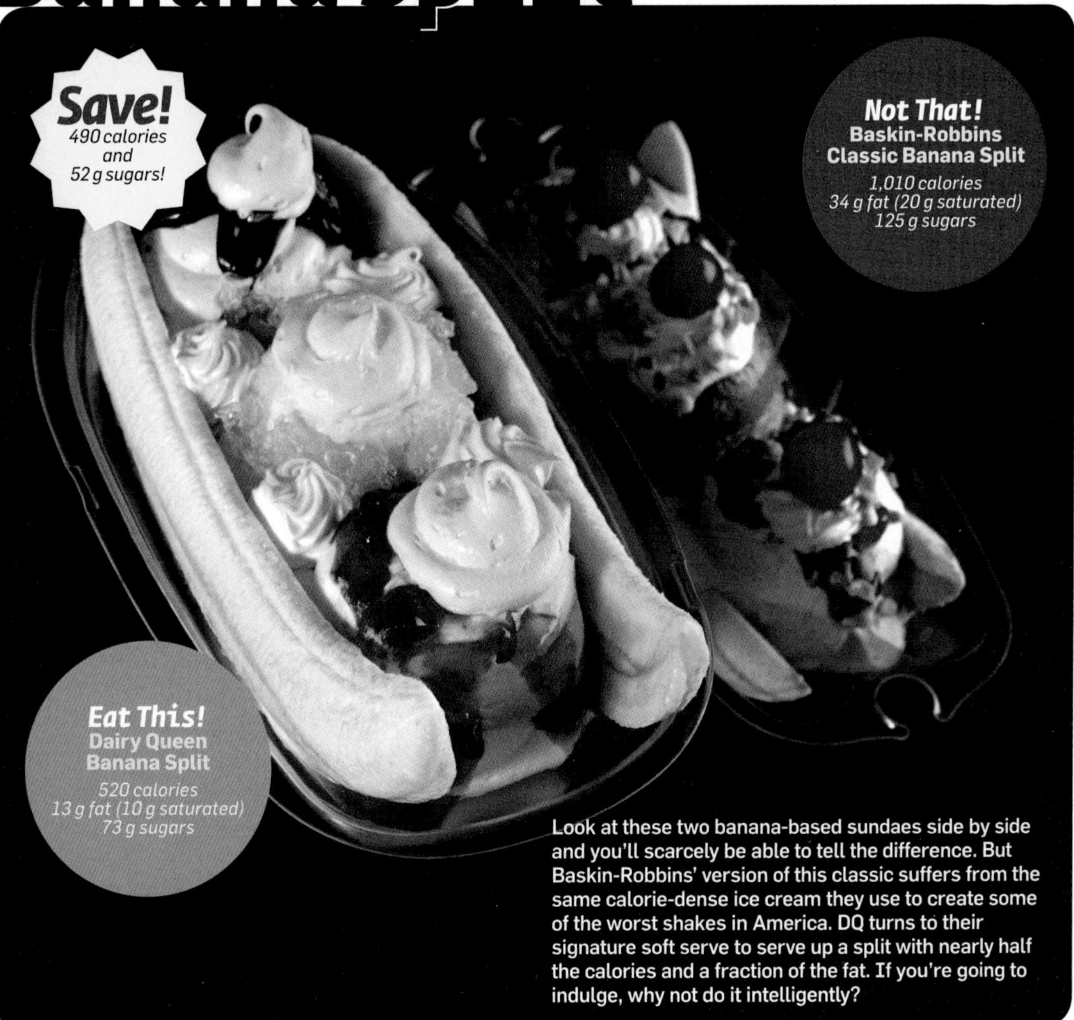

Look at these two banana-based sundaes side by side and you'll scarcely be able to tell the difference. But Baskin-Robbins' version of this classic suffers from the same calorie-dense ice cream they use to create some of the worst shakes in America. DQ turns to their signature soft serve to serve up a split with nearly half the calories and a fraction of the fat. If you're going to indulge, why not do it intelligently?

1

Eat This, Not That!

THE TRUTH ABOUT YOUR FOOD

As with the banking industry,

the Russian political system, and the romantic liaisons on Gossip Girl, all is not as it seems in the world of food and drink.

Misnomers and confusing labels have been with us for generations—at least since our hungry ancestors devoured the first hamburger (with no actual ham in it) and snarfed down the first hot dog (with no actual dog in it). And how many diners and takeout places in your neighborhood claim to sell "world-famous" coffee or pizza? (Wouldn't you think being "world famous" might allow them to upgrade to neon signs that aren't missing a few letters?)

What a food seller chooses to call his product or how he chooses to advertise it has always been as much a matter of fiction and salescraft as anything else. And everybody's in on the joke. Nobody believes that Count Chocula really comes from Transylvania. Or that Aunt Jemima is out there somewhere, making pancakes. Or that there's a salty, bearded Gorton's fisherman overseeing the day's catch up in Gloucester. These silly marketing claims and characters are just part of the commercial spin of modern life, and if they make one box of frozen fish sticks look somehow more appealing than the next, so be it.

But the hype and the spin get a little more serious—and a lot more unfair—when food starts to carry words that seem to make one food "healthier" than another. Words and phrases like "lower in fat" or "all natural" or "multigrain" sure sound appealing. Who wouldn't choose the all-natural multigrain product that's lower in fat?

Problem is, none of these words and phrases really mean anything. The food that's "lower in fat" simply has less fat than the original version of the product—the "lower in fat" version is probably still bulging with unnecessary calories. (And as you'll learn in the coming chapters, the type of fat you're eating matters more than the amount.) "All natural"? So are crude oil, snake venom, and botulism, but I wouldn't want to pay to eat any of those. And "multigrain" means nothing more than "made from more than one grain"—it sounds healthy, but if all those many grains have been stripped of their fiber and nutrients, you might as well be eating a teaspoon of pure sugar.

And therein lies the rub—and the reason for this book.

While the government has made some significant strides in getting nutrition information to the public—like requiring food packaging to carry nutrition labels—there's still so much room for obfuscation and outright mendacity that knowing what's in our food is never a matter of certainty.

WHY FOOD IS DIFFERENT TODAY

Two out of every three American adults are now overweight. How is this possible? You might say it's because we've all stopped exercising—except, there's a Curves or a Bally in every strip mall and downtown block in the United States and a Dick's or Sports Authority in every shopping plaza. You might say it's because we stopped watching what we eat—except that on any given week, half of the best sellers on the *New York Times* list are diet or cookbooks. You might say it's because we all just stopped caring—except that liposuction and belly band surgery are practically an epidemic. And you know and I know that the two most common phrases in the American lexicon are "I'm trying to watch my weight" and "Does this make me look fat?"

So what's causing all this weight gain? Well, here's a clue: The Centers for Disease Control and Prevention found that American men eat 7 percent more calories than they did in 1971; American women eat a whopping 18 percent more calories (an additional 335 calories a day—enough to pack on a pound of extra flab every 11 days!). And American kids average 150 daily calories more than they did just 20 years ago. Did our stomachs get larger? Did our mouths expand? Do we have more teeth than previous generations?

Of course not. *We* haven't changed. The food has changed.

- **WE'VE ADDED EXTRA CALORIES TO TRADITIONAL FOODS.** In the early 1970s, food manufacturers, looking for a cheaper ingredient to replace sugar, came up with a substance called high-fructose corn syrup (HFCS). Today, HFCS is in an unbelievable array of foods—everything from breakfast cereals to bread, from ketchup to pasta sauce, from juice drinks to iced teas. (Indeed, just try going to your local convenience store and buying a drink that doesn't contain HFCS!) According to the FDA, the average American consumes 82 grams of added sugars every day, which contribute 317 empty calories to our daily diet. HFCS might not be any worse for our bodies than normal table sugar, but it's dirt-cheap cost and prevalence in processed foods has only served to intensify America's collective sweet tooth in recent years.

- **WE'RE SUPERSIZING OUR LIVES.** Of course we want to be smart with our money, especially in this economy. So of course when we see the word "value," especially as it pertains to a "meal," we're going to want to go for it. Supersizing it at your local fast-food restaurant gives you an average of 73 percent more calories for a mere 17 percent more in cost. Sounds like a bargain, until you realize that you don't need the 73 percent more calories! Like clothes you bought on sale that you'll never wear, they look like a bargain, but they're really just a waste of money. (Except that you will wear those extra calories—on your belly, on your butt, or around your waist—perhaps for the rest of your life.)

- **WE'RE EATING THINGS OUR BODIES AREN'T SUPPOSED TO EAT.** A generation ago, it was hard for food manufacturers to create baked goods that would last on the store shelves. Most baked goods require oils, and oil runs and leaks at room temperature. But since the 1960s, manufacturers have been baking with—and restaurants have been frying with—something called "trans fat." Trans fat is cheap and effective: It makes potato chips crispier and Oreo cookies tastier; and it lets fry cooks make pound after pound of fries without smoking up their kitchens. But trans fat has been shown to have a horrific effect on our bodies: It raises our LDL (bad) cholesterol, lowers our HDL (good) cholesterol, and greatly increases our risk of heart disease and obesity. (If you see the words "partially hydrogenated" on the list of ingredients, you've got trans fat.)

The result of all this manipulation—manipulation of our food, to make it more appealing to our taste buds, and manipulation of our minds, to make us want to spend money on this crap—is that we absorb more calories than would have been humanly possible just a few decades ago. Our food and beverages are so calorie dense that it's nearly impossible to eat healthy. And the way that foods are sold, in both grocery stores and restaurants, has made smart nutritional choices harder and harder to discern.

That's why ***EAT THIS, NOT THAT!*** is such an invaluable resource for those who want to eat their favorite foods and not be ambushed by hidden fat, sugar, and calories.

The ETNT! Encyclopedia

UNPACKING THE MOST MISLEADING CLAIMS OF THE FOOD INDUSTRY

LIGHTLY SWEETENED
A frequently abused claim with no formal definition, this appears most often in the cereal aisle, and many of the boxes it adorns are actually loaded with various sweeteners. Need proof? Look at Kellogg's Smart Start. It claims to be "lightly sweetened," yet it has more sugar per cup than a full serving of Oreo cookies!

GOOD SOURCE OF . . .
This packaging claim is of slightly less importance than "excellent source of." It means that the product contains between 10 and 19 percent of your daily requirement for the mentioned nutrient. In other words, you would have to eat between 5 and 10 servings to get your full day's value.

REDUCED FAT
Splashed across too many packaged goods to count, this term means that the total fat grams have been reduced by at least 25 percent. Sounds great, right? Problem is, that reduction in fat often comes with an increase in sugar and sodium and ultimately, no net nutritional gain to speak of.

MULTIGRAIN
This simply means that more than one type of grain was used in processing (e.g., wheat, rye, barley, and rice). It doesn't, however, make any claim about the degree of processing used on those grains. Also, beware of the equally ambiguous "wheat bread," a claim that simply means the loaf was made from wheat flour, which might very well be refined and colored with molasses to appear darker. The only trustworthy claim for whole grains is "100 percent whole grain."

LIGHTLY BREADED
The phrase most restaurants use to

distract diners from the fact that the food they're about to eat has been rolled in flour, egg, and bread crumbs and let loose in a vat of bubbling fat. Doesn't matter how light the breading is; it's the oil part that will get you.

NATURAL

This term is used almost entirely at the discretion of food processors. With the exception of meat and poultry products, the USDA has set no definition and imposes no regulations on the use of this term, making it essentially meaningless.

COMPLIMENTARY

Usually attached to one of the following words: chips, bread, desserts, refills. In any case, the act of giving away low-cost, high-calorie foods is a common tactic restaurants use to add value to the "customer experience." Remember, just because it's free doesn't mean it won't cost you—these empty calories add up fast.

REDUCED SODIUM

Used when the sodium level is reduced by 25 percent or more, regardless of the total amount. "Low sodium," on the other hand, can be used only when the product contains no more than 140 milligrams per serving.

TRANS FAT–FREE

Food processors can make this claim so long as their product contains less than 0.49 gram of trans fat per serving. Considering the American Heart Association recommends capping daily intake at 2 grams, this is no small amount. So even if the label reads "0 g trans fat," that's no guarantee that you're in the clear. Instead, read the ingredients list; if shortening or partially hydrogenated oil is listed, then you need to find another product.

13 Restaurant Industry Secrets

When we first launched ***EAT THIS, NOT THAT!***, we uncovered 16 dirty little secrets the restaurant industry was keeping hidden under countertops and tucked behind boardroom doors. We exposed certain chains for refusing to disclose their nutritional content, and others for refusing to remove trans-fatty acids from their foods, in spite of a flood of scientific evidence that shows how harmful partially hydrogenated oils can be. The good news is that, once exposed, some of the shamed chains moved to rectify these secrets. The bad news is that some didn't. And the even more disappointing news is that in the years since, we've discovered a slew of new secrets that the restaurant industry would rather you never hear about. Too bad for them.

We're sick of false advertising, misleading health claims, and fast-food chains that refuse to acknowledge (and mitigate) their role in America's current obesity epidemic. We understand that business is business, but tricking your customers into believing your foods are healthy or free of trans fat when they aren't isn't just a dirty trick—it should be downright criminal. Hopefully, this round of secrets can help motivate the restaurant industry to make changes for the better. Until then, we'll be here to help you read between the lines, recognize the hype, and choose the best options for your wallet and waistline.

JACK IN THE BOX

Doesn't Want You to Know . . .

that it's the Trans-Fattiest Restaurant in America. Why? Because of items like the Bacon Cheddar Potato Wedges, which have 13 grams of trans-fatty acids—nearly six times the amount the American Heart Association recommends you consume in a single day! In fact, it doesn't want you to know that more than 83 percent of its food items still contain the heart-damaging processed fat (out of the 102 items listed, only 18 are trans fat–free)!

Check out the trans fat menu breakdown here (and keep in mind, this is only the list of foods with 3 grams or more of the stuff—there are still plenty more Jack in the Box menu items with 1, 1.5, or 2 grams of the stuff).

3 grams trans fat • Asian Chicken Salad with Crispy Chicken Strips • Southwest Chicken Salad with Crispy Chicken Strips • Bacon Ultimate Cheeseburger • Homestyle Ranch Chicken Club • Jack's Spicy Chicken • Jack's Spicy Chicken with Cheese • 3 Egg Rolls • 24-ounce Chocolate Ice Cream Shake • 24-ounce Oreo Cookie Ice Cream Shake • 24-ounce Strawberry Ice Cream Shake • 24-ounce Vanilla Ice Cream Shake • Homestyle Chicken Biscuit • 2 Grilled Chicken Breast Strips Kids' Meal • 2 Crispy Chicken Strips, Kids' Meal • Kids' Portion Natural Cut Fries

3.5 grams • 5 Mini Churros • Chicken Club Salad with Crispy Chicken Strips • Steak and Egg Burrito • 6 Mozzarella Cheese Sticks • Supreme Croissant

4 grams • Sausage Croissant

4.5 grams • 7 Stuffed Jalapeños • small Natural Cut Fries • 5 Hash Brown Sticks

5 grams • small Seasoned Curly Fries • 4 Original French Toast Sticks

6 grams • Sampler Trio • 4 Crispy Chicken Strips

7 grams • medium Natural Cut Fries • medium Seasoned Curly Fries • 10 Mini Churros • Denver Breakfast Bowl • Hearty Breakfast Bowl

9 grams • large Natural Cut Fries

10 grams • small Fish and Chips • 8 Onion Rings • large Seasoned Curly Fries

13 grams • Bacon Cheddar Potato Wedges

COLD STONE

Doesn't Want You to Know . . .
that every drink on its regular line of shakes contains 1,000 calories or more, 92 grams of sugar, and 1.5 grams of trans fat. Key word "small"—the larger varieties have up to 2,010 calories and 2 days' worth of fat (we're looking at you, Gotta-Have-It size PB&C Shake).

DUNKIN' DONUTS

Doesn't Want You to Know . . .
that its muffins are worse than its doughnuts. Even the reduced-fat blueberry muffin still has 450 calories —more than all but two doughnuts on the menu.

KFC

Doesn't Want You to Know . . .
that it still uses partially hydrogenated oils. One look at the KFC nutrition information would have you believe

that you'll only find trans fat if you eat the gravy. What's worse, KFC boasts on its Web site that KFC Chicken contains 0 grams of trans fat per serving. But partially hydrogenated oils appear 83 times on its menu's ingredients list—in a range of menu items, from chicken dishes to sauces to potatoes and rice! Technically, their nondisclosure isn't totally illegal: The FDA says that if a product contains less than 0.5 gram of trans fat per serving, you're allowed to say it's "trans fat–free." Other restaurants like McDonald's and Wendy's follow suit, touting the use of trans fat–free frying oil, while ignoring the load of trans fats in their burgers. We applaud these places for cutting back significantly on the trans fat over the past few years, but do us all a big favor and go the whole way.

ROMANO'S MACARONI GRILL

Doesn't Want You to Know . . .

that you can make spaghetti and meatballs at home for 1,040 calories less and at nearly one-fifth the price. One dinner plate of spaghetti and meatballs with tomato basil sauce at the Grill packs 1,500 calories and costs about $10.79 (depending on the location). But you can make a 460-calorie version for $2.28 per serving at home. Here's how.

YOU'LL NEED

- **¾ lb ground turkey breast**
- **¾ lb 90 percent lean ground beef**
- **1 egg**
- **½ cup bread crumbs**
- **½ cup chopped parsley**
- **1 onion, minced**
- **3 garlic cloves, minced**
- **¾ tsp salt**
- **½ tsp black pepper**
- **1 Tbsp olive oil**
- **1 (28-oz) can Muir Glen Fire Roasted Crushed Tomatoes**
- **12 oz DeCecco Whole Wheat Spaghetti**

Traditional meatballs are made with a mixture of beef, pork, and veal. Turkey, lean and tender, will taste just as good and save you major calories.

Consider this Goldilocks dilemma: 95 percent is too lean to make a tasty meatball, and 80 percent is too fatty to make a healthy one. So, 90 percent is just right.

"Fire roasted" means that this velvety tomato sauce will taste like it's been cooking all day.

7 grams of fiber and 8 grams of protein per serving make a strong case for wheat over white pasta.

HOW TO MAKE IT

Mix the meat, egg, bread crumbs, parsley, half of the onion and garlic, and the salt and pepper. Form into 18 golf balls.

Heat half of the oil in a large nonstick skillet and cook the meatballs over medium heat until well browned. Set aside.

Heat the remaining oil in a saucepan and cook the remaining onion and garlic over medium heat until translucent. Add the tomatoes and bring to a simmer. Add the meatballs and cook for 15 to 20 minutes.

Cook the pasta according to the package instructions. Dish out on plates and top with a few meatballs and sauce.

Makes 6 servings; cost per serving: $2.28

THE CHEESECAKE FACTORY
Doesn't Want You to Know . . .
its nutritional information. As quoted from the Factory's Web site: "At this point, we do not provide nutritional information for our menu selections. We pride ourselves on using only the freshest and finest ingredients available. Everything on our menu is made in-house on a daily basis so that we can maintain the highest food quality standards." It goes on: "Our menu items are known for their generous portion sizes and, consequently, we have always encouraged 'sharing' at the table. However, we will happily wrap left-overs for guests to take home and enjoy for another meal." We're pleased the ingredients they use are fresh and fine and that they offer doggie bags along with their hulking portions. But are they packed with fat, calories, sugar, and sodium? Until they tell us, we're going to assume the worst.

Neither Does
IHOP OR T.G.I.FRIDAY'S . . .
From their Web site, in response to the FAQ "Is nutritional information available?": "IHOP offers a wide variety of food that should allow most people to choose a meal that suits their dietary needs." Sure, but how are they supposed to do that—close their eyes and pick an item at random? Friday's is no better. When asked, a T.G.I.Friday's rep said he wasn't aware of any such misleading link. "We don't provide nutritional information unless required by law," he said. Thankfully, New York City law requires both of these restaurants to provide calorie counts on their menus, and the numbers we've seen confirm our suspicions that these two titans of the restaurant industry are serving some of America's unhealthiest food.

APPLEBEE'S
Doesn't Want You to Know . . .
that their vaunted Weight Watchers menu has come under scrutiny during multiple nutritional investigations. It started in late 2008, when E.W. Scripps news service sent a number of the dishes on the Weight Watchers menu, taken from eight different locations, to a lab to be analyzed. Results found that certain "healthy" entrées packed double the calories and up to eight times the fat that Applebee's claims they do. Class action lawsuits followed from four different states and continue today. In a separate case from the

summer of 2009, an Ohio woman is suing Applebee's over claims that their Cajun Lime Tilapia dish is worse than the restaurant discloses.

RUBY TUESDAY

Doesn't Want You to Know . . .
that the Veggie Burger isn't as healthy as it sounds. With 952 calories, 53 grams of fat, and 95 grams of carbohydrates, there's nothing "healthy" about this deceptive dish. It's no Colossal burger, to be fair (the former coup de grâce of Ruby's menu rang in at a diet-sinking 2,014 calories), but even without the belt-buckling Colossal on the menu, an average RT burger packs an appalling 1,103 calories.

SBARRO

Doesn't Want You to Know . . .
that its nutritional information Web page has been "under construction" for at least 20 months. It must just be taking them a long time to add up all those calories, carbs, grams of fat, and milligrams of sodium—when we called a Sbarro in New York City, where calorie counts are required by law to be displayed prominently on menu boards, we learned that *1 slice* of stuffed pepperoni pizza has 960 calories!

STARBUCKS

Doesn't Want You to Know . . .
that most of its lattes pack more sugar than a two-scoop ice cream sundae. The Starbucks nutrition Web site boasts that one Grande Latte provides "half the dairy you need for the day"; what it doesn't say is that some of those calcium-packed beverages also provide almost your entire day's worth of sugars. Check it out: A no-whip Grande Gingersnap Latte packs 34 grams of the sweet stuff, a no-whip Grande Cinnamon Dolce Latte offers 38 grams, and the healthy-sounding Grande Black Tea Latte includes 31 grams. Add whipped cream, add sugar. And cutting back from 2 percent milk to skim doesn't help, either—in fact, the fat-free versions are even sweeter.

SUBWAY

Doesn't Want You to Know . . .
that you'll eat more calories there than you would at McDonald's. It's not exactly Subway's fault—most of their offerings are healthy, nutritious, and low calorie. But a 2007 study at Cornell University found that when shown two 1,000-calorie dishes, people underestimate the load by about 159 calories in food they consider healthy. The

researchers also found that when people eat at "healthy" restaurants, like Subway, they tend to order 131 percent more calories in side items than they do at known "unhealthy" restaurants. They call this meal-compromising phenomenon a "health halo." Not that calorie count alone tells the whole story about the nutritional quality of the foods you're eating, but if you're already going out of your way to eat as healthfully as possible, it's important to remember that it's still possible to overdo it, even at "good" restaurants.

UNO CHICAGO GRILL

Doesn't Want You to Know . . .
that the nutrition information it lists on its Web site is only a fraction of what you're actually eating. That's because they list the nutrition contents for one "serving" of the dish—but if you look at the top right corner of the page, you'll see that each dish comes with two, three, four, or even five servings. Since you typically aren't going to split your burger or mac 'n' cheese among four people, you can go ahead and multiply the already eye-popping calories and fat grams by the number of servings listed. Quadruple yikes.

SIT-DOWN RESTAURANTS

Don't Want You to Know . . .
that their food is considerably worse for you than fast food. Fast-food chains might get all the bad press (remember *Super Size Me*?), but our research has uncovered that it's the places with the foldable menus and the pleather banquettes that we really need to be concerned about. Consider this: Our menu analysis of 24 national chains revealed that the average entrée at a sit-down restaurant contains 867 calories, compared with 522 calories in the average fast-food entrée. And that's before appetizers, sides, and desserts—selections that can easily double your total calorie intake. Blame enormous portion sizes, to start. The reason a McDonald's cheeseburger has only 300 calories is because it's little. But a cheeseburger from Outback is roughly five times the size and packs up to six times the calories. Tack on the free loaves of brown bread and butter at Outback (or the chips and salsa at On the Border, or the breadsticks at Oliver Garden, or the . . .) and the impact of eating at a sit-down restaurant really starts to take shape. Maybe being caught in the drive-thru isn't such a bad thing after all . . .

The Truth about Your Food

Just as the titans of the restaurant industry seek to obscure the reality behind their most dubious products and practices, so do the package-goods producers partake in active campaigns of secrecy, embellishment, and outright deception. What does that mean to you, dear reader? It means you're spending your hard-earned cash and calories on foods you thought were great for you but that may secretly be undermining your health. Eating well is hard enough, but when companies start complicating matters with false marketing and ambiguous label claims, that's when you need to arm yourself with a few simple, savvy methods for outsmarting the food powers that be. What follows is just that, a guide to 9 of the most misunderstood foods in America that will help you separate fact from fiction in a quest to getting exactly what you bargained for every time you take to the supermarket.

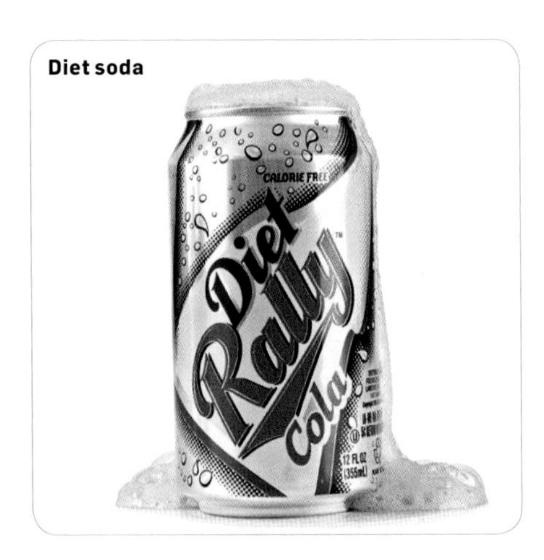

Diet soda

The Truth about . . .
DIET SODA

When confronted with the growing tide of calories from sweetened beverages, the first response is, "Why not just drink diet soda?" Well, there are plenty of reasons why not.

THE TRUTH: Just because diet soda is low in calories doesn't mean it can't lead to weight gain. It may have only 5 or fewer calories per serving, but emerging research suggests that consuming sugary-tasting beverages—even if they're artificially sweetened

—may lead to a high preference for sweetness overall. That means sweeter (and more caloric) cereal, bread, dessert—everything. Whatever the reason, it's clear that people who drink a ton of diet soda aren't doing themselves any favors: New research found that people who drink diet on a daily basis have an increased risk of developing type 2 diabetes and metabolic syndrome. To top it all off, diet soda is 100 percent nutrition free—and it's just as important to actively drink the good stuff as it is to avoid the bad stuff. The more diet soda you drink, the less healthful beverages, like water and tea, you're also consuming. This can ultimately hinder your health.

WHAT YOU REALLY WANT: If it's the caffeine boost you're looking for, switch to unsweetened tea or coffee. Both are packed with antioxidants and have known health benefits, from boosting your memory and metabolism to helping protect you against dementia and Alzheimer's. Certainly beats diabetes.

The Truth about . . .

REDUCED-FAT PEANUT BUTTER

Nothing makes a PB&J feel less indulgent like a scoop of low-fat Jif.

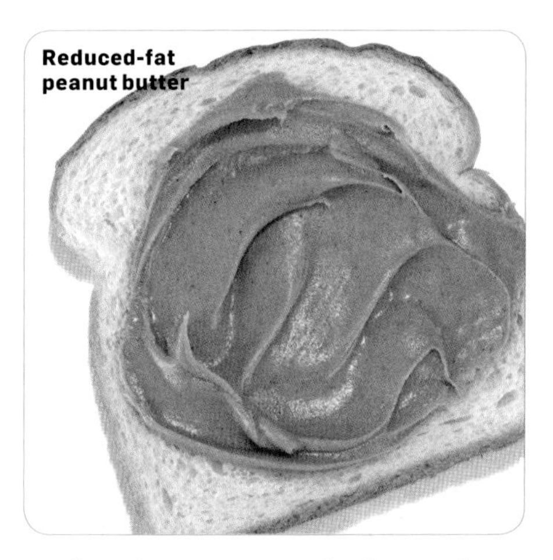

It's low fat, so it must be better for you . . . right?

THE TRUTH: A tub of reduced-fat peanut butter indeed comes with a fraction less fat than the full-fat variety—they're not lying about that. But what the food companies don't tell you is that they've replaced that healthy fat with maltodextrin, a carbohydrate used as a filler in many processed foods. This means you're trading the *healthy* fat from peanuts for empty carbs, double the sugar, and a savings of a meager 10 calories.

WHAT YOU REALLY WANT: The real stuff: no oils, fillers, or added sugars. Just peanuts and salt. Smucker's Natural fits the bill, as do many other peanut butters out there. We especially like

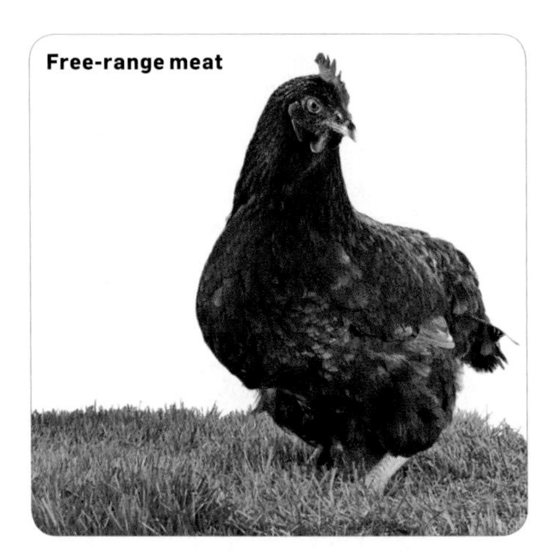
Free-range meat

Peanut Butter & Co. Original Smooth Operator and Original Crunch Time.

The Truth about . . .
FREE-RANGE MEAT

The claim sounds idyllic enough to reassure even the most ethical omnivore. But don't breathe easy yet: This popular buzzword might not live up to the peaceful, rolling-hills freedom it evokes.

THE TRUTH: Technically, free-range chickens must have access to the outdoors for at least 51 percent of their lives, but the USDA, which approves each manufacturer's "free-range" claim on a case-by-case basis, does not strictly define "outdoors." The term could mean anything from idyllic open acreage to a puny pen. Guess which is true for the majority of free-range chickens available in supermarkets?

WHAT YOU REALLY WANT: Even though it can mean any number of things, free-range is certainly an improvement over meat that doesn't bear the label. For an extra health boost, consider choosing meat that boasts "raised without antibiotics." This applies to poultry, not beef—big chicken producers have begun to curtail the use of antibiotics in recent years, addressing concerns that bacteria dangerous to humans could be developing drug resistance. Still, Tyson, Perdue, and others have been unable to wean their birds entirely off antibiotics, so this claim is worth something.

The Truth about . . .
100 PERCENT FRUIT JUICE

You may be a savvy enough grocery shopper to be able to spot the juice impostors (we're looking at you, sugar-jacked cranberry cocktail). But when you smugly pull a Tropicana Pure 100% Juice Pomegranate Blueberry off the shelf, do you know what kind of juice you're actually buying?

THE TRUTH: Drinks may be labeled 100 percent pure juice, but that doesn't mean they're made exclusively with the advertised juice. With respect to the Tropicana in question, pomegranate and blueberry get top billing, even though the ingredient list reveals that pear, apple, and grape juices are among the first four ingredients. These juices are used because they're cheap to produce and because they're super

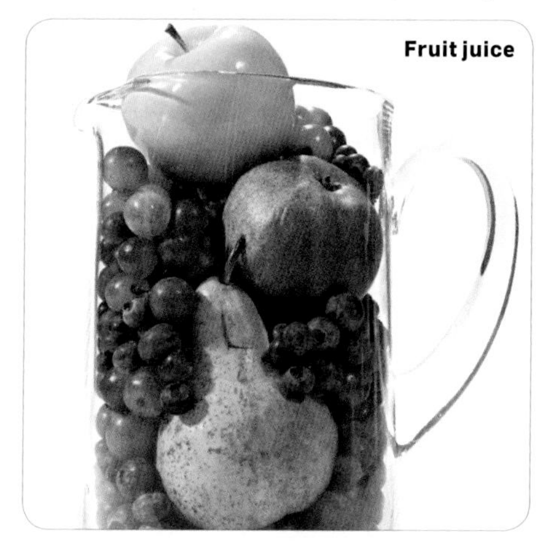
Fruit juice

sweet—likely to keep you coming back for more. Labels loaded with of-the-moment superfoods like açai and pomegranate are especially susceptible to this type of trickery. Beware.
WHAT YOU REALLY WANT: To avoid the huge sugar surge, pick single-fruit juices. POM, Lakewood Organic, and R.W. Knudsen all make some reliably pure products.

The Truth about . . .
ENERGY DRINKS

These ubiquitous beverages boast exotic-sounding supplements and make superhuman claims: Long-lasting energy! Steel-trap concentration! Peak athletic prowess! But do they really rev up your body and sharpen your mind?
THE TRUTH: The jolt you'll feel from downing an energy elixir comes from a combination of sky-high caffeine levels and staggering sugar content. Added extras, like ginseng, guarana, and taurine, make minimal difference (if any). Ginseng, for example, won't give you an energy blast, although it might boost your brainpower—researchers from Australia's Swinburne University of Technology found that people who swallowed 200 milligrams of the extract an hour before taking a cognitive test scored significantly better than when they skipped the supplement. Guarana's benefit comes from its caffeine content—a guarana seed contains 4 to 5 percent caffeine (about twice as much as a coffee bean). And taurine (the boasted additive in Red Bull) actually might make you feel sluggish, not hyperactive, according to researchers at Weill Cornell Medical College. As for that "long-lasting" energy? If your drink is packed with sugar (and most

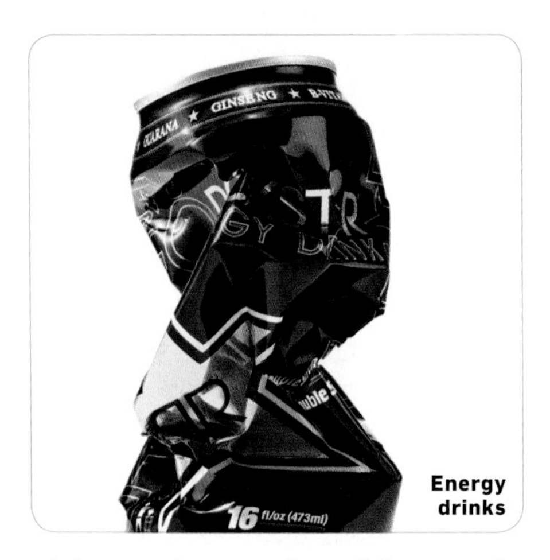

Energy drinks

of them are), you're bound for a crash. Seems counterproductive, doesn't it?

WHAT YOU REALLY WANT: Coffee, preferably black. The caffeine content in one cup of coffee should guarantee you about 5 hours of alertness (give or take, depending on how much sleep you've been getting and your own personal chemistry). Even better, researchers have found that coffee is packed with antioxidants, and studies have shown it enhances short-term memory and helps protect against dementia and cancer.

The Truth about . . . **ORGANIC FOOD**

"Organic" is another one of those nutrition buzzwords repeated so often it's hard to remember what it even means. Don't brush it off as the overpriced impractical food fare of hippies—but don't accept it as the answer to all your nutritional prayers without some careful consideration.

THE TRUTH: It all depends on your priorities. Organic food is better for the earth, at least when grown and sold locally: The certification criteria of the National Organic Standards Board specifically outline that organic food must be grown with methods that promote biodiversity, minimize pollution, and use cultural, biological, and mechanical methods of agriculture in place of synthetic materials. This goes beyond cutting out pesticides and fertilizers that can be harmful to people and animals. It involves methods that actually improve the soil—for those agrophiles out there, this means using cover crops, manure, and crop rotations; grazing animals on mixed forage pastures; using renewable resources; and conserving soil and water.

As for whether organic food is actually better for you from a health perspective—the jury's still out. For every study that says organic food has higher concentrations of nutrients, there's another that denies it. Consider: Researchers at the University of

Organic food

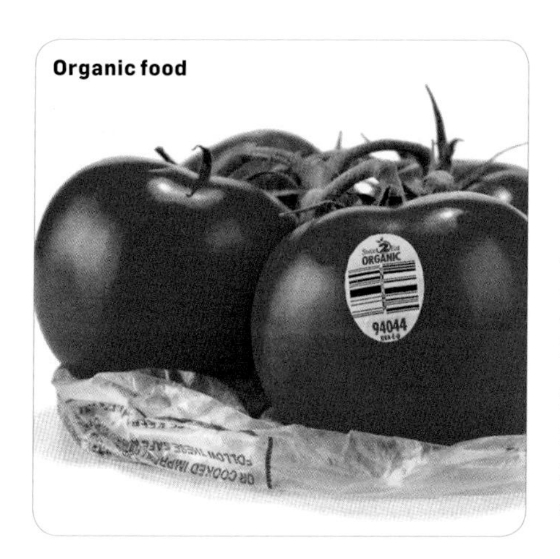

California at Davis found that organic kiwis had substantially more disease-fighting polyphenols than conventionally grown kiwis. But in the fall of 2009, a team of British researchers, after reviewing fifty years of studies and data, concluded that organic produce offers no unique nutritional benefit.

Finally, when it comes to packaged and processed foods, "organic" does not equal "healthy." As Michael Pollan quips in his eater's manifesto *In Defense of Food*, "Organic Oreos are not a health food"—they're still a heavily processed cookie filled with fat and sugar, and your body metabolizes organic fat and sugar the same way it does conventional.

WHAT YOU REALLY WANT: Trust only organic claims certified by a seal from the Secretary of Agriculture or, with regard to meat, from the USDA. That confirms that the animals were fed organic feed and had access to pasture. And if you're going to buy organic, don't waste your money on the organic packaged and processed foods. Stick to produce from your local farmers' markets—any out-of-region organic fare has negated its positive environmental impact with greenhouse gas emissions in the transport.

The Truth about . . .

FRUIT-ON-THE-BOTTOM YOGURT

It seems like the ideal breakfast or snack for a man or woman on the go—a perfect combination of yogurt and antioxidant-packed fruits, pulled together in one convenient little cup. But are these low-calorie dairy aisle staples really so good for you?

THE TRUTH: While the yogurt itself offers stomach-soothing live cultures and a decent serving of protein, the sugar content of these seemingly healthy products is sky-high. The fruit itself is swimming in thick syrup—so much of it, in fact, that high-fructose corn syrup (and other such sweeteners) often shows up on the ingredients list well before the fruit

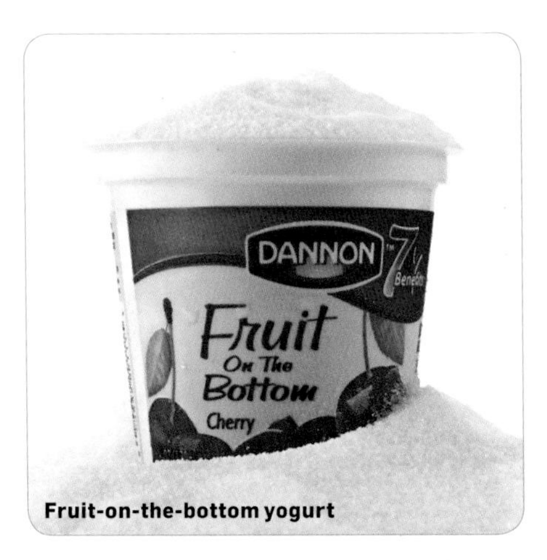

Fruit-on-the-bottom yogurt

itself. And these low-quality refined carbohydrates are the *last* thing you want for breakfast—Australian researchers found that people whose diets were high in carbohydrates had lower metabolism than those who ate proportionally more protein. Not to mention, spikes in your blood sugar can wreck your short-term memory, according to a study in the *European Journal of Clinical Nutrition.* Not what you need just before your urgent 9 a.m. meeting with the boss!

WHAT YOU REALLY WANT: Plain Greek-style yogurt, mixed with real blueberries. We like Oikos and Fage brands—they're jacked with about 15 to 22 grams of belly-filling protein, so they'll help you feel satisfied for longer. And blueberries are another great morning add—scientists in New Zealand found that when they fed blueberries to mice, the rodents ate 9 percent less at their next meal.

The Truth about . . .
PREMADE GUACAMOLE

When you buy premade guacamole, it seems reasonable to expect real guacamole. But is it?

THE TRUTH: Most guacamoles with the word "dip" attached to the label suffer from a lack of real avocado. Take Dean's Guacamole, for example. This guacamole dip is composed of less than 2 percent avocado; the rest of the green goo is a cluster of fillers

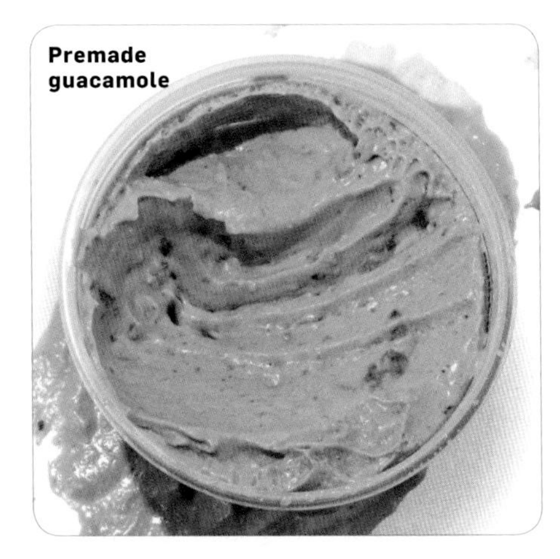
Premade guacamole

and chemicals, including modified food starch, soybean oils, locust bean gum, and food coloring. Dean's is not alone in this offense. In fact, this avocado caper was brought to light when a California woman filed a lawsuit against Kraft after she noticed "it just didn't taste avocadoey." Along the same lines, a British judge ruled that Pringles are not technically "chips," being that they only have 42 percent potato in them (though the ruling was recently reversed).

WHAT YOU REALLY WANT: If you want the heart-healthy fat, you'll need avocado. Wholly Guacamole makes a great guac or mash up a bowl yourself. Scoop out the flesh of two avocados, combine with two cloves of minced garlic, a bit of minced onion, the juice of one lemon, chopped cilantro, one medium chopped tomato, and a pinch of salt.

The Truth about . . .

TURKEY BACON

Pork bacon's got a bad rap for wreaking havoc on your cholesterol. But is turkey bacon really any better?

THE TRUTH: Stick with the pig. As far as calories go, the difference between "healthy" turkey bacon and "fatty" pig is negligible—and depending on the slice, turkey might sometimes tip the scales a touch more. Additionally, while turkey is indeed a leaner meat, turkey bacon isn't made from 100 percent bird: One look at the ingredients list will show a long line of suspicious additives and extras that can't possibly add anything of nutritional value. And finally, the sodium content of the turkey bacon is actually higher than what you'll find in the kind that oinks—so if you're worried about your blood pressure, opting for the original version is usually the smarter move.

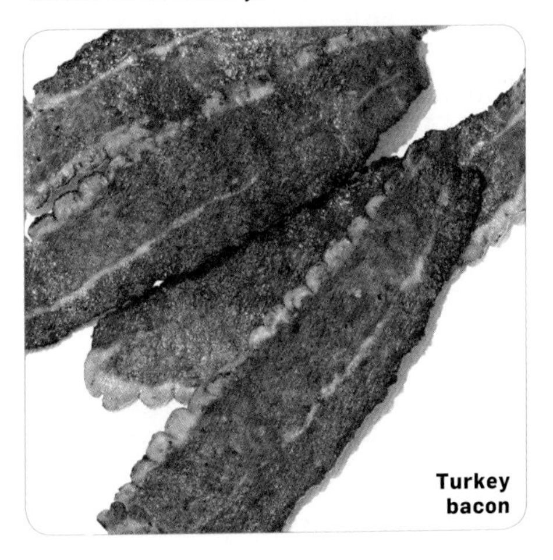
Turkey bacon

WHAT YOU REALLY WANT: Regular bacon. We like Hormel Black Label and Oscar Mayer Center Cut bacon for some low-cal, low-additive options.

The Best and Worst Changes in the Food Industry

Lots has changed to our food supply and policies since we first published ***EAT THIS, NOT THAT!*** in late 2007. Some of these changes have made healthy eating easier than ever, while others continue to put industry interests in front of our collective need to slim down. Here are some of the most notable.

NEW YORK CITY (AND CALIFORNIA) PASS CALORIE COUNT LAWS
In June 2007, New York City began to require that all its chain restaurants list calorie counts for each of their menu items. The decision was (predictably) met with outrage from the restaurant industry. In our opinion, this was a critical piece of legislation, in part because it helps to educate the people of New York City about diet and nutrition—a socially responsible act, considering the rising rates of obesity (and, not to mention, the rising costs), but also because this groundbreaking legislation inspired other cities and states to follow suit. Most notably, the state of California recently required restaurant chains to fork over their calorie counts, in addition to total carbs, sodium, and saturated fat in each item.

MACARONI GRILL IMPROVES THEIR MENU
Over the past two years, Romano's Macaroni Grill has consistently clawed for the title of Worst Restaurant in America. While other restaurants began to take the hint and add fitter fare to their menus, Mac Grill changed nothing, reflecting a baffling indifference to the potential harm they were causing to their customers' health. We're talking 1,630-calorie desserts (the New York Cheesecake with Fudge Sauce) and outrageous 1,810-calorie dinners (the comfort-food classic, Spaghetti with

Meatsauce), stuffed with as much sodium as you'd find in five, six, or seven large orders of McDonald's French fries . . . and not a single reasonable entry item in sight.

Recently, however, we were thrilled to see that Mac Grill has finally made some long-overdue additions. Many of the old and calorific staples have been strategically slimmed down, while two new sections on their menu—Mediterranean Grill and Amore de la Grill—offer reasonable-size meals that won't bust your belt buckles, including the 294-calories Jumbo Shrimp Spiedini. There's still a slew of nutritionally void danger items littering their lineup, but we're pleased to see the progress. Other restaurants should take note.

OLIVE GARDEN AND RED LOBSTER REVEAL NUTRITIONAL INFORMATION

Until this year, both Olive Garden and Red Lobster were among the delinquent restaurant chains that clung to their nutrition facts like they were state secrets. Finally, though, the parent company (both belong to Darden) decided to do away with the obstructionist policy. To our delight, we learned that the Red Lobster menu was actually among the best we've seen—that's why their grade has improved from the big fat F to a pride-worthy A- (the highest we've awarded any sit-down restaurant so far). Unfortunately, Olive Garden didn't fare as well as its seafood-serving cousin—blame the carbohydrate-loaded plates of pasta with more calories than 5 glazed doughnuts. Still, a D+ beats a failing grade . . . We hope Applebee's, IHOP, T.G.I. Friday's, and other nutritional holdouts follow the Darden lead.

THE FIRST FAMILY PLANTS A GARDEN

In March 2009, Michelle Obama planted an organic vegetable garden in the South Lawn of the White House, the first since Eleanor Roosevelt's victory garden during World War II. The immediate purpose of the garden was to help feed the First Family; the extended purpose was to demonstrate the value of locally grown fruits and vegetables. Whether the majority of Americans agree with the president's politics or not, lifestyle changes in the White House have a direct

WORST FOODS GRAVEYARD

Let's be honest: There are few **EAT THIS, NOT THAT!** fans within the restaurant industry. Since we published our first list of the 20 Worst Foods in America over two years ago, a full 10 of those dishes have either disappeared or have been altered significantly. And in the time since, a number of other caloric calamities have come and gone, making America a safer place to live and eat. Here are a few of our favorite vanishing acts.

WORST STARTER
Chili's Awesome Blossom
- *2,710 calories*
- *203 g fat*
- *194 carbs*
- *6,360 mg sodium*

WORST BURGER
Ruby Tuesday Colossal Burger
- *2,014 calories*
- *141 g fat*
- *95 g carbohydrates*

WORST KIDS' MEAL
Macaroni Grill Double Macaroni 'n' Cheese
- *1,210 calories*
- *62 g fat*
- *3,450 mg sodium*

WORST NACHOS
On the Border Stacked Border Nachos
- *2,740 calories*
- *166 g fat*
- *191 g carbs*
- *5,280 mg sodium*

WORST DRINK
Baskin-Robbins Large Heath Bar Shake
- *2,310 calories*
- *108 g fat*
- *266 g sugars*

WORST SUPERMARKET MEAL
Pepperidge Farm Roasted Chicken Pot Pie
- *1,020 calories*
- *64 g fat*
- *86 g carbs*

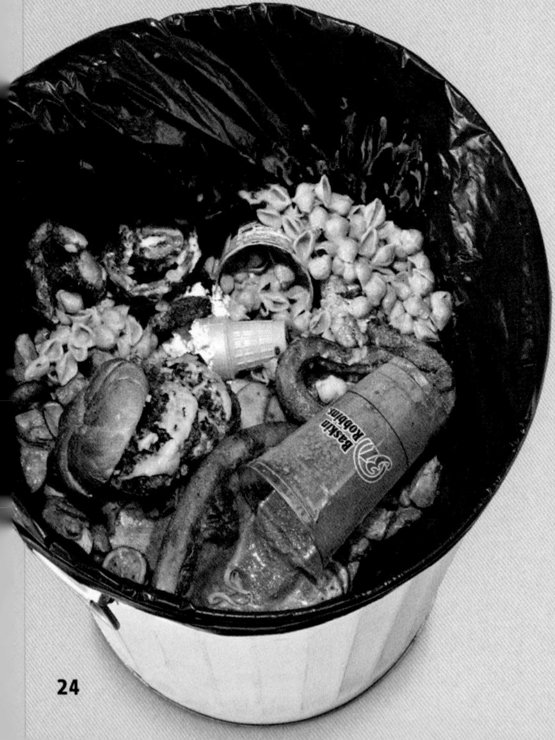

impact on lifestyle changes for the average American. A First Family that's openly conscientious about nutritious and environmentally friendly food can only have a positive impact on combating the increasing overweight and obesity rates we're facing.

BASKIN-ROBBINS SCRAPS THEIR PREMIUM SHAKE LINE

Until recently, Baskin-Robbins was home to the Worst Drink in America: The 2,600-calorie Large Chocolate Oreo Shake from its jaw-dropping premium shake line. This Oreo shake had an ingredient list that read like an O-chem final. Those 70-plus ingredients conspired to pack this shake with more sugar than 29 Fudgsicles, as much fat as a stick and a half of butter, and more calories than 48 actual Oreos. Oh, it also had 3 days' worth of saturated fat and, most bizarre of all, as much salt as you'd find in 9 bags of Lay's Classic potato chips. Understandably, we lambasted B-R for this busted beverage every opportunity we got. To our huge relief, they finally gave up: Not only did Baskin remove the Chocolate Oreo Shake from its menu, it removed the entire premium shake line. Good riddance.

THE RECESSION SHAPES OUR EATING HABITS

One byproduct of the shoddy economy is that people are cooking at home more and eating out less. The upside is that people typically eat substantially more calories at restaurants than they do when they prepare their own meals. The downside is that when money's tight, people are also more likely to skip increasinbly more expensive (and more healthful) produce, lean protein, and dairy products in favor of cheap and nutritionally void packaged foods. Whether our country's economic problems will have any impact, good or bad, on our waistlines has yet to be seen. In the meantime, though . . .

THE OVERWEIGHT AND OBESITY RATES CONTINUE TO RISE

Between 2008 and 2009, obesity rates rose in 23 out of 50 states, and remained troublingly steady in all the others, according to a report issued by advocacy groups Trust for America's Health and the Robert Wood Johnson Foundation. Not a single state saw their obesity rate fall. Mississippi topped the list for the fifth year in a row with a 32.5 percent obesity rate, and Colorado came out on top with the lowest, 18.5 percent. The only good news is that some states are imposing stricter regulations on the nutrition content of food served in schools, and a number are requiring kids to be screened for high body mass index. The report recommended that states work to make healthy, nutritious food options more readily available. In reality, of course, it's not that simple—which is why we offer an alterative option: Education about simple food swaps that can eliminate hundreds of calories from your daily diet without impacting your happiness or restricting you from eating the foods you love.

2

Eat This, Not That!

FOODS THAT CURE

You might think,

after skimming a few chapters in this book, that we'd like nothing more than to have you stop eating food altogether. And you might think, after surveying the American dietary landscape, that that's not such a bad idea.

After all, it's hard to escape the reality of America's obesity crisis—especially after a day at the shore, when you watch a crowd of environmentally conscious children trying to save a beached whale, only to discover it's just a pale, middle-aged guy in a Speedo who's had one too many margaritas. Or after an evening on the couch watching the news, when you listen intently to the debate over national health care and realize that if our food supply weren't so tainted by calorie-laden junk, we wouldn't be spending one in every five health care dollars supporting Americans who suffer from diabetes. You might think the solution is to put the whole country on a diet and make everybody stop eating so many meals and so many snacks.

But eating too much food isn't the problem. The problem is that we're eating too many things that aren't actually food—the additives, the preservatives, the chemically enhanced foodlike substances. And when we do eat real food, those meals and snacks are often served in such calorie-laden portions that even our old-fashioned grandmothers who always told us to "eat, eat" would step back, aghast, and yell, "Take that out of your mouth!"

But in reality, food—real food—is a good thing. Real food—the kind that comes from the earth, not a science lab—is about more than just calories and carbs, salts and sugars. Real food can have nearly magical properties—amazing abilities to prevent or even heal many of our

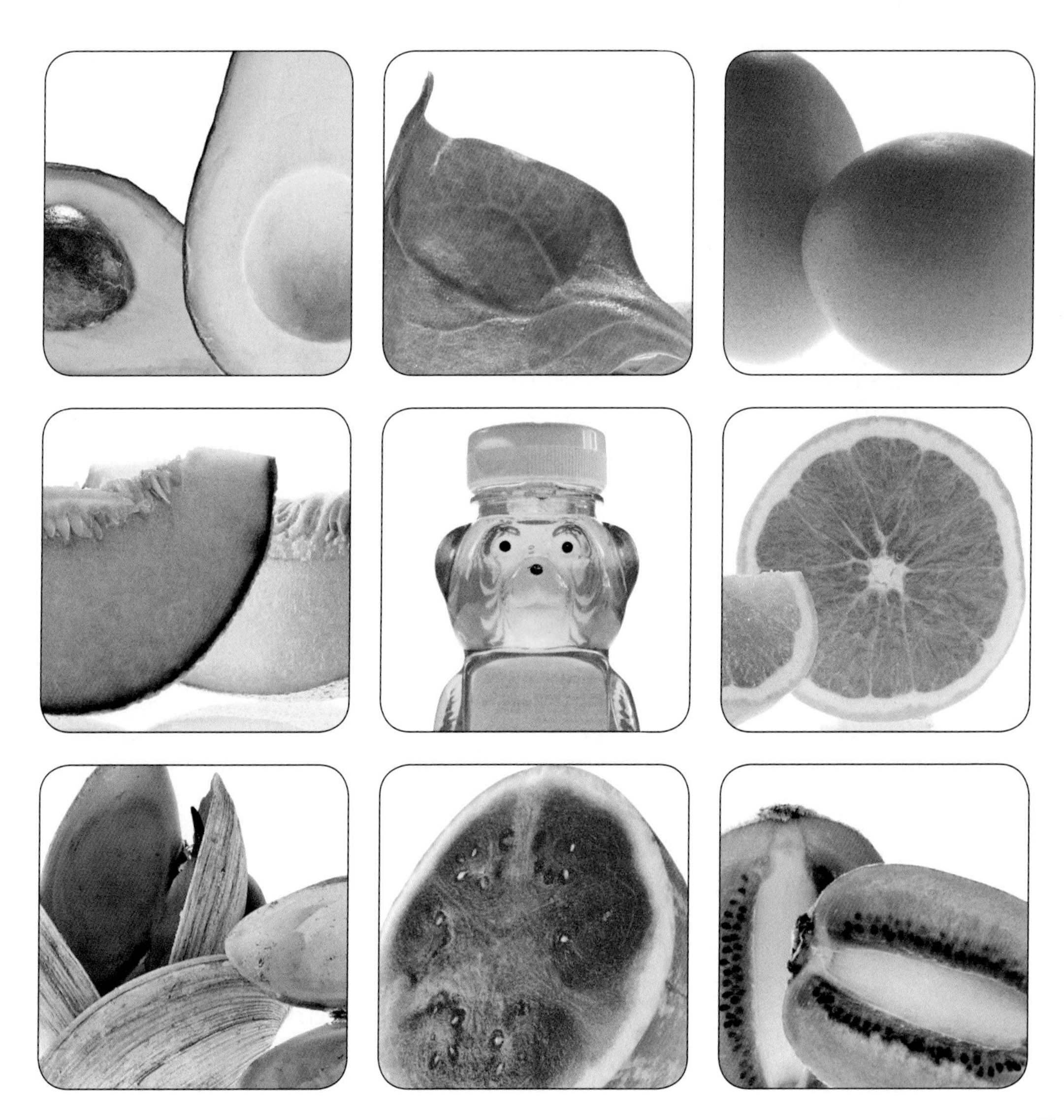

physical and emotional woes.

Indeed, our bodies are designed to function at their optimum levels and to look and feel lean, strong, and vibrant when they're fed the vitamins and minerals and healthy fats and micronutrients in real food. In fact, we could all just get along, if we all just ate a little bit better.

Imagine, if you will, a world with less stress, less insanity, and less self-loathing. It would look a lot like today's world, except for two things: (1) Lewis Black wouldn't have a job, and (2) the rest of us would be dining on salmon, washing it down with a glass of wine, and snacking on dark chocolate for dessert. Those three things have been shown in studies to brighten our moods and beat back the fatigue, depression, and anxiety so many of us labor under.

But chances are, the screaming, frothing comedian will still have plenty of angst to get out in coming years, as long as he and the rest of us keep chowing down on foods that are high in carbs, high in fat, and high in preservatives. And we will continue to battle weight issues as well because all of those bad-for-you foodstuffs set us up for even more hunger and even more weight gain.

But eating lots and lots of healthy foods can help you lose weight—in fact, it's a much better way to keep off extra pounds than not eating anything at all.

That's because our bodies are designed not only to enjoy real food and to thrive on the nutrients within, but also to burn off the calories in real food and drink. Indeed, eating smart throughout the day revs up your body's metabolism—the internal fat furnace that turns calories into energy (including the calories you've got stored in your love handles) and gives you all-day get-up-and-go. Stop feeding yourself good food and your body goes into starvation mode, saving calories like a Depression-era miser—except instead of saving them under a mattress, you'll be saving them in your belly, your butt, and other unsightly hiding places.

So in this chapter, we're outlining the best foods for whatever ails you and explaining exactly how these mealtime miracle workers will improve your looks, your life, and even your attitude. Consider this your nutritional prescription program to cure anything—and you don't even need preapproval from your HMO!

When You're Stressed

Eat This
FRIED EGGS

Go ahead, crack under pressure: Eating fried eggs may help reduce high blood pressure. In a test-tube study, scientists in Canada discovered that the breakfast standby produced the highest levels of ACE inhibitory peptides, amino acids that dilate blood vessels and allow blood to flow more easily.

WINE

It's true: A glass of wine really does take the edge off. But you may want to stop there. Researchers from the University of Toronto discovered that one alcoholic drink caused people's blood vessels to relax, but two drinks began to reverse the benefits. That's because when your blood alcohol content reaches a certain level, your central nervous system releases noradrenaline—the same hormone released when you're in high stress.

GUM

When you find yourself feeling overwhelmed at work, reach for the Wrigley's: Chewing gum can help tame your tension, according to Australian researchers. People who chewed gum while taking multitasking tests experienced a 17 percent drop in self-reported stress. This might have to do with the fact that we associate chewing with positive social interactions, like mealtimes.

Not That!
COFFEE

A cup of joe can cut through your morning mental fog, but too much coffee may exacerbate your work anxiety, according to researchers from the University of Oklahoma. The scientists found that when people downed the caffeine equivalent of three cups of java, their symptoms of psychological stress increased. Caffeine triggers a rise in your blood level of cortisol, the hormone released when you feel threatened.

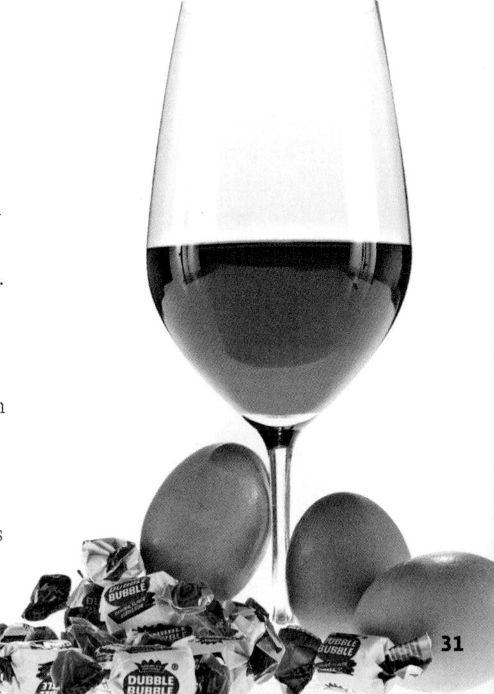

When You're Feeling Down

Eat This

SALMON

Omega-3s may calm your neurotic side, according to a study in the journal *Psychosomatic Medicine*. Researchers found that adults with the lowest blood levels of eicosapentaenoic acid (EPA) and docosahexaenoic acid (DHA) were more likely to have neuroses, which are symptoms for depression. EPA and DHA are key brain components, and higher levels of each can bolster the potent mood enhancers serotonin and dopamine. Salmon is loaded with EPAand DHA, as are walnuts, flaxseeds, and even cauliflower.

GARLIC

Tuck a few extra cloves into your next stir-fry or pasta sauce: Research has found that enzymes in garlic can help increase the release of serotonin, a neurochemical that makes you feel relaxed. Plus, garlic may have the added benefit of improving memory. Pakistani researchers found that rats fed a puree of garlic and water performed better on a memory test than rats that weren't fed the mixture.

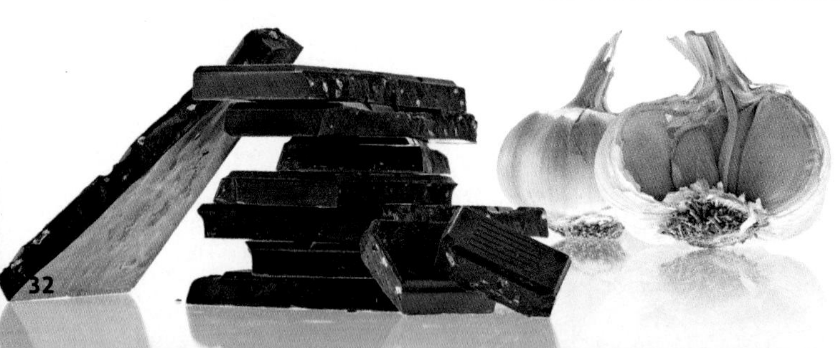

DARK CHOCOLATE

Research shows that dark chocolate can improve heart health, lower blood pressure, reduce LDL cholesterol, and increase the flow of blood to the brain. It also boosts serotonin and endorphin levels, which are associated with improved mood and greater concentration. Look for chocolate that is 60 percent cocoa or higher.

Not That!

WHITE CHOCOLATE

White chocolate isn't technically chocolate, since it contains no cocoa solids. Instead, it's made mostly with fats and sugar, lacking any of the nutritional vigor of the real stuff. That means it also lacks the ability to stimulate the euphoria-inducing chemicals that real chocolate does, especially serotonin.

When You Want to Boost Your Metabolism

Eat This

CHILE PEPPERS

It turns out that capsaicin, the compound that gives chile peppers their mouth-searing quality, can also fire up your metabolism. Eating about 1 tablespoon of chopped red or green chiles boosts your body's production of heat and the activity of your sympathetic nervous system (responsible for our fight-or-flight response), according to a study published in the *Journal of Nutritional Science and Vitaminology*. The result is a metabolism spike 42 percent higher than in those who didn't take capsaicin.

CAFFEINATED COFFEE

A study published in the journal *Physiology & Behavior* found that the average metabolic rate of people who drank caffeinated coffee increased 16 percent over those who drank decaf. Caffeine stimulates your central nervous system by increasing your heart rate and breathing.

YOGURT

The probiotics in yogurt may speed weight loss. British scientists found that these active organisms boosted the breakdown of fat molecules in mice, preventing the rodents from gaining weight. Try the Horizon brand of yogurt—it contains the probiotic L. casei, the same organism used in the study.

Not That!

NOTHING

That's right: There's no better way to grind your metabolism to a halt than skipping a meal. When your body goes without food, it switches into survival mode, storing calories rather than burning them. Breakfast is most important, since your body is still in shutdown mode and your metabolism needs a strong protein- and fiber-based jump start.

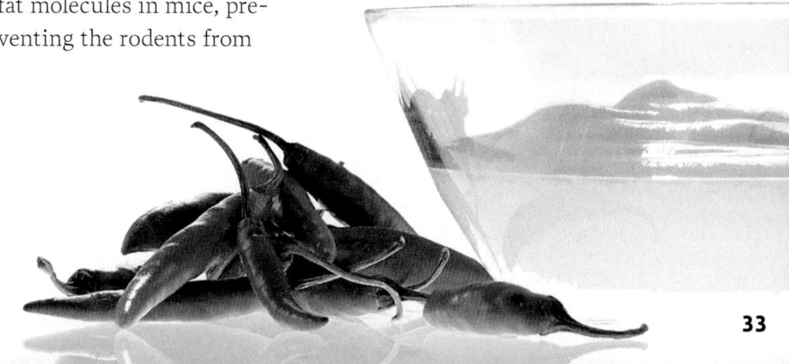

When You Need More Energy

Eat This

CLAMS

Clams stock your body with magnesium, which is important in metabolism, nerve function, and muscle function. When magnesium levels are low, your body produces more lactic acid—the same fatigue-inducing substance that you feel at the end of a long workout.

GRILLED CHICKEN BREAST

The protein in lean meat like chicken, fish, or pork loin isn't just vital in squashing hunger and boosting metabolism, it's also a top source of energy. University of Illinois researchers found that people who ate higher amounts of protein had higher energy and didn't feel as tired as people with proportionally higher amounts of carbs in their diet.

KIDNEY BEANS

These legumes are an excellent source of thiamin and riboflavin. Both vitamins help your body use energy efficiently, so you won't be nodding off mid PowerPoint.

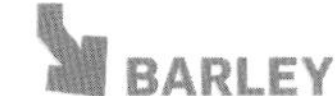

BARLEY

Swedish researchers found that if you eat barley for breakfast, the fibrous grain cuts blood sugar response by 44 percent at lunch and 14 percent at dinner. And the less your sugar spikes, the more stable your energy levels will be.

Not That!

BAGELS

MIT researchers analyzed blood samples from people who had eaten either a high-protein or a high-carbohydrate breakfast. Two hours after eating, the carb eaters had tryptophan levels 11 percent higher than before, and the people who had eaten protein dropped their tryptophan levels by 37 percent. The higher your tryptophan level, the more likely you are to feel tired and sluggish. That means fewer waffles, pancakes, and muffins and more eggs and oatmeal.

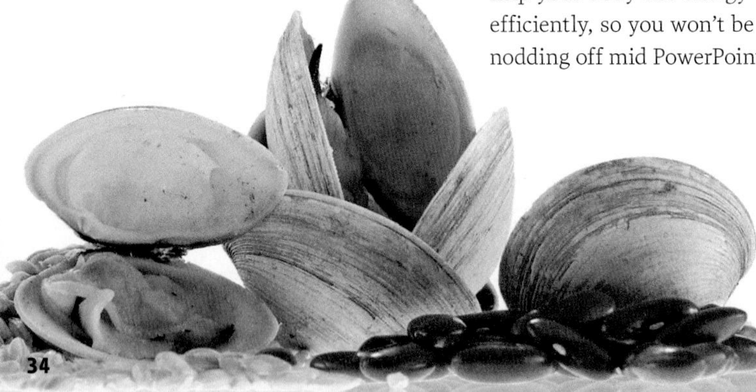

When You're Sick

Eat This
ROOIBOS TEA

Some animal research suggests that this South African tea may provide many health benefits, such as boosting immunity. Large human studies have yet to be conducted, though.

HONEY

Penn State scientists have discovered that honey is a powerful cough suppressant—so next time you're hacking up a lung, head for the kitchen. When parents of 105 sick children doled out honey or dextromethorphan (the active ingredient in over-the-counter cough medicines like Robitussin), the honey was better at lessening cough frequency and severity. (Try a drizzle in your rooibos tea!)

KIWI

The vitamin C in kiwi won't prevent the onslaught of a cold, but it might decrease the duration of your symptoms. One kiwifruit provides nearly 100 percent of your daily recommended intake of vitamin C.

OLIVES

Foods rich in healthy fats help reduce inflammation, a catalyst for migraines. One study found that the anti-inflammatory compounds in olive oil suppress the same pathway as ibuprofen.

Not That!
CAFFEINATED BEVERAGES AND ENERGY DRINKS

Excessive caffeine screws with your sleep schedule and suppresses functions of key immunity agents. And insufficient sleep opens the door to colds, upper respiratory infections, and other ills. What's more, caffeine can dehydrate you, and hydration is vital during illness: Fluids not only transport nutrients to the illness site but also dispose of toxins.

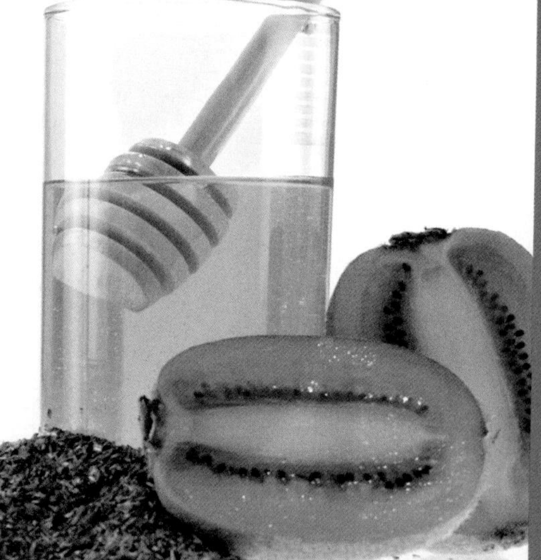

When You Want to Get in the Mood

Eat This
DARK CHOCOLATE

Chocolate is full of anandamide and phenylethylamine, two compounds that cause the body to release the same feel-good endorphins triggered by sex and physical exertion. Cocoa also contains methylxanthines, which make skin more sensitive to touch.

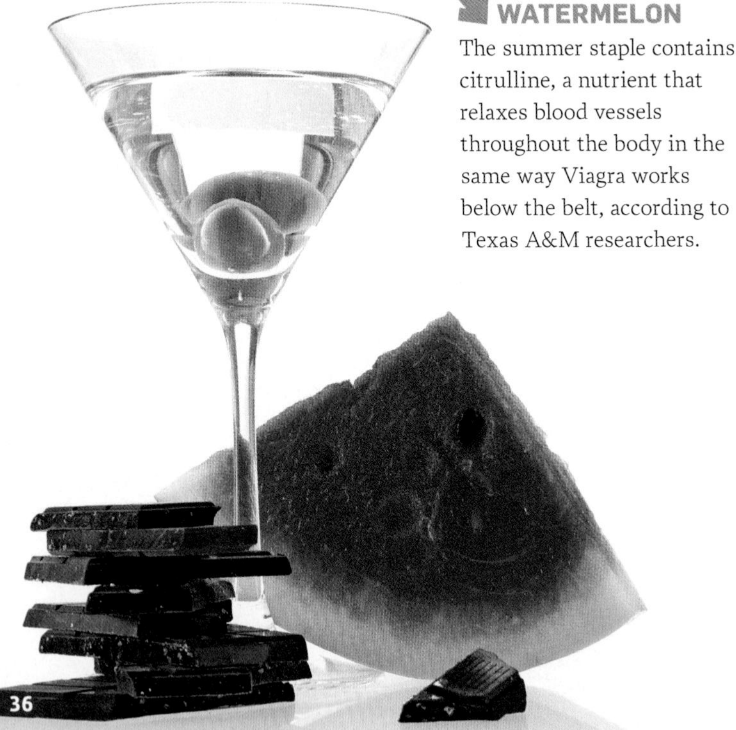

WATERMELON

The summer staple contains citrulline, a nutrient that relaxes blood vessels throughout the body in the same way Viagra works below the belt, according to Texas A&M researchers.

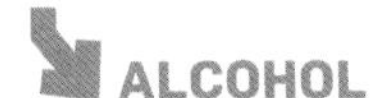

ALCOHOL

Booze acts as a depressant in the brain's cerebral cortex, lowering inhibitions that could otherwise restrain arousal. When men consumed too much, though, their erections weren't as strong as if they'd limited themselves to one or two drinks.

Not That!
OYSTERS

Okay, they won't exactly inhibit your bedroom behavior, but these legendary "aphrodisiacs" have never been proven to actually boost libido. While zinc, abundant in oysters of all shapes and sizes, is linked to male fertility, the connections to actual arousal have never been borne out in clinical research.

When You Work Out

Eat This

SPINACH

In a test-tube study, Rutgers researchers discovered that treating human muscle cells with a compound found in spinach increased protein synthesis by 20 percent. The compound allows muscle tissue to repair itself faster, the researchers say.

GREEN TEA

Brazilian scientists found that participants who consumed three cups of the beverage every day for a week had fewer markers of the cell damage caused by resistance to exercise. That means that green tea can help you recover faster after an intense workout.

CHOCOLATE MILK

That's right, nothing like a little dessert after a long workout. British researchers found that chocolate milk does a better job than sports drinks at replenishing the body after a workout. Why? Because it has more electrolytes and higher fat content. And scientists at James Madison University found that the balance of fat, protein, and carbs in chocolate milk makes it one-third more effective at replenishing muscles than other recovery beverages. And, of course, don't forget H_2O: Even as little as 1 percent decrease in your body water can impair exercise performance.

FISH OIL

Australian researchers found that cyclists who took fish oil for 8 weeks had lower heart rates and consumed less oxygen during intense bicycling than a control group did.

Not That!

RED BULL

Caffeine is a proven training aid, but drinking a Red Bull won't provide enough stimulation to affect your workouts, according to Canadian studies. Seventeen fit adults who drank up to two cans of the drink an hour before a sprint workout didn't experience a performance boost. The beverage just doesn't provide enough of a jolt.

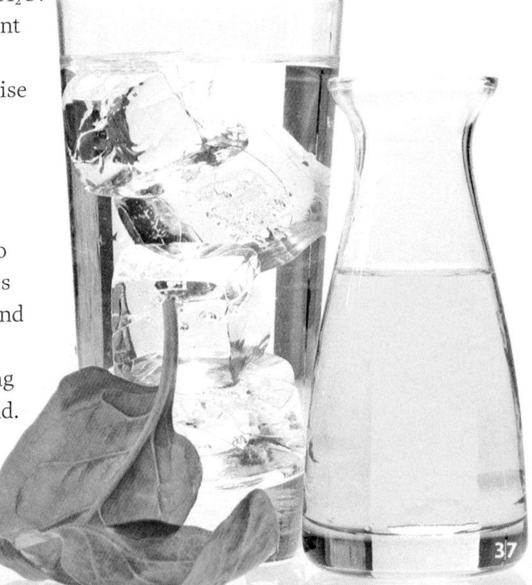

When You Need a Brain Boost

For Focus

Eat This
SARDINES

According to research published in *Nutrition Journal,* fish oil can help increase your ability to concentrate. Credit EPA and DHA, fatty acids that bolster communication among brain cells and help regulate neurotransmitters responsible for mental focus. Can't stomach sardines at your desk? Try a handful of omega-3 rich walnuts instead.

Not That!
CANDY

Sugary foods provoke sudden surges of glucose that result in energetic highs and lows. Unfortunately, the lows outlast the highs, as do the possible headaches and lack of concentration.

For Memory

Eat This
GARLIC

Researchers in Pakistan found that rats fed a puree of garlic and water performed better on a memory test than rats that weren't fed the mixture. That's because garlic increases the brain's levels of serotonin, which has been shown to enhance memory function.

BANANAS

The antioxidants in bananas, apples, and oranges may help protect you from Alzheimer's, report Korean scientists. In a test-tube study, the researchers discovered that plant chemicals known as polyphenols helped shield brain cells from oxidative stress, a key cause of the disease.

Not That!
SODA AND JUICE

Spikes in blood sugar can wreck your short-term memory, states a study in the *European Journal of Clinical Nutrition*. When scientists conducted memory tests on adults who had just downed a sugary drink, those with the highest blood glucose levels had the worst recall. Soda's an obvious offender, but even many "juice" drinks are loaded down with a rush of added sugars and high-fructose corn syrup.

ENERGY DRINKS AND VENTI LATTES

Like a politician whose smile is just a little too eager, caffeine has a dark side, too. Too much of it can make you jittery, anxious, and unsure of yourself. It can also derail your sleep schedule, meaning that extra cup of coffee today can blunt your cognitive powers tomorrow.

For Long-Lasting Brainpower

Eat This
STEAK

Vitamin B_{12}, an essential nutrient found in meat, milk, and fish, may help protect you against brain loss, say British scientists. The researchers found that older people with the highest blood levels of the vitamin were six times less likely to have brain shrinkage than those with the lowest levels.

CARROTS

Researchers from Harvard found that men who consumed more beta-carotene over 15 years had significantly delayed cognitive aging. Carrots are a tremendous source of the antioxidant, as are other orange foods like butternut squash, pumpkin, and bell peppers.

For Sharper Senses

GROUND FLAXSEED

Flax is the best source of alpha-linolenic acid (ALA)—a healthy fat that improves the workings of the cerebral cortex, the area of the brain that processes sensory information, including that of pleasure. To meet your quota, sprinkle 1 tablespoon flaxseed on salads daily or mix it into a smoothie or shake.

Not That!
ALCOHOL

This one's obvious, but worth stressing anyway. While a drink or two can increase arousal signals, more than a few drinks will actually depress your nervous system. This will dull sensations and make you tired, not sharp—in your brain and throughout the rest of your body.

Cut Your Carbohydrate Footprint

FIGHT BACK AGAINST DIABETES—AND OBESITY—BY ELIMINATING SNEAKY SUGARS FROM YOUR DIET.

Americans consume an average of 82 grams of added sugar a day. That's more than you'd find in six Breyers Oreo Ice Cream Sandwiches. But truth is, a good part of the excess sweet stuff isn't coming from ice cream or cookies or even soft drinks—it's coming from the sources we'd least expect. Open your pantry and start scanning ingredient lists. We're willing to bet that nearly every food you buy contains at least one of these blood sugar–spiking elements: modified food starch, maltodextrin, cane sugar, crystallized cane juice, evaporated cane juice, honey, tapioca syrup, brown sugar, brown rice syrup, barley, or anything with "ose" at the end of it. Food manufactures have an arsenal of empty carbohydrates at their disposal, and they're not shy about using them to make everything we eat taste like candy. Read on for eight of the most surprisingly sugar-riddled foods in your pantry.

CEREAL

Just because your favorite cereal doesn't have a cartoon character on the box doesn't mean it isn't still loaded with sugar. Not even heart-smart logos and bloated health claims can salvage the contents of boxes like Post Raisin Bran, General Mills Basic 4, or Multi-Bran Chex, all of which have more sugar than the same-size bowl of Froot Loops. Stick to cereals with high fiber to sugar ratios ensure a wholesome start to your morning.

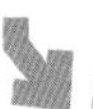
Eat This

Post Shredded Wheat Original (1 cup)

- *170 calories*
- *1 g fat*
- *0 g sugars*
- *6 g fiber*

There's one ingredient in this box: whole wheat. Either eat it as is or add cinnamon and ground flaxseed—together they will give your blood sugar the smoothest ride possible.

Not That!

Kellogg's Smart Start Original Antioxidants (1 cup)

- *190 calories*
- *0.5 g fat*
- *14 g sugars*
- *3 g fiber*

The numbers don't lie; this box has more blood sugar–spiking impact than Apple Jacks and about the same as Frosted Flakes. That's because sugar in its various forms shows up no fewer than 10 times on the ingredient list.

GRANOLA

Shoppers stop questioning a food the second it earns the unofficial seal of approval from the food-and-fitness community. In reality, that's when they should become most suspicious. This is what's happened to granola, and it's the reason why it's now near impossible to find a box with less sugar per serving than a plate of cookies. Deflect granola's unruly sugar load by scanning the cereal aisle for cereal-and-granola hybrids, like this one from Kashi.

Eat This

Kashi U 7 Whole Grain Flakes & Granola with Black Currants & Walnuts (1 cup)

- *200 calories*
- *3.5 g fat (0 g saturated)*
- *10 g sugars*
- *7 g fiber*

This box is fortified with omega-3 fats and has 7 grams of fiber to help keep your blood sugar steady. Still, you don't want to eat it alone like you would cereal. Instead, try a homemade parfait by sprinkling a little U over a cup of unsweetened yogurt.

Not That!

Quaker Natural Granola, Oats, Honey, & Raisins (1 cup)

- *420 calories*
- *12 g fat (7 g saturated)*
- *30 g sugars*
- *6 g fiber*

How do they get away with calling this granola "natural"? It has as much added sugar as a Snicker's bar. And Quaker's low-fat version is almost as bad—it has 27 grams of sugar.

WHEAT BREAD

American palates are used to the relatively bland flavor of white bread, which is why so many of us have trouble accepting wheat's more robust and earthy tones. But instead of allowing our taste buds to work through the new flavors on their own terms, manufacturers use sugar to mask wheat's true identity and make it more familiar to those unaccustomed to eating whole foods. The result? Aside from perpetually confused taste buds, these sticky loaves of "wheat bread" are spiking our blood glucose levels nearly as badly as the white loaves we're trying to leave behind.

Eat This

Food for Life Ezekiel 4:9 Bread Sprouted Grain (2 slices)

- *160 calories*
- *1 g fat*
- *0 g sugars*
- *6 g fiber*

If you were to find a loaf of bread that had been fossilized for 1,000 years, it probably wouldn't be much different from this one from Food for Life. Looking to shave a few more calories? Try Nature's Own Sugar Free 100% Whole Grain Bread. It uses a small shot of sugar alcohol to give it a light sweetness while capping the energy load at 50 calories a slice.

Not That!

Sara Lee Hearty & Delicious 100% Whole Wheat Bread (2 slices)

- *240 calories*
- *3 g fat (1 g saturated)*
- *10 g sugars*
- *6 g fiber*

Ten grams of sugars isn't uncommon for full-size sandwich breads, but it is more sugar than a single Twix bar. In this loaf, Sara Lee reaches dismal heights with a combination of brown sugar, molasses, and raisin juice concentrate. That last one might sound healthy, but your body won't be able to tell it apart from pure table sugar.

CRACKERS

Yes, even crackers are now sweetened. It's not that there's an extremely large amount of sugar going in, but ironically the most sugar is being added to crackers that are made almost entirely from refined grains. The result is a one-two punch to your pancreas: First, manufacturers strip the cracker down to nothing but fast-digesting starches, and then they finish it off with a nice dose of corn sweeteners. In a healthy body, the resulting flood of glucose will be met by an equally massive tide of insulin, but as your body edges closer to diabetes, the insulin won't be able to keep up. Switch to an unsweetened cracker to flush this whole volatile scenario out of your body.

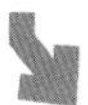

Eat This

Triscuit Thin Crisps Original (15 crackers)

- *130 calories*
- *5 g fat (1 g saturated)*
- *0 g sugars*
- *3 g fiber*

A cracker as it should be: nothing but whole wheat held together with a little oil and seasoned with salt. The Thin Crisps are perfect for those who aren't fans of Triscuit's usual heavy design.

Not That!

Wheat Thins Reduced Fat (16 crackers)

- *130 calories*
- *4 g fat (0.5 g saturated)*
- *3.5 g sugars*
- *1 g fiber*

Wheat thins are held together with three different sweeteners and a sprinkling of cornstarch, which basically affects your blood glucose in exactly the same way as pure sugar.

NUTRITION BARS

Few foods create more nutritional anxiety than the still relatively new concept of meal replacement bars. Should you be looking for high protein? High fiber? What's the ideal amount of calories? Unfortunately, sugar seems to be the one thing that all meal replacement bars have in common. And to get around it, they hide the sugar under highfalutin monikers like crystalline fructose, brown rice syrup, or—in Powerbar's case—C2 MAX Carbohydrate Blend. Your goal: Eat only those bars that earn the large majority of their calories from protein, fiber, and healthy fats. That will ensure your blood sugar stays at safe levels.

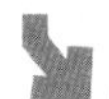

Eat This

Odwalla Sweet & Salty Almond (1 bar)

- *220 calories*
- *11 g fat (1 g saturated)*
- *8 g sugars*
- *6 g fiber*
- *7 g protein*

This bar has every one of the big three essential elements: protein, fiber, and healthy fats. These are the nutrients responsible for filling your belly and keeping your internal sugars in the healthy range. Now you know why we call almonds a superfood.

Not That!

Powerbar Energize Tangy Tropical Fruit Smoothie (1 bar)

- *220 calories*
- *3.5 g fat (0.5 g saturated)*
- *30 g sugars*
- *<1 g fiber*
- *6 g protein*

No fiber and more sugar than two scoops of Edy's Slow Churned Rocky Road Ice Cream? Yikes. Powerbar makes this bar for quick-burn energy, but it's not the kind of energy you need unless you just turned the third leg of an Ironman Triathlon.

YOGURT

Here's an interesting fact: Milk is the only animal product to be naturally sweetened. That's probably why most people don't think it's odd to lift a creamy spoonful of yogurt to their lips and get a dessert-like blast of flavor in return. But the truth is that nature's treats are more subtle. In fact, if you haven't been skimming ingredient lists, you might never have tasted real, unadulterated yogurt. The stuff you've been eating is a candified version of the real thing, and it's probably jacking your blood sugar ever higher with each cup you eat.

Eat This

Stonyfield Farm Oikos Organic Greek Yogurt, Plain (1 container, 5.3 oz)

- *80 calories*
- *0 g fat*
- *6 g sugars*
- *15 g protein*

At the very least, you should convert to plain yogurt and sweeten it at home with real fruit, but if you want to do one better, switch over to creamier Greek yogurt. It has three times as much slow-digesting protein as the regular version.

Not That!

Yoplait 99% Fat Free Cherry Orchard (1 container, 4 oz)

- *170 calories*
- *1.5 g fat (1 g saturated)*
- *27 g sugars*
- *4 g protein*

The marketing brains at Yoplait are hoping that by painting 99% Fat Free on the label, they will divert your attention from the ingredient list, which exposes this yogurt for the dangerous snack that it is. By using more sugar, than fruit, they gave this cup as much sugar as three Pillsbury Cinnamon Rolls.

"HEALTHY" DRINKS

Few people truly realize the dramatic effect that sugary beverages have on blood sugar. Bottlers wrangle you in with overblown promises of increased energy, improved immune function, or instant and long-lasting stress release, but what they neglect to tell you is that the sugar in most of these drinks far outweighs any unproven health benefit that might result from sucking down a bottle. At best, you'll feel a placebo-like boost, but you can be certain that inside your body there's a frenetic rush to cope with the unnatural influx of glucose. The reason is simple: Sweetened drinks don't provide the safety net that real food does. There's no fat, fiber, or protein, which leaves nothing but a torrent of pure sugar sloshing through your body. Want a real health drink? Water and tea are your best bets.

Drink This

Honest Tea Just Green Tea (16 oz)

- *0 calories*
- *0 g fat*
- *0 g sugars*

Think that green tea is too simple to be a bona fide antioxidant powerhouse? Wrong. It does more good for your body than any smart or functional beverage on the market.

Not That!

Snapple Protect Antioxidant Water Tropical Mango (20 oz)

- *150 calories*
- *0 g fat*
- *30 g sugars*

New rule for choosing a beverage: Read the ingredient list before you read the claims on the front of the bottle. If you did this with Snapple's Tropical Mango Antioxidant Water, you'd realize straight away that it is made from water and sugar. That makes those antioxidant and electrolyte claims on the front label absolutely meaningless.

TOMATO SAUCE

Have you ever been to an Italian restaurant and had the waiter come by with a cup of sugar and ask if you'd like some sprinkled over your spaghetti? No, of course you haven't. So why would you let the food scientists at Ragu or Prego add sugar to your marinara? The answer is you wouldn't, not if you knew they were doing it. Half a cup of spaghetti sauce ought to have around 5 grams of sugar—that's how much you'll find naturally in the tomatoes. Any more than that is cause for concern, especially considering how many Americans rely on bottled tomato sauce for easy weeknight meals.

Eat This

Classico Tomato & Basil (1/2 cup)

- *50 calories*
- *1 g fat*
- *5 g sugars*
- *380 mg sodium*

Classico makes some of the best sauces on the shelf, but that doesn't mean the company is without fault. Even they sometimes succumb to the low standard of high sugar levels. Not this jar though—the only sugars here are all natural.

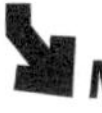

Not That!

Newman's Own Tomato & Basil Bombolina (1/2 cup)

- *90 calories*
- *4.5 g fat (0.5 g saturated)*
- *12 g sugars*
- *620 mg sodium*

All considered, this jar has 72 grams of sugar—42 of which don't belong. The culprit is the 10 added teaspoons of sugar, which hold down a spot on the ingredient list between soybean oil and salt.

10 Foods for a Longer, Healthier Life

We talk a lot about the foods you can't eat in these books, foods so infused with calories, fat, and sodium they should come with Surgeon General warnings like cigarette packs. And often times the better choice for you when eating on the run still isn't textbook nutritious stuff—it's the lesser of two formimidable fast-food or sit-down evils. But these 10 foods highlighted below are as perfect as food on this planet gets, capable not just of helping you boost metabolism and melt fat, but also fight disease, lower cholesterol, stabilize blood sugar, and live a longer, better life. And did we mention that they're delicious? Make it your goal to work these edible all-stars into your diet every day.

EGGS

When it comes to breakfast, you can't beat eggs. (That was too easy, wasn't it?) Seriously though, at a cost of only 72 calories, each large egg holds 6.3 grams of high-quality protein and a powerhouse load of vital nutrients. A study published in the *International Journal of Obesity* found that people who replace carbs with eggs for breakfast lose weight 65 percent quicker. Researchers in Michigan were able to determine that regular egg eaters enjoyed more vitamins and minerals in their diets than those who ate few or no eggs. By examining surveys from more than 25,000 people, the researchers found that egg eaters were about half as likely to be deficient in vitamin B_{12}, 24 percent less likely to be deficient in vitamin A, and 36 percent less likely to be deficient in vitamin E. And here's something more shocking: Those who ate at least four eggs a week had significantly lower cholesterol levels than those who ate fewer than one. Turns out the dietary cholesterol in the yolk has little impact on your serum cholesterol.

Substitutes: Egg Beaters egg substitute

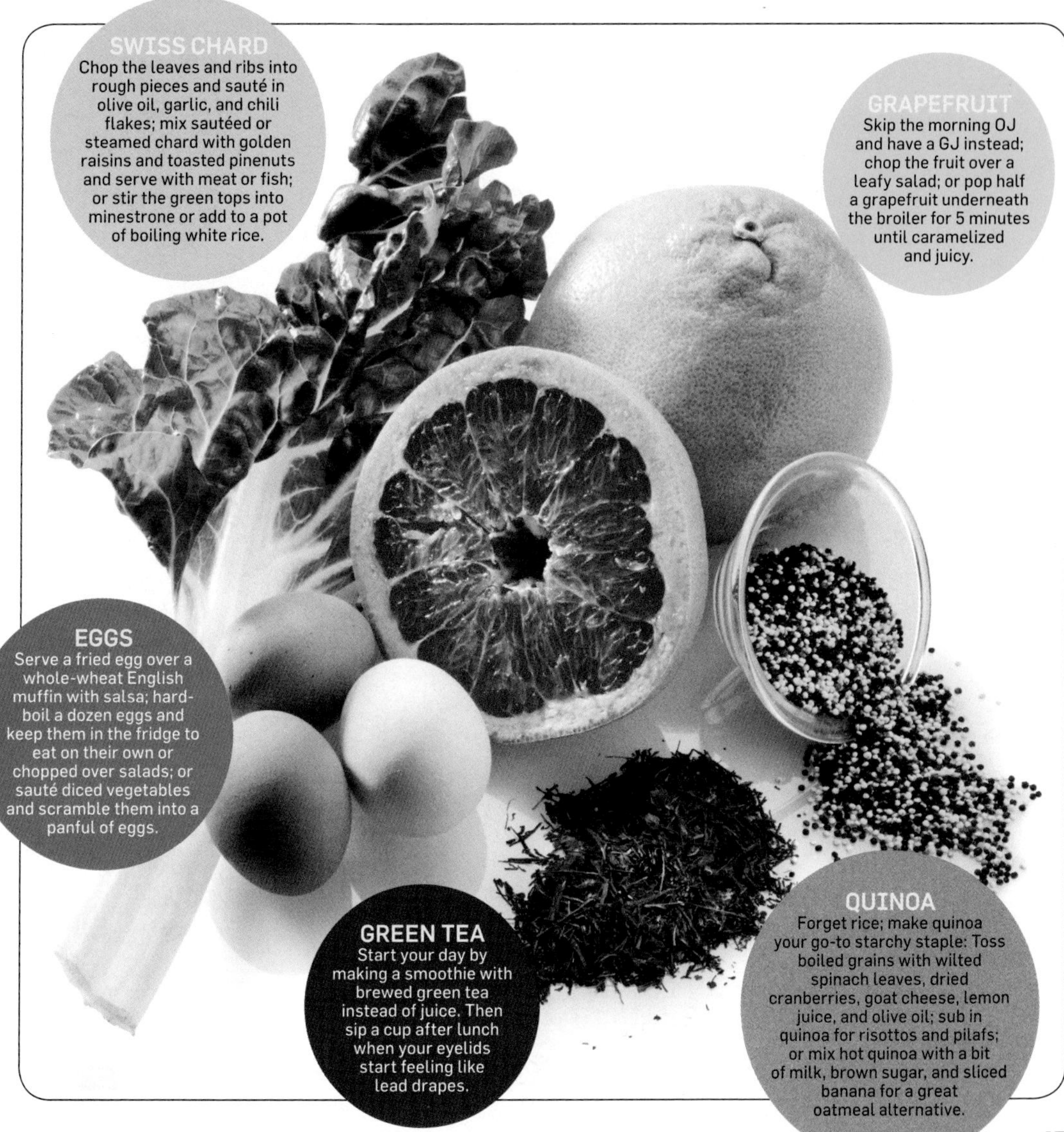
SWISS CHARD
Chop the leaves and ribs into rough pieces and sauté in olive oil, garlic, and chili flakes; mix sautéed or steamed chard with golden raisins and toasted pinenuts and serve with meat or fish; or stir the green tops into minestrone or add to a pot of boiling white rice.
GRAPEFRUIT
Skip the morning OJ and have a GJ instead; chop the fruit over a leafy salad; or pop half a grapefruit underneath the broiler for 5 minutes until caramelized and juicy.
EGGS
Serve a fried egg over a whole-wheat English muffin with salsa; hard-boil a dozen eggs and keep them in the fridge to eat on their own or chopped over salads; or sauté diced vegetables and scramble them into a panful of eggs.
GREEN TEA
Start your day by making a smoothie with brewed green tea instead of juice. Then sip a cup after lunch when your eyelids start feeling like lead drapes.
QUINOA
Forget rice; make quinoa your go-to starchy staple: Toss boiled grains with wilted spinach leaves, dried cranberries, goat cheese, lemon juice, and olive oil; sub in quinoa for risottos and pilafs; or mix hot quinoa with a bit of milk, brown sugar, and sliced banana for a great oatmeal alternative.

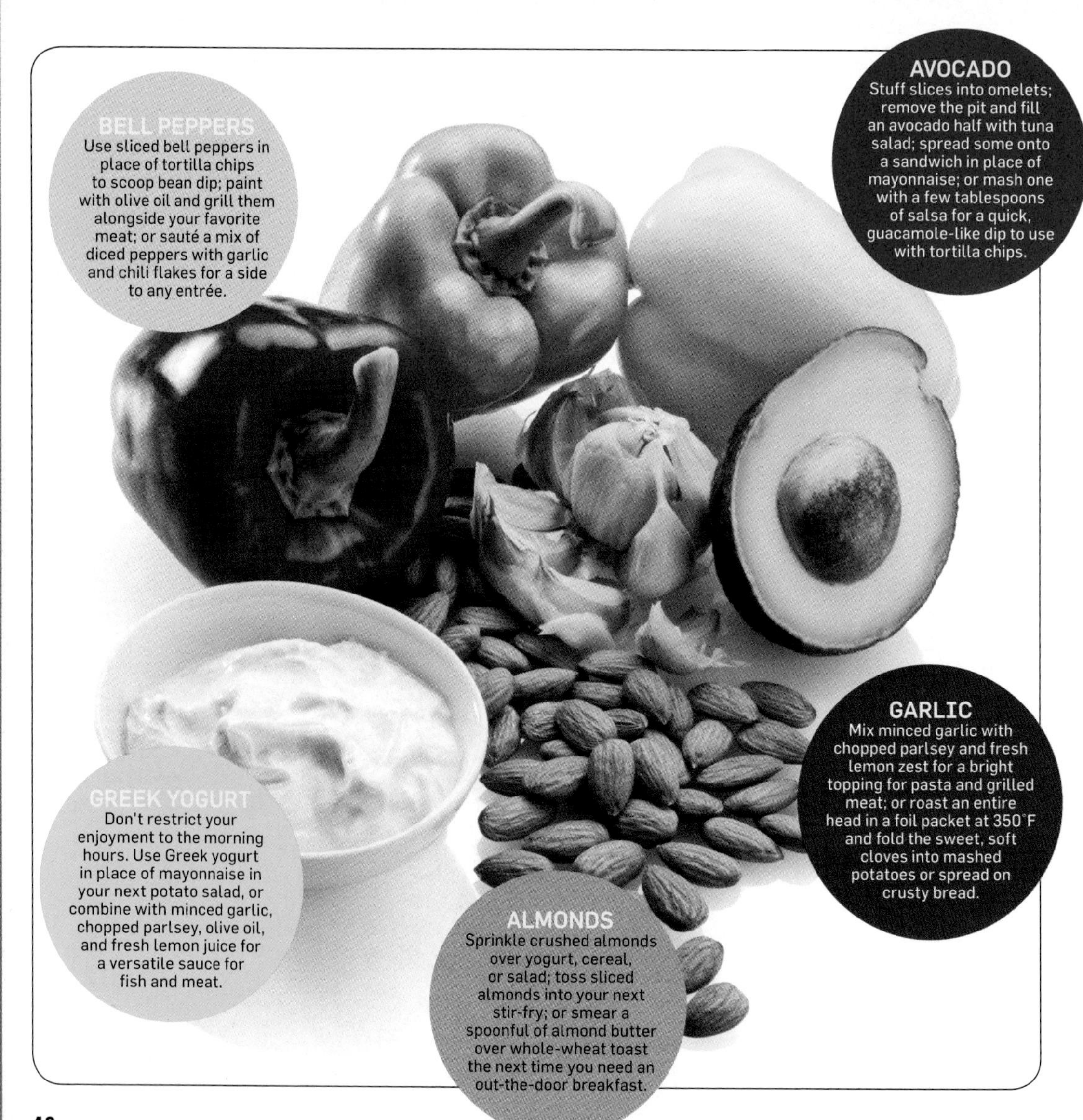
BELL PEPPERS
Use sliced bell peppers in place of tortilla chips to scoop bean dip; paint with olive oil and grill them alongside your favorite meat; or sauté a mix of diced peppers with garlic and chili flakes for a side to any entrée.
AVOCADO
Stuff slices into omelets; remove the pit and fill an avocado half with tuna salad; spread some onto a sandwich in place of mayonnaise; or mash one with a few tablespoons of salsa for a quick, guacamole-like dip to use with tortilla chips.
GARLIC
Mix minced garlic with chopped parlsey and fresh lemon zest for a bright topping for pasta and grilled meat; or roast an entire head in a foil packet at 350°F and fold the sweet, soft cloves into mashed potatoes or spread on crusty bread.
GREEK YOGURT
Don't restrict your enjoyment to the morning hours. Use Greek yogurt in place of mayonnaise in your next potato salad, or combine with minced garlic, chopped parlsey, olive oil, and fresh lemon juice for a versatile sauce for fish and meat.
ALMONDS
Sprinkle crushed almonds over yogurt, cereal, or salad; toss sliced almonds into your next stir-fry; or smear a spoonful of almond butter over whole-wheat toast the next time you need an out-the-door breakfast.

GREEN TEA

Literally hundreds of studies have been carried out to document the health benefits of catechins, the group of antioxidants concentrated in the leaves of tea plants. Among the most startling studies was one published by the American Medical Association in 2006. The study followed more than 40,000 Japanese adults for a decade, and at the 7-year follow-up, those who had been drinking five or more cups of tea per day were 26 percent less likely to die of any cause compared with those who averaged less than a cup. Looking for more immediate results? Another Japanese study broke participants into two groups, only one of which was put on a catechin-rich green-tea diet. At the end of 12 weeks, the green-tea group had achieved significantly smaller body weights and waistlines than those in the control group. Why? Because researchers believe that catechins are effective at boosting metabolism.

Substitutes: Yerba mate, white tea, oolong tea, rooibos (red) tea

GARLIC

Allicin, an antibacterial and antifungal compound, is the steam engine pushing forward garlic's myriad health benefits. The chemical is produced by the garlic plant as a defense against pests, but inside in your body it fights cancer, strengthens your cardiovascular system, decreases fat storage, and fights acne inflammation. To activate the most possible allicin, you've first got to crush the garlic as finely as possible. Peel the cloves, then use the side of a heavy chef's knife to crush the garlic before carefully mincing. Then be sure not to overcook it, as too much heat will render the compound completely useless (and your food totally bitter).

Substitutes: Onions, chives, leeks

GRAPEFRUIT

Just call it the better-body fruit. In a study of 100 obese people at The Scripps Clinic in California, those who ate half a grapefruit with each meal lost an average of 3.6 pounds over the course of 12 weeks Some lost as much as 10 pounds. The study's control group, in contrast, lost a paltry ½ pound. But here's something even better: Those who ate the grapefruit also exhibited a decrease in insulin levels, indicating that their bodies had improved upon the ability to metabolize sugar. If you can't stomach a grapefruit-a-day regime, try to find as many ways possible to sneak grapefruit into your diet. Even a moderate increase in grapefruit intake should yield results, not to mention earning you a massive dose of lycopene—the cancer-preventing antioxidant found most commonly in tomatoes.

Substitutes: Oranges, watermelon, tomatoes

GREEK YOGURT

If it's dessert you want, you go with regular yogurt, but if it's protein, you go Greek. What sets the two apart? Greek yogurt has been separated from the watery whey that sits on top of regular yogurt, and the process has removed excessive sugars such as lactose and increased the concentration of protein by as much as three times. That means it fills your belly more like a meal than a snack. Plus a single cup has about a quarter of your day's calcium, and studies show that dieters on calcium-rich diets have an easier time losing body fat. In one of these studies, participants on a high-calcium dairy diet were able to lose 70% more body weight than those on a calorie-restricted diet alone. If only everything you ate could make a similar claim.

Substitutes: Kefir and yogurt with "live and active cultures" printed on the product label

AVOCADO

Here's what often gets lost in America's fat phobia: Some of them are actually good for you. More than half the calories in each creamy green fruit comes from one of the world's healthiest fats, a kind called monounsaturates. These fats differ from saturated fats in that they have one double-bonded carbon atom, but that small difference at the molecular level amounts to a dramatic improvement to your health. Numerous studies have shown that monounsaturated fats both improve you cholesterol profile and decrease the amount of triglycerides (more fats) floating around in your blood. That can lower your risk of stroke and heart disease. Worried about weight gain? Don't be. There's no causal link between monounsaturated fats and body fat.

Substitutes: Olive, canola and peanut oils, peanut butter, tahini

QUINOA

Although not yet common in American kitchens, quinoa boasts a stronger distribution of nutrients than any grain you'll ever get a fork into. It has about twice as much fiber and protein as brown rice, and those proteins it has consist of a near-perfect blend of amino acids, the building blocks that your body pulls apart to reassembles into new proteins. And get this, all that protein and fiber—in conjunction with a handful of healthy fats and a comparatively small dose of carbohydrates—help insure a low impact on your blood sugar. That's great news for pre-diabetics and anyone watching their weight. So what's the trade off? There is none. Quinoa's soft and nutty taste is easy to handle for even picky eaters and it cooks just like rice, ready in about 15 minutes.

Substitutes: Oats, amaranth, millet, pearl barley, bulgur wheat

BELL PEPPERS

All peppers are loaded with antioxidants, but none so much as the brightly colored reds, yellows, and oranges. These colors result from carotenoids concentrated in the flesh of the pepper, and it's these same carotenoids that give tomatoes, carrots, and grapefruits their healthy hues. The range of benefits provided by these colorful pigments include improved immune function, better communication between cells, protection against sun damage, and a diminished risk for several types of cancer. And if you can take the heat, try cooking with chili peppers. The bell pepper cousins are still loaded with carotenoids and vitamin C, but have the added benefit of capsaicins, temperature-raising phytochemicals that have been shown to fight headache and arthritis pain as well as boost metabolism.

Substitutes: Carrots, sweet potatoes, watermelon

ALMONDS

An ounce of almonds a day, about 23 nuts, provides nearly 9 grams of heart-healthy oleic acid, which is more than peanuts, walnuts, or cashews. This monounsaturated fat is known to be responsible for a flurry of health benefits, the most recent of which is improved memory. Rats in California were better able to navigate a maze the second time around if they'd been fed oleic acid, and there's no reason to assume that the same treatment won't help you navigate your day-to-day life. If nothing else, snacking on the brittle nuts will take your mind of your hunger. Nearly a quarter of an almond's calories come from belly-filling fiber and protein. That's why when researchers at Purdue fed subjects nuts or rice cakes, those who ate the nuts felt full for a full hour and a half longer than the rice cake group.

Substitutes: Walnuts, pecans, peanuts, sesame seeds, flaxseeds

SWISS CHARD

Most fruits and vegetables are role players, supplying us with a monster dose of a single nutrient. But Swiss chard is nature's ultimate multivitamin, delivering substantial amounts of 16 vitamins and vital nutrients, and it does so at a rock bottom caloric cost. For a mere 35 calories worth of cooked chard, you get more than 300% of your recommended daily intake of bone—strengthening vitamin K, 100% of your day's vitamin A, shown to help defend against cancer and bolster vision, and 16% of hard-to-get vitamin E, which studies have shown may help sharpen mental acuity. Plus, emerging research suggests that the combination of phytonutrients and fiber in chard may provide an effective defense against colon cancer.

Substitutes: Spinach, mustard greens, collard greens, watercress, arugula, romaine lettuce

3

Eat This, Not That!

AT YOUR FAVORITE RESTAURANTS

On television, being a restaurant chef looks so romantic.

You could go one-on-one with Gordon Ramsay on *Hell's Kitchen,* cook yourself to victory over Bobby Flay on *Iron Chef America,* find a recipe to melt Padma Lakshmi's heart on *Top Chef,* or travel the world feasting on critters like Anthony Bourdain on *No Reservations.* Foodie television makes it seems as though anyone with a ladle and a spatula is a swashbuckling pirate prince.

The reality is very, very different. The vast majority of professional cooks in the United States don't work under wild-eyed slave drivers, whipping up ingenious new recipes out of scrod liver, bull testicles, and bok choy and wowing their customers with stunning new taste sensations. The average cook works in your local Olive Garden, or T.G.I.Friday's, or Applebee's, and the *last* thing his boss or his customers want is for him to get *creative.* Indeed, the line cooks at the IHOP in Tucson are cooking the exact same ingredients in the exact same way as their compatriots in Tuscaloosa. Uniformity, not creativity, is the key to modern restaurant success.

So when it comes to knowing exactly what's in your restaurant meal—and how many calories you're consuming when you eat it—you'd think getting the facts would be pretty easy. After all, it's not like the Tucson chefs are hunting the desert for cactus leaves and the Tuscaloosa cooks are picking berries on the banks of the Black Warrior River. They're using the same stuff in every Bacon Temptation Omelette from Arizona to Alabama, from Connecticut to California.

Yet many restaurant chains—IHOP included—refuse to tell their customers what it is, exactly, that they're putting into their bodies, claiming that it's just too hard to figure out. And one thing we've learned is this: Nobody hesitates to tell you *good* news. As we began researching our first edition of ***EAT THIS, NOT THAT!***, we asked IHOP repeatedly for nutritional information—and we were turned down time and again. It was only after New York City imposed a law forcing chain restaurants operating within the city to reveal their calorie counts that we learned the terrible truth about that Bacon Temptation Omelette: That little breakfast treat packs more than 1,400 calories, or about two-thirds of what the average adult should eat in an entire day. Indeed, IHOP is the land of 1,000-calorie crepes, 1,200-calorie breakfast combos, and 1,800-calorie chicken dishes. Put an *e* on the end of that restaurant's name, and *hope* it's located close to a 24-hour fitness center.

On the other hand, many restaurants have heeded our call to action and started taking their customers' right to know seriously. A great example: Red Lobster. While the seafood purveyor at first withheld its nutritional information, they recently relented and gave ***EAT THIS, NOT THAT!*** an inside look at their menu. The result: We give Red Lobster an A for their array of healthy menu options.

Still, trusting a multinational corporation to put things into your body—and not let you know what exactly those things contain—sounds like a foolhardy enterprise (and maybe the plot to a Philip K. Dick novel). So for this chapter, we have dug deep and revealed the secrets that many top restaurants don't want you to know. Whether you're Outback, On the Border, or in the Subway, everything you need to know is in these pages.

The 20 Worst Foods in America

WORST KIDS' MEAL

20 Chili's Pepper Pals Little Chicken Crispers with Ranch Dressing and Homestyle Fries

- *1,010 calories*
- *75 g fat (13 g saturated)*
- *1,780 mg sodium*
- *46 g carbohydrates*

Most kids, if given the choice, would live on chicken fingers for the duration of their lives. If those chicken fingers happened to come from Chili's, it might be a pretty short life. A moderately active 8-year-old boy should eat around 1,800 calories a day. This single meal plows through 75 percent of that allotment. So unless he plans to eat carrots and celery sticks for the rest of the day (and we know he doesn't), find a healthier chicken alternative.

Eat This Instead!

Pepper Pals Grilled Chicken Platter with Cinnamon Apples

• 340 calories • 8 g fat (2.5 g saturated)
• 755 mg sodium • 38 g carbohydrates

WORST SUPERMARKET MEAL

19 Stouffer's White Meat Chicken Pot Pie (large)

- *1,160 calories*
- *66 g fat (26 g saturated)*
- *1,780 mg sodium*

Whether ordered in restaurants or eaten straight from the microwave, potpies are seriously problematic. Why? The flaky, oil-soaked crust and the viscous, cream-based filling, to start with. Stouffer's creation suffers because of its size, packing within its carbo-walls as much saturated fat as you'll find in 6 scoops of Breyers All Natural Butter Almond ice cream.

Eat This Instead!

Stouffer's Grilled Herb Chicken

• 250 calories • 6 g fat (1 g saturated)
• 740 mg sodium

WORST "HEALTHY" SANDWICH

18 Blimpie Special Vegetarian (12")

- *1,186 calories*
- *60 g fat (19 g saturated)*
- *3,532 mg sodium*

Sure, a Special Vegetarian sandwich sounds healthy, but this foot-long monster comes with 3 different kinds of cheese and a thick slick of oil. Hard to believe you'd be better off with 2 Big Macs.

Eat This Instead!

Mediterranean Ciabatta

• 447 calories • 8 g fat (2 g saturated)
• 1,719 mg sodium

WORST STEAK

17 Outback Steakhouse Rib Eye Steak

- *1,190 calories*

Start with a 14-ounce hunk of beef, and you're already skating on thin nutritional ice. To make matters worse, rib eye is one of the most heavily marbled cuts of beef on the cow. Factor in the whole meal—

2,115 calories

California Pizza Kitchen
Thai Crunch Salad

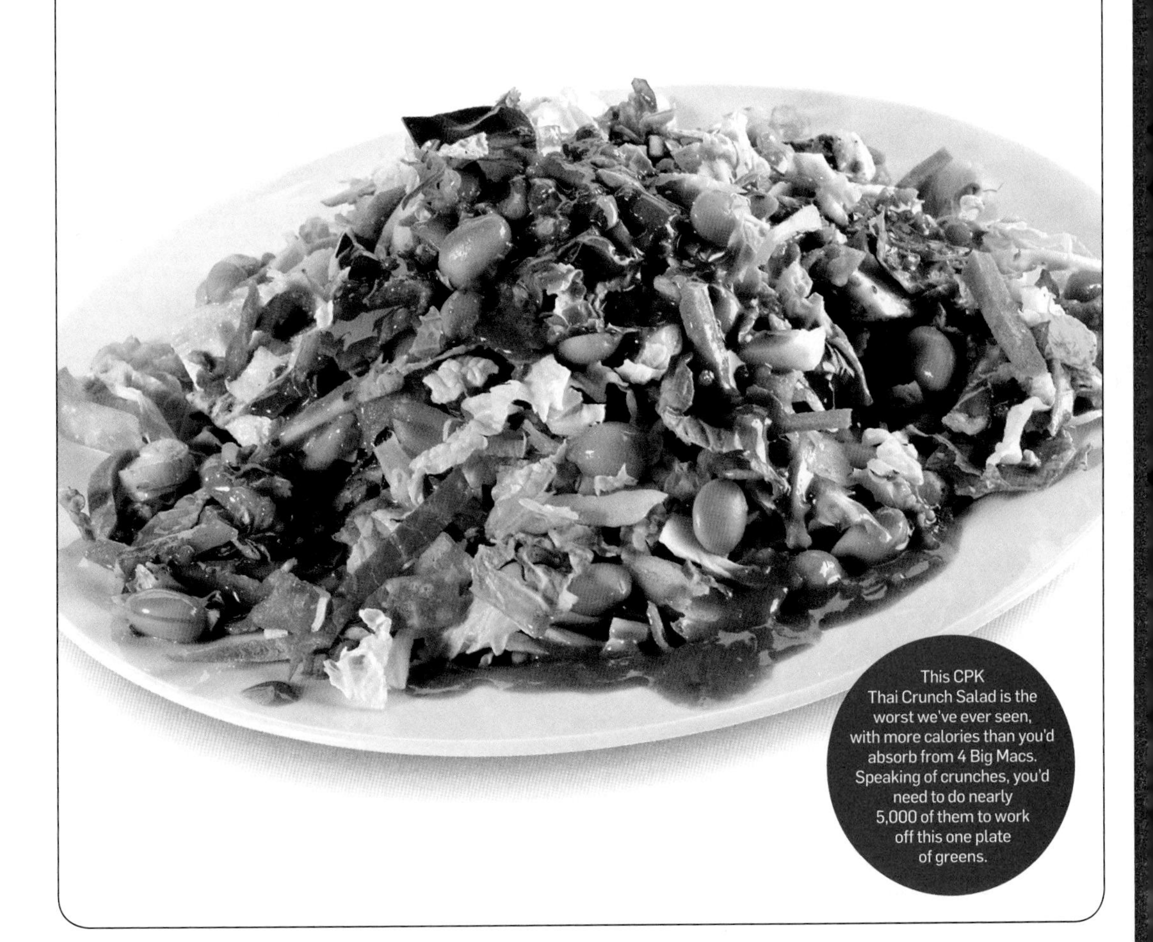

This CPK Thai Crunch Salad is the worst we've ever seen, with more calories than you'd absorb from 4 Big Macs. Speaking of crunches, you'd need to do nearly 5,000 of them to work off this one plate of greens.

including bread, salad, baked potato, and seasonal veggies—and you're looking at a 2,195-calorie steak dinner! Cut that number by a third by sticking to leaner cuts of beef (Outback does offer a few steaks worth ordering—think sirloin and petite fillets), slicing the serving size in half, and passing on the bread.

Eat This Instead!

Prime Rib (8 oz)

• 540 calories

*Outback refuses to disclose complete nutritional data for their dishes.

WORST FAST-FOOD BREAKFAST

16 McDonald's Deluxe Breakfast (large biscuit) with syrup and margarine

- 1,150 calories
- 60 g fat (20 g saturated)
- 2,260 mg sodium
- 116 g carbohydrates

This breakfast comes with the works—scrambled eggs, sausage, biscuit, hash browns, you name it. Problem is, it also comes with more than half your day's allotment of calories and an entire day's worth of sodium. It's the caloric equivalent of 4 McDonald's cheeseburgers—can you imagine starting your day off like that? Embrace the McMuffin,* but steer clear of sausage.

Eat This Instead!

Egg McMuffin

• 300 calories • 12 g fat (5 g saturated) • 820 mg sodium • 30 g carbohydrates

WORST CHINESE ENTRÉE

15 P.F. Chang's Combo Lo Mein

- 1,476 calories
- 72 g fat (9 g saturated)
- 4,395 mg sodium

Lo mein is normally looked at as a side dish, a harmless pile of noodles to pad your plate of orange chicken or broccoli beef. This heaping portion (to be fair, Chang's does suggest diners share an order) comes spiked with chicken, shrimp, beef, and pork, not to mention an Exxon Valdez–size slick of oil. The damage? A day's worth of calories, more than a day's worth of fat, and nearly 2 days' worth of sodium. No meat-based dish beats out the New York strip.

Eat This Instead!

Asian Marinated New York Strip

• 558 calories • 30 g fat (12 g saturated) • 864 mg sodium

WORST BREAKFAST

14 Bob Evans Stacked & Stuffed Caramel Banana Pecan Hotcakes

- 1,493 calories
- 70 g fat (21 g saturated, 9 g trans)
- 110 g sugars
- 2,265 mg sodium

It's not a good sign when it takes you nearly 5 seconds to spit out the name of your breakfast. This bad boy packs in more than 75 percent of your calories for the day, along with more sugar and almost as much fat as 8 glazed Dunkin' Donuts and nearly as much sodium as 5 Bloody Marys. That's why it's back on our list of the 20 Worst Foods in America again this year.

Eat This Instead!

3 Scrambled Egg Lites with bacon (2 slices) and fresh fruit

• 502 calories • 19 g fat (7 g saturated) • 19 g sugars • 832 mg sodium

WORST ICE CREAM DESSERT

13 Così Double Trouble Brownie Sundae

- 1,594 calories
- 95 g fat
- 1,039 mg sodium
- 163 g carbohydrates

This dessert is dubbed "Double Trouble" for a reason.

Così doesn't provide sugar content, but the 163 grams of carbohydrates suggests that this sundae racks up at least 100 grams of the sweet stuff, easily. That's the sugar equivalent of 10 Krispy Kreme original glazed doughnuts. And there could be even more. Add to that enough calories to fill you up for almost an entire day (not to mention a disturbingly high level of sodium), and this dessert is sure to absolutely trash your diet.

Eat This Instead!

S'Mores

- *361 calories • 10 g fat*
- *234 mg sodium • 61 g carbohydrates*

WORST CHICKEN ENTRÉE

12 Dairy Queen Chicken Strip Basket (6-piece) with Country Gravy

- *1,640 calories*
- *74 g fat (12 g saturated, 1 g trans)*
- *3,690 mg sodium*
- *121 g carbohydrates*

It's astonishing how many calories DQ can pack into 6 strips of chicken. Don't blame the trans-fatty gravy alone—it adds only about 400 extra calories. This disastrous basket will send your blood pressure soaring with the sodium equivalent of 112 saltine crackers, and it'll drag you down for the rest of the day with its crippling carbohydrate overload.

Eat This Instead!

Grilled Flamethrower Chicken Sandwich

- *590 calories • 36 g fat (9 g saturated)*
- *1,480 mg sodium*
- *34 g carbohydrates*

WORST SANDWICH

11 Quiznos Tuna Melt (large)

- *1,760 calories*
- *133 g fat (25 g saturated, 1.5 g trans)*
- *2,120 mg sodium*
- *92 g carbohydrates*

When we first published *Eat This, Not That!*, we singled out this troublesome tuna sandwich for its massive caloric load. In response, Quiznos claims to have shaved a good 300 calories from the filling. But incredibly enough, it's still the most atrocious sandwich we found in our latest round of menu scouring. Blame the gobs of calorie- and fat-packed mayo, the endless inches of carb-heavy bread, and the full day's worth of sodium.

Eat This Instead!

Small Honey Bourbon Chicken on Wheat Bread

- *320 calories • 4.5 g fat (0.5 g saturated)*
- *920 mg sodium • 50 mg carbohydrates*

WORST ITALIAN ENTRÉE

10 Romano's Macaroni Grill Spaghetti and Meatballs with Meat Sauce

- *1,810 calories*
- *118 g fat (54 g saturated)*
- *4,900 mg sodium*
- *109 g carbohydrates*

With nearly three times your recommended daily intake of saturated fat and 2 days' worth of salt, these ain't your mama's meatballs (at least we hope not). This dish debuted on our 2008 list with even more calories, but there's still no other pasta that delivers this bad a blow.

Eat This Instead!

Capellini Tre Pomodoro

- *470 calories • 25 g fat (3 g saturated)*
- *949 mg sodium • 87 g carbohydrates*

WORST BURGER

9 Outback Steakhouse Blooming Burger

- *1,880 calories*

What do you get when you cross one of America's worst appetizers with one of America's most imprudent purveyors of high-calorie

2,030 calories

Cold Stone Creamery PB&C Shake

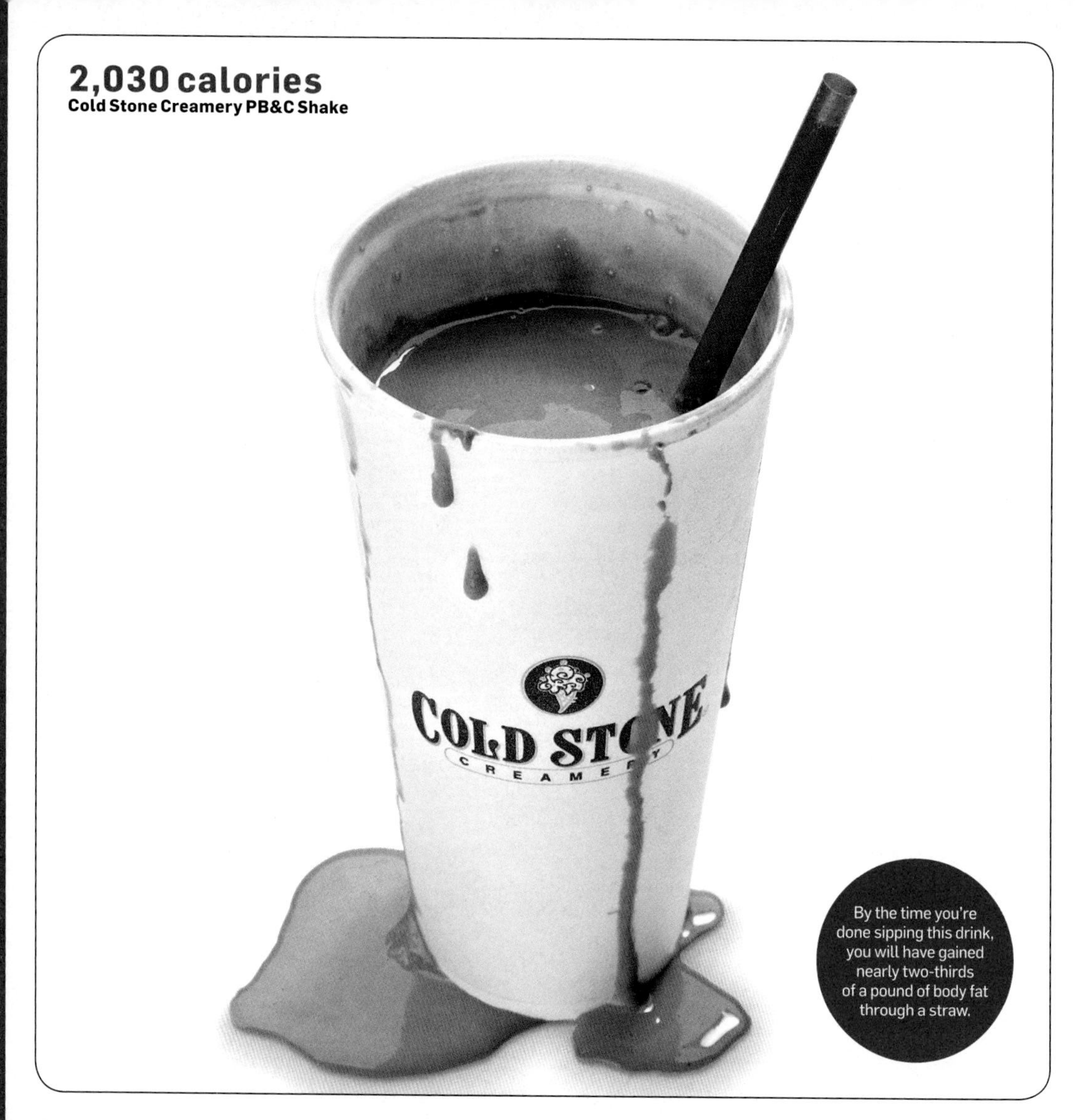

By the time you're done sipping this drink, you will have gained nearly two-thirds of a pound of body fat through a straw.

beef products? A burger with 690 more calories than the worst steak on Outback's menu. Even a plain Outback burger contains 1,530 calories, so if you want something handheld to eat here, make it a simple chicken sandwich.

Eat This Instead!

Grilled Chicken and Swiss Sandwich

- 760 calories

WORST DRINK

8 Cold Stone Creamery PB&C Shake (Gotta Have It size)

- 2,030 calories
- 131 g fat (68 g saturated)
- 153 g sugars

Now that Baskin-Robbins has cleaned up its beleaguered beverage program and exorcised the devlish line of premium shakes, Cold Stone sits in the dubious position of housing America's most deleterious line of drinks. Not a single regular shake on their menu contains fewer than 1,000 calories, and this atrocious peanut butter and chocolate concoction is the source of 340 percent of your day's recommended saturated fat intake.

Drink This Instead!

Sinless Oh Fudge! Shake (Like It size)

- 490 calories • 2 g fat (2 g saturated)
- 44 g sugars

WORST SALAD

7 California PIzza Kitchen Thai Crunch Salad

- 2,115 calories

The menu description reads like a textbook definition of healthy eating: "Shredded Napa cabbage, chilled grilled chicken breast, julienne cucumbers, edamame." But somehow this simple salad packs more calories than America's worst burger, pasta dish, and milkshake. Blame falls primarily on the massive serving size and the use of 2 different dressings. The good news is you can eat 3 slices of pizza instead and save more than 1,500 calories. How's that for an encouraging weight loss message?

Eat This Instead!

The Original Barbecue Chicken Pizza (3 slices)

- 525 calories

WORST FISH ENTRÉE

6 Romano's Macaroni Grill Parmesan-Crusted Sole

- 2,190 calories
- 141 g fat (58 g saturated)
- 2,980 mg sodium
- 145 g carbohydrates

Fish is normally a safe bet, but this entrée proves that it's all in the preparation. If you fry said fish in a shell of cheese, be prepared to pay the consequences. In this case, that means meeting your daily calorie, fat, saturated fat, and sodium allowances in one sitting.

Eat This Instead!

Simple Salmon

- 590 calories • 32 g fat (6 g saturated)
- 1,800 mg sodium
- 15 g carbohydrates

WORST TEX-MEX ENTRÉE

5 Chili's Fire Grilled Bacon Chicken Ranch Quesadilla with rice and beans and condiments

- 2,280 calories
- 142.5 g fat (50 g saturated)
- 5,900 mg sodium

Chili's has managed to right some of their previous wrongs, either by getting rid of them entirely (good riddance, Awesome Blossom!) or scaling them back considerably (most of their still-shockingly bad fajitas and burgers). But they continue to introduce new mayhem to the menu, this time in the form of a quesadilla so outlandishly oversize that it gobbles up an entire day's caloric allotment, plus more than 2 days' worth of fat and sodium. If it comes in a tortilla from Chili's, keep it off of your plate!

Eat This Instead!

Guiltless Carne Asada Steak

- *370 calories • 10 g fat (8 g saturated)*
- *1,440 mg sodium*
- *11 g carbohydrates*

WORST PIZZA

4 Uno Chicago Grill Chicago Classic Deep Dish Pizza

- *2,310 calories*
- *165 g fat (54 g saturated)*
- *4,920 mg sodium*

This pie contains a horrific 254 percent of your daily allowance of fat and more than 200 percent of your daily allowance of sodium. It also wipes out your whole day's caloric allotment. It may be a Chicago classic, but so was Al Capone.

Eat This Instead!

Cheese and Tomato Flatbread Pizza (half) and a house side salad

- *485 calories*
- *21.5 g fat (8.5 g saturated)*
- *1115 mg sodium*

WORST STARTER

3 Uno Chicago Grill Pizza Skins

- *2,400 calories*
- *155 g fat (45 g saturated)*
- *3,600 mg sodium*
- *195 g carbohydrates*

Eating a full order of this appetizer is like eating a Large Domino's Hand-Tossed Sausage Pizza all by yourself. Split among 4 people, it's still a full dinner's worth of calories. Order the Thai Vegetable Pot Stickers—the only starter with fewer than 800 calories.

Eat This Instead!

Thai Vegetable Pot Stickers

- *400 calories • 20 g fat (2 g saturated)*
- *1,080 mg sodium • 46 g carbohydrates*

WORST MEXICAN ENTRÉE

2 On the Border Dos XX Fish Tacos with Chipotle Sauce and Refried Beans and Rice

- *2,550 calories*
- *151 g fat (31 g saturated)*
- *4,790 mg sodium*

This dish is an astonishing example of a restaurant defying all preconceived notions about so-called healthy food. No food is sacred, not even fish—at least not when it's breaded, fried, and served to you containing more calories than you'd get in 3 sticks of butter.

Eat This Instead!

Pico Shrimp Tacos

- *490 calories • 5 g fat (1 g saturated)*
- *1,650 mg sodium*

THE WORST FOOD IN AMERICA

1 Outback Steakhouse Baby Back Ribs (full rack)

- *2,580 calories*

Imagine this: You start your meal by splitting a plate of Aussie Cheese Fries with 3 dining companions. Next, you have a bit of complimentary brown bread and a house salad. You wash down dinner with a few Diet Cokes. When it comes time for dessert, you prudently pass on the Chocolate Thunder from Down Under. When the bill comes, guess what the damage is? 3,860 calories. That's why this is the Worst Food in America.

Eat This Instead!

Prime Rib (8 ounces) with Fresh Seasonal Veggies

- *690 calories*

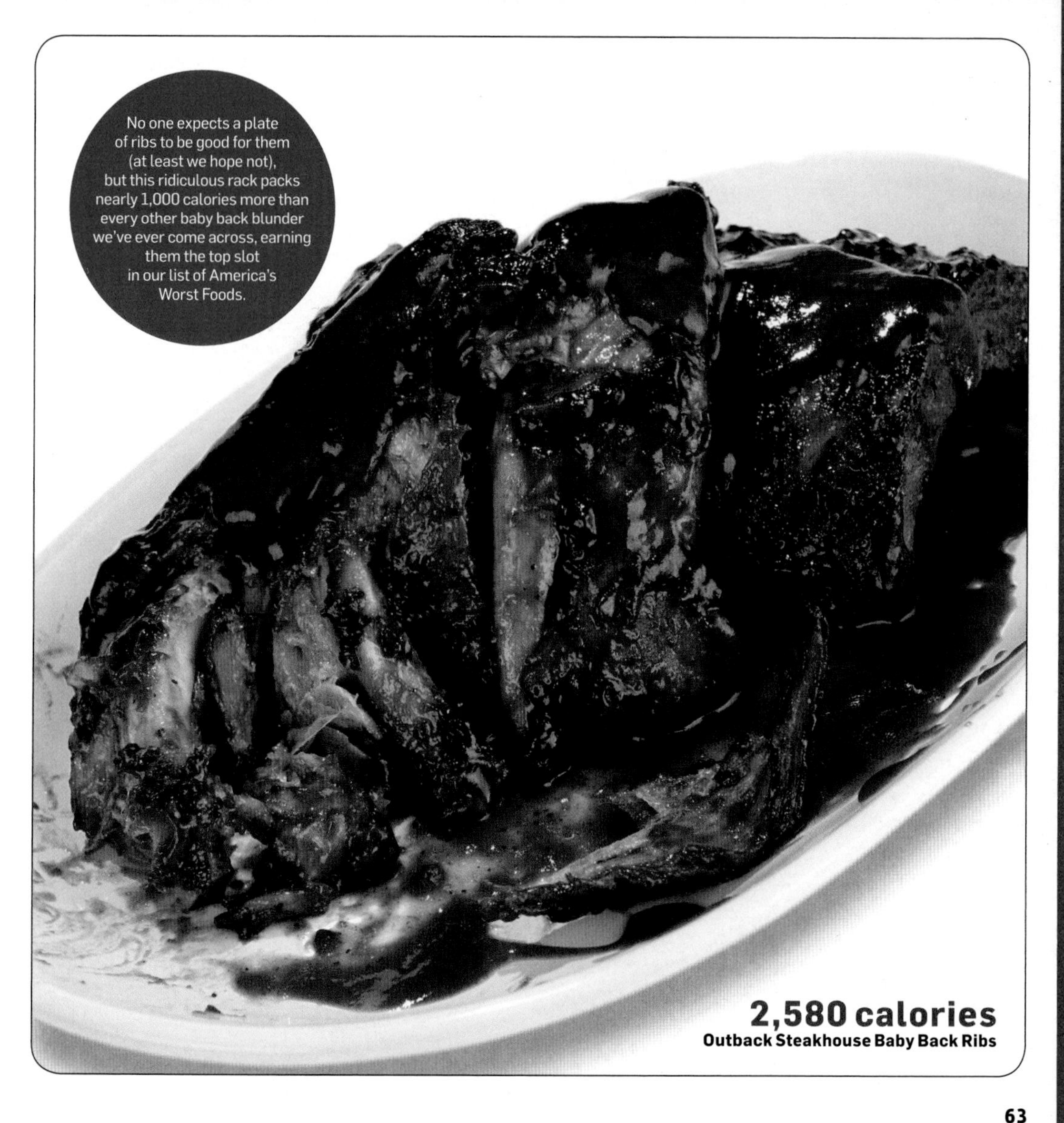

No one expects a plate of ribs to be good for them (at least we hope not), but this ridiculous rack packs nearly 1,000 calories more than every other baby back blunder we've ever come across, earning them the top slot in our list of America's Worst Foods.

2,580 calories
Outback Steakhouse Baby Back Ribs

A&W

C-

The issue with A&W isn't one of egregious calorie gouging, but rather the absence of any discernible level of true nutrition to be found anywhere on the menu. Every side is deep-fried; there is but one entrée that isn't a burger, a hot dog, or fried chicken; and more than half the menu is dedicated to shakes, floats, and sundaes. Oh, and A&W is one of the last fast-food joints still clinging to the use of trans fat.

SURVIVAL STRATEGY

The best item on the entire menu is the Grilled Chicken Sandwich. Start with that or a small burger, skip the sides and the regular root beer, and finish (if you must have something sweet) with a small sundae or a vanilla cone.

Eat This

Papa Single Burger

470 calories
25 g fat (8 g saturated, 0.5 g trans)
1,000 mg sodium

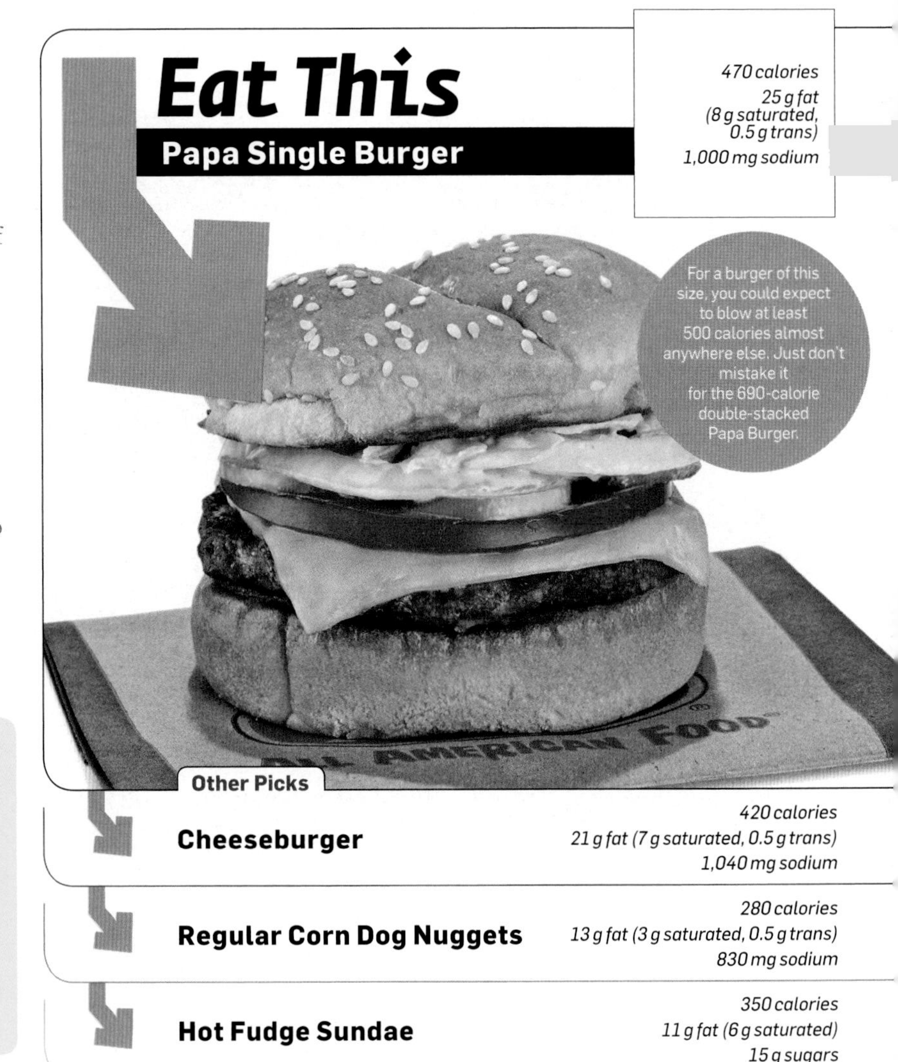

For a burger of this size, you could expect to blow at least 500 calories almost anywhere else. Just don't mistake it for the 690-calorie double-stacked Papa Burger.

Other Picks

Cheeseburger
420 calories
21 g fat (7 g saturated, 0.5 g trans)
1,040 mg sodium

Regular Corn Dog Nuggets
280 calories
13 g fat (3 g saturated, 0.5 g trans)
830 mg sodium

Hot Fudge Sundae
350 calories
11 g fat (6 g saturated)
15 g sugars

660 calories
46 g fat
(7.5 g saturated, 2 g trans)
1,290 mg sodium

Not That!

Chicken Strips

(3), with ranch

Blame the partially hydrogenated oil in the fryer for the day's worth of trans fat found in these skinny strips.

Other Passes

550 calories
25 g fat (4.5 g saturated, 1.5 g trans)
1,130 mg sodium

Crispy Chicken Sandwich

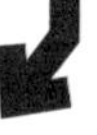

350 calories
16 g fat (3.5 g saturated, 4.5 g trans)
710 mg sodium

Large Breaded Onion Rings

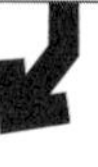

880 calories
36 g fat (23 g saturated, 2 g trans)
75 g sugars

Chocolate Milkshake

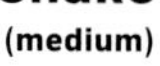

(medium)

WEAPON OF MASS DESTRUCTION
Cheese Curds

570 calories
40 g fat
(21 g saturated, 1 g trans)
1,220 mg sodium

Wildly popular in the Wisconsin dairy lands and now available at A&Ws across the country, these tiny squiggles are actually fried puffs of white Cheddar cheese. *Fromage*-ophiles beware: A single order of curds contains your entire day's allotment of saturated fat.

MENU DECODER

CONEY DOG: Despite the name, this dog has nothing to do with the famous New York hot dog haven. The Coney is a popular midwestern creation that denotes a dog that's been topped with chili, diced onion, and yellow mustard. With just 340 calories, it's one of A&W's better options.

Applebee's

F

We've tried repeatedly to get Applebee's to cough up the nutritional info on their menu items, but they won't deliver. Without full disclosure, we have no choice but to give them a flunking grade. (And while Applebee's takes its sweet time coming clean, we found out a bit of what they're hiding by taking advantage of New York City's legislation requiring chain restaurants to publish calorie counts.)

SURVIVAL STRATEGY
Skip the meal-wrecking appetizers, pastas, and fajitas, and be very careful with salads, too; half of them pack more than 1,000 calories with dressing. Instead seek out lean protein—either from one of the Weight Watchers items or the 9-ounce sirloin (just 310 calories).

Eat This

Italian Chicken Portobello Sandwich

*360 calories**

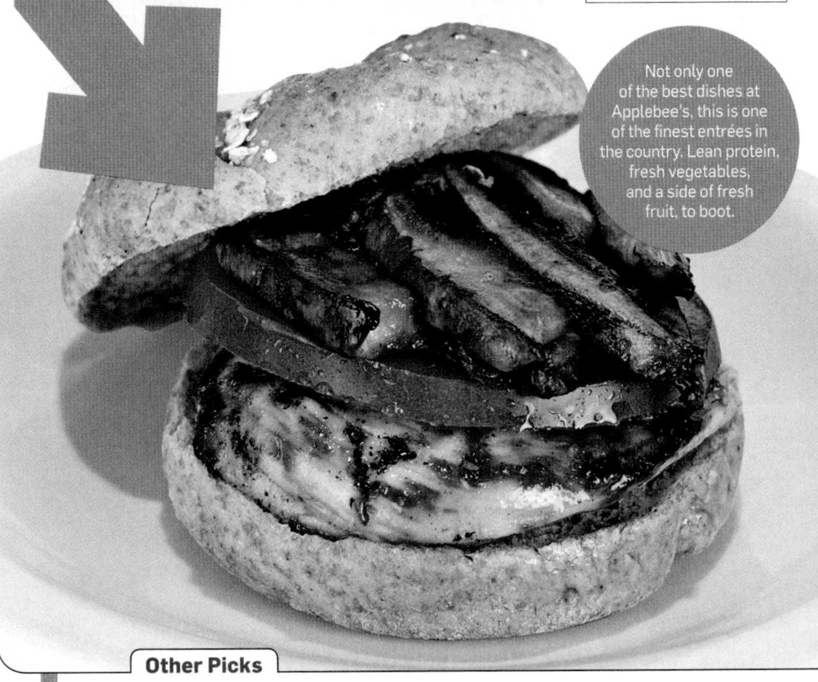

Not only one of the best dishes at Applebee's, this is one of the finest entrées in the country. Lean protein, fresh vegetables, and a side of fresh fruit, to boot.

Other Picks

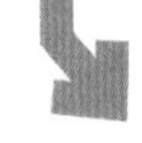

Garlic Herb Chicken — *370 calories*

House Sirloin (9 oz) — *310 calories*

1,050 calories*

Not That!

Chicken Fajita Rollup

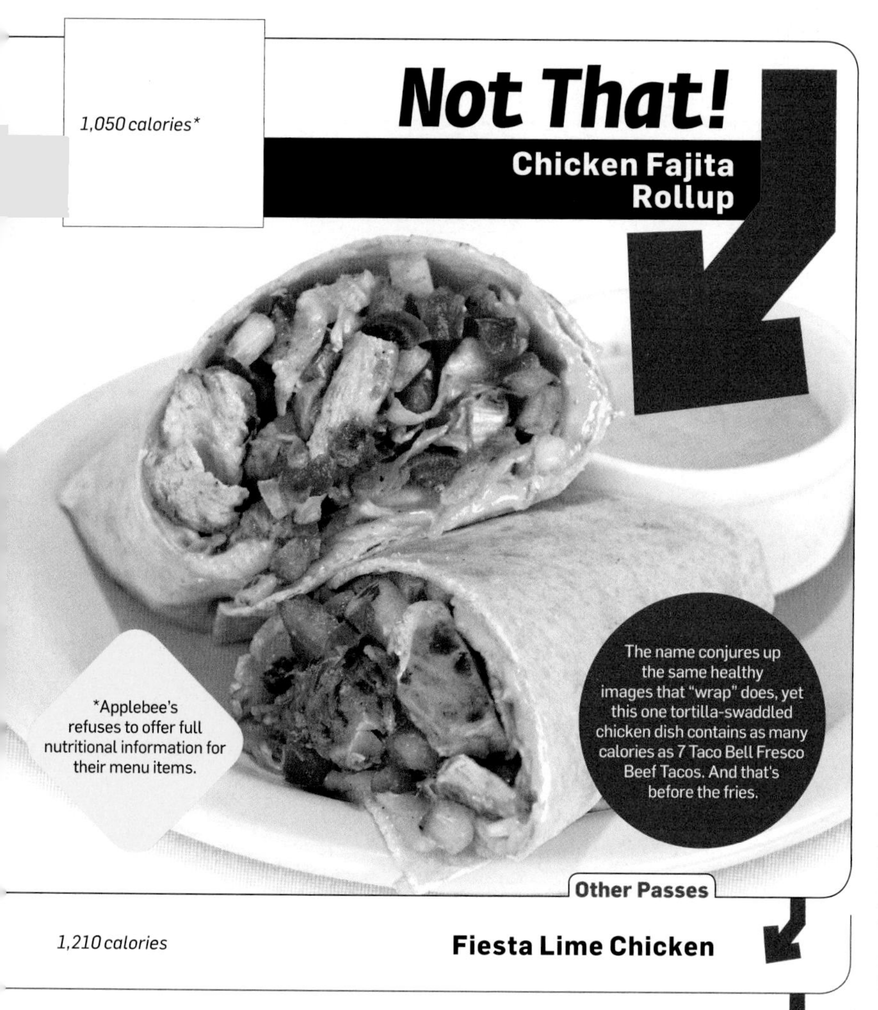

The name conjures up the same healthy images that "wrap" does, yet this one tortilla-swaddled chicken dish contains as many calories as 7 Taco Bell Fresco Beef Tacos. And that's before the fries.

*Applebee's refuses to offer full nutritional information for their menu items.

Other Passes

1,210 calories **Fiesta Lime Chicken**

1,330 calories **Chicken Broccoli Pasta Alfredo Bowl**

GUILTY PLEASURE

Steak & Fried Shrimp Combo

630 calories

So they may not win the "Health Food of the Year" award, but Applebee's steak combos pair one of their leanest menu items with a small portion of their less-than-diet-friendly fare. Just make sure you swap the potato that comes alongside the meat for a helping of seasonal vegetables—it'll save you 300 calories.

MENU DECODER

SHOOTERS: Tasty layered desserts served up in small whiskey glasses. Part of a (thankfully!) growing trend toward downsized desserts, they average around 300 calories.

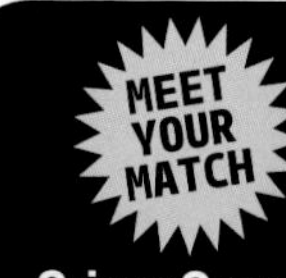

Crispy Orange Chicken Bowl

(1,880 calories)

15 scoops of chocolate ice cream

Arby's

C+

Arby's offers a long list of sandwiches with fewer than 500 calories. Problem is, there's an even longer list of sandwiches with considerably more than 500 calories, many with warm, virtuous-sounding names. Credit Arby's for nixing the trans fat from their frying oil back in 2006, but it seems they might be just a little too proud of that fact; the restaurant doesn't offer a single side that hasn't had a hot oil bath.

SURVIVAL STRATEGY

Don't think you're doing yourself any favors by ordering off the Market Fresh menu. You're far better off with a regular roast beef or Melt Sandwich, which will save you an average of nearly 300 calories over a Market Fresh sandwich or wrap.

Eat This

Arby's Melt

298 calories
12 g fat (4 g saturated, 0.5 g trans)
922 mg sodium

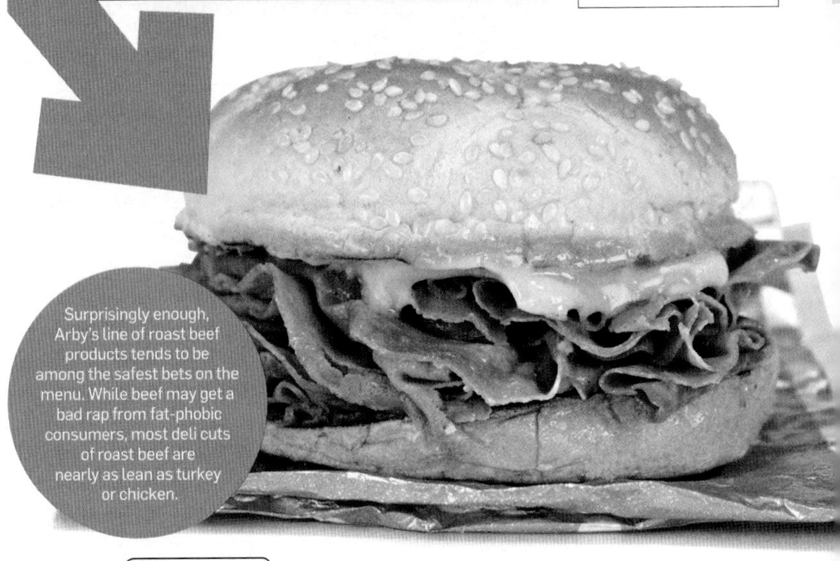

Surprisingly enough, Arby's line of roast beef products tends to be among the safest bets on the menu. While beef may get a bad rap from fat-phobic consumers, most deli cuts of roast beef are nearly as lean as turkey or chicken.

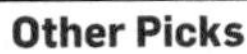

Other Picks

Roast Chicken Fillet Sandwich

383 calories
16 g fat (3 g saturated)
921 mg sodium

Chopped Turkey Club Salad

410 calories
28 g fat (9 g saturated, 0.5 g trans)
1,041 mg sodium

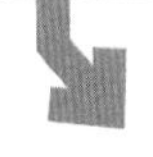

Potato Cakes
(2)

250 calories
18 g fat (3.5 g saturated, 1 g trans)
390 mg sodium

710 calories
30 g fat (8 g saturated, 1 g trans)
1,680 mg sodium

Not That!

Market Fresh Roast Turkey and Swiss

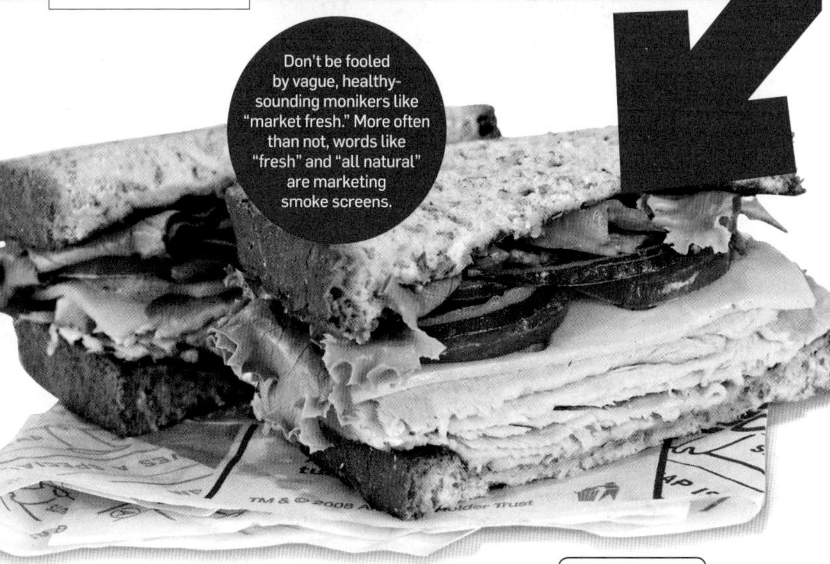

Don't be fooled by vague, healthy-sounding monikers like "market fresh." More often than not, words like "fresh" and "all natural" are marketing smoke screens.

Other Passes

691 calories
31 g fat (8 g saturated, 0.5 g trans)
1,952 mg sodium

Roast Ham & Swiss Sandwich

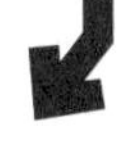

620 calories
43 g fat (10.5 g saturated, 1 g trans)
1,250 mg sodium

Chopped Farmhouse Crispy Chicken Salad
with buttermilk ranch

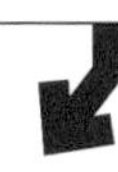

360 calories
21 g fat (4 g saturated, 0 g trans)
840 mg sodium

Curly Fries
(small)

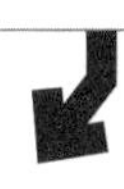

FOOD MYTH

Wheat bread is always healthier than white bread.

Unless the bread is "100% whole grain," you might be getting extra sugar and calories, but not extra fiber and other nutrients. Case in point: 2 slices of Honey Wheat Bread pack an unruly 361 calories and 14 grams of sugar.

BAD BREED

"Sides and Sidekickers"

We know it's hard to resist the curly fries, but the Arby's sides menu reads like a list of America's Most Wanted—it's all deep-fried and stuffed with potatoes and/or cheese. At best you're looking at 250 calories and 18 grams of fat (for the small potato cakes). If you need *something* to go with that sandwich, see if they'll give you an order of applesauce from the kids' menu.

MENU DECODER

ROASTBURGER: A roast beef sandwich piled high with burger-esque toppings. The best? The 420-calorie All American.

Atlanta Bread Company

B-

The bad news is that the breakfast menu is riddled with unnecessary fats and refined carbohydrates, and most of the sandwiches are a little too high in calories for comfort. The good news is that there's also a robust selection of healthy soups and salads to offset these problems, so focus your appetite there and you'll escape relatively unscathed.

SURVIVAL STRATEGY

Atlanta Bread Company lets you order a half sandwich with a half salad or a cup of soup, which is the perfect compromise for those who prefer a handheld lunch. Hold the mayo on your sandwich and this is a pretty safe bet. Oh, and avoid the pizzas, pastas, and calzones at all costs.

Eat This

Turkey on Nine Grain Sandwich

370 calories
6 g fat (2 g saturated)
29 g protein
1,240 mg sodium

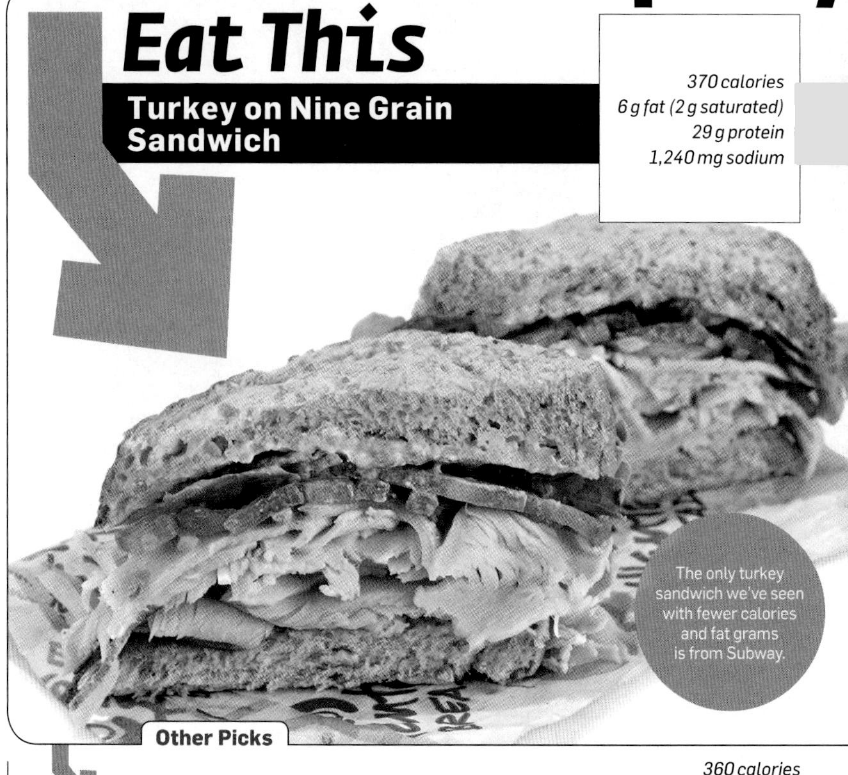

The only turkey sandwich we've seen with fewer calories and fat grams is from Subway.

Other Picks

Tomato Bacon Omelette

360 calories
27 g fat (12 g saturated)
1,000 mg sodium

BBQ Chicken Pizza
(½ pizza)

320 calories
5 g fat (2.5 g saturated)
1,110 mg sodium

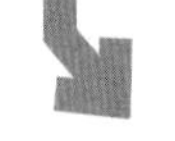

Chopstix Chicken Salad
with Asian sesame dressing

360 calories
20 g fat (3 g saturated)
850 mg sodium

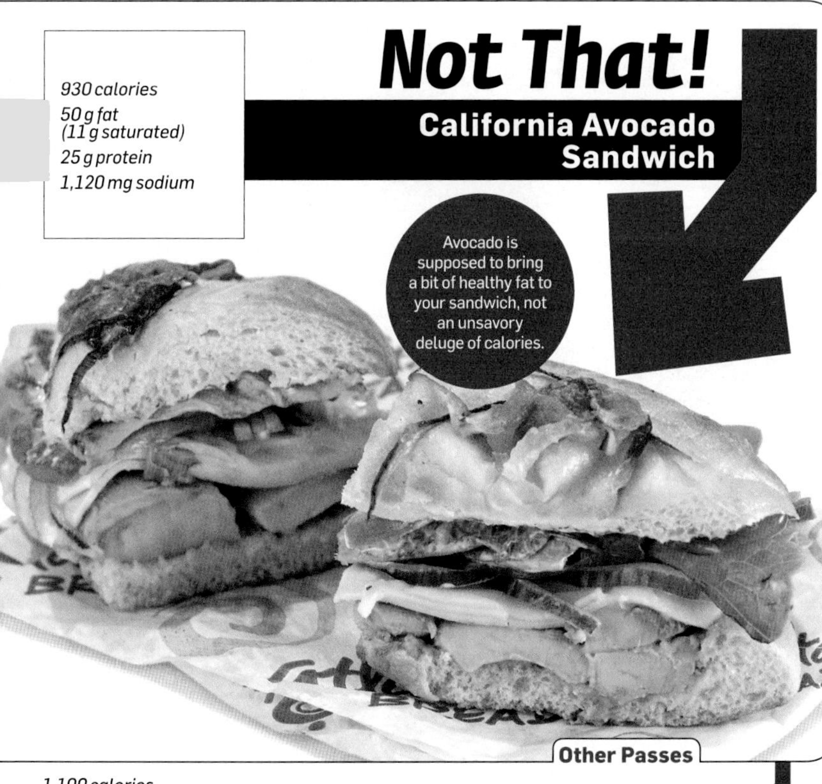

Not That!

California Avocado Sandwich

930 calories
50 g fat (11 g saturated)
25 g protein
1,120 mg sodium

Avocado is supposed to bring a bit of healthy fat to your sandwich, not an unsavory deluge of calories.

Other Passes

Three Cheese Omelette

1,100 calories
85 g fat (44 g saturated)
1,990 mg sodium

White Pizza
(½ pizza)

460 calories
22 g fat (10 g saturated)
1,400 mg sodium

Salsa Fresca Salmon Salad
with balsamic vinaigrette

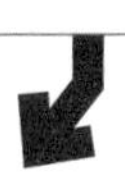

740 calories
48 g fat (7.5 g saturated)
840 mg sodium

LITTLE TRICK

Choose your bread wisely and you could save more than 200 calories. Try the low-cal nine grain or a French baguette—both contain fewer than 25 grams of carbohydrates per slice.

HIDDEN DANGER

Turkey Club Panini

Turkey may be lean, but paninis rarely are. That's because pressed sandwiches run heavy on the cheese (to maximize the melting effect) and condiments, making it nearly impossible to find a panini that comes in under 600 calories. Try a regular turkey sandwich instead, and you'll save 680 milligrams of sodium and nearly 340 calories.

710 calories
24 g fat (9 g saturated)
1,920 mg sodium

Au Bon Pain

A- There are plenty of ways you could go wrong here, but Au Bon Pain couples an extensive inventory of healthy items with an unrivaled standard of nutritional transparency. Each store has an on-site nutritional kiosk to help customers find a meal to meet their expectations, and the variety of ordering options provides dozens of paths to a sensible meal.

SURVIVAL STRATEGY

Many of the café sandwiches come in around 650 calories, so make a lean meal instead by combining soup with one of the many low-calorie options on the All Portions menu. And if you're in the mood to indulge, pass up the baked goods in favor of a cup of fruit and yogurt or a serving of chocolate-covered almonds.

Eat This

Spicy Tuna Sandwich

470 calories
16 g fat (3 g saturated)
1,180 mg sodium

Tuna normally comes drowning in a sea of fatty mayo, but Au Bon Pain keeps their rendition light, relying on the fish's healthy natural fat and a dose of heat to carry the flavor.

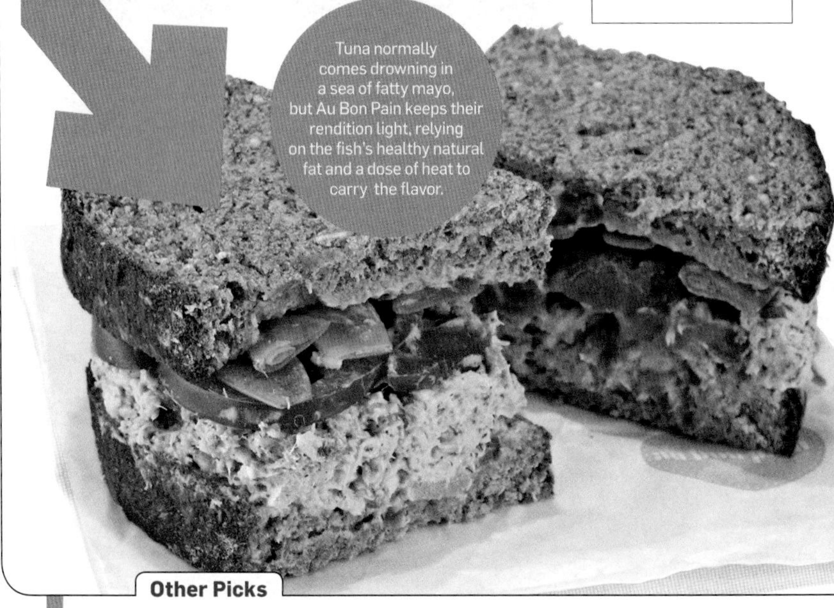

Other Picks

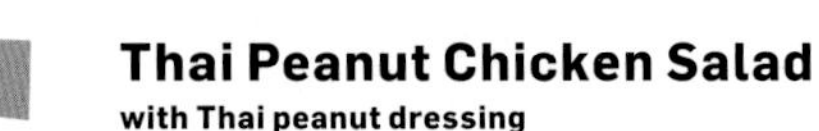

Thai Peanut Chicken Salad
with Thai peanut dressing

400 calories
16 g fat (1 g saturated)
1,020 mg sodium

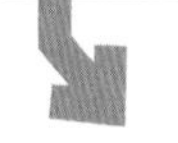

Apple Croissant

270 calories
11 g fat (6 g saturated)
20 g sugars
160 mg sodium

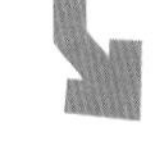

Chicken Gumbo Soup
(12 oz)

80 calories
8 g fat (1 g saturated)
880 mg sodium

680 calories
32 g fat (15 g saturated)
1,200 mg sodium

Not That!

Caprese Sandwich

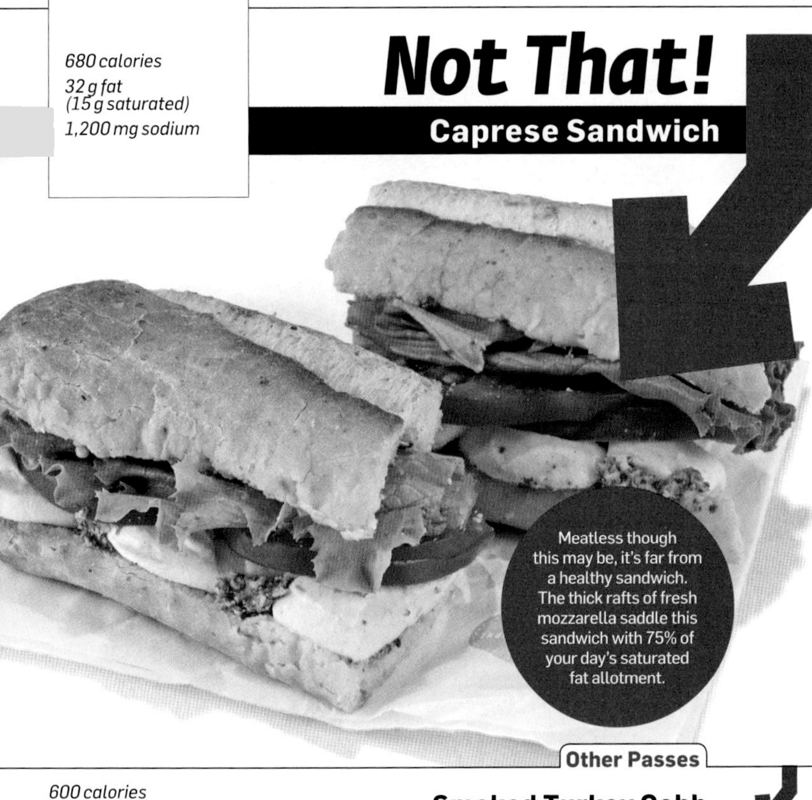

Meatless though this may be, it's far from a healthy sandwich. The thick rafts of fresh mozzarella saddle this sandwich with 75% of your day's saturated fat allotment.

Other Passes

Smoked Turkey Cobb with hazelnut vinaigrette

600 calories
44 g fat (12 g saturated)
1,360 mg sodium

Almond Croissant

600 calories
38 g fat (14 g saturated, 0.5 g trans)
16 g sugars
300 mg sodium

Corn Chowder (12 oz)

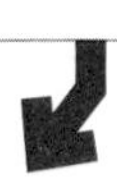

350 calories
18 g fat (8 g saturated)
1,120 mg sodium

HIDDEN DANGER

Bread Bowl

There's no quicker way to sink a bowl of soup than by housing it in a massive refined-carb container. The bread bowl alone packs more than a meal's worth of calories and as much salt as you'd find in 6 medium orders of McDonald's French fries.

620 calories
3 g fat
(1 g saturated)
1,720 mg sodium
123 g carbohydrates

SMART SIDES

More than just a side, we like to use Au Bon Pain's savvy All Portions menu to create exciting, nutritionally diverse meals. Everything on this menu, which includes salads, sides, and even desserts, weighs in under 200 calories. Pick 1 for a snack, 2 for a light lunch, or 3 for a more substantial meal. Our favorite combos: Chicken Pesto Salad with Brie, Fruit and Crackers (360 calories) and Thai Peanut Chicken and Mango Coconut Mousse (310 calories).

Auntie Anne's

C+

Is there anything redeeming on Auntie Anne's menu? Not really. The average pretzel is about 360 calories of refined carbohydrates, and they supplement the twisted-bread menu with a long list of sweetened beverages and smoothies. But you can find far worse indulgences on just about any dessert menu in the country, so go here in search of relatively healthy indulgences, not genuinely nutritious food.

SURVIVAL STRATEGY

Cut most of the fat and half of the sodium by skipping the butter and salt they put on most pretzels, relying instead on a healthier dipping sauce such as marinara or sweet mustard for big flavor.

Eat This

Jalapeño Pretzel with Marinara

(no salt)

350 calories
5.5 g fat (3 g saturated)
810 mg sodium

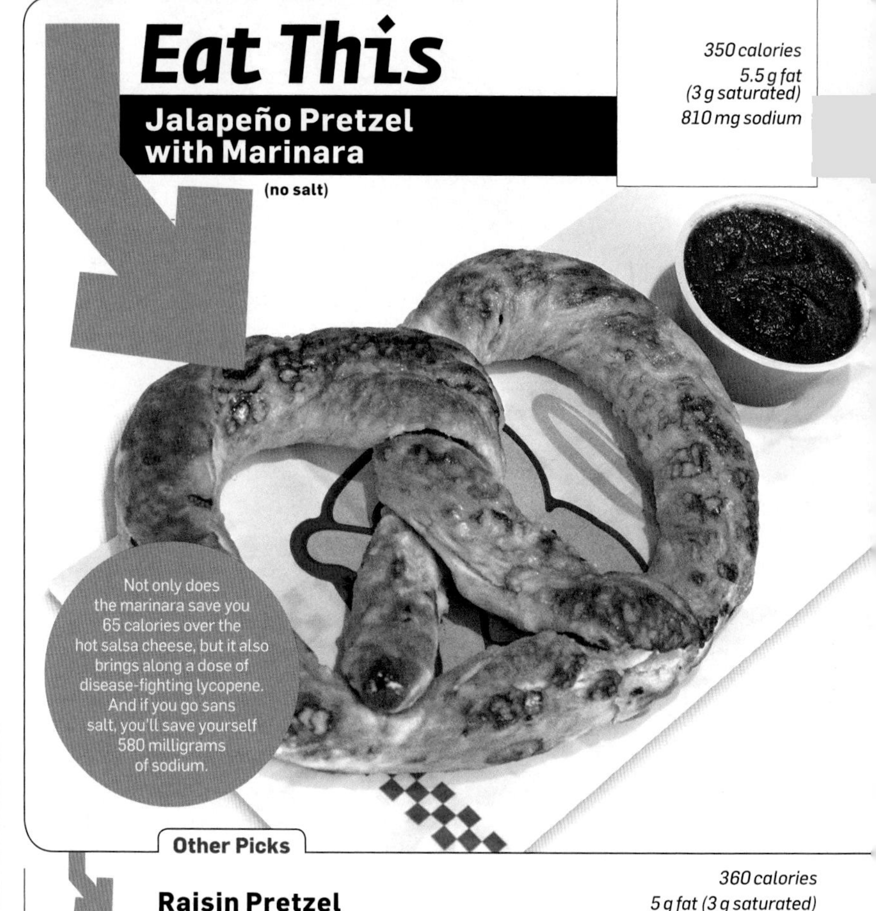

Not only does the marinara save you 65 calories over the hot salsa cheese, but it also brings along a dose of disease-fighting lycopene. And if you go sans salt, you'll save yourself 580 milligrams of sodium.

Other Picks

Raisin Pretzel

360 calories
5 g fat (3 g saturated)
16 g sugars

Strawberry Dutch Ice
(14 oz)

160 calories
0 g fat
37 g sugars

Not That!

Sesame Pretzel with Hot Salsa Cheese

510 calories
18 g fat (7 g saturated)
1,440 mg sodium

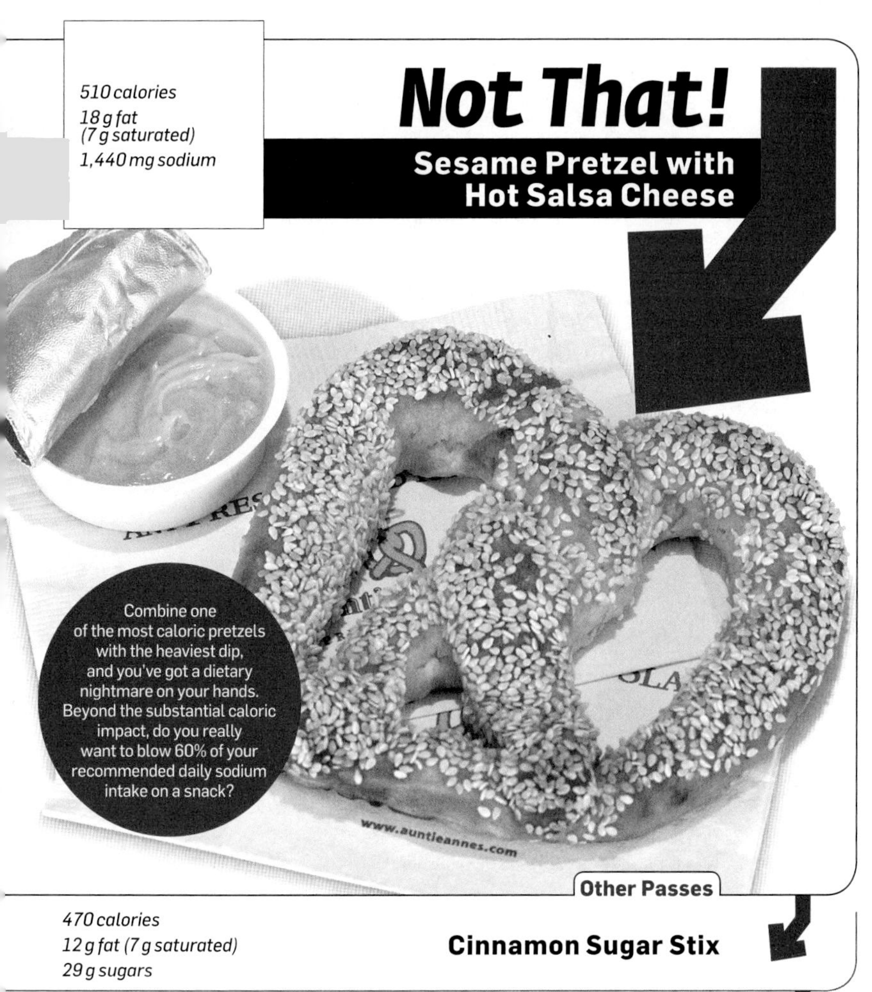

Combine one of the most caloric pretzels with the heaviest dip, and you've got a dietary nightmare on your hands. Beyond the substantial caloric impact, do you really want to blow 60% of your recommended daily sodium intake on a snack?

Other Passes

Cinnamon Sugar Stix

470 calories
12 g fat (7 g saturated)
29 g sugars

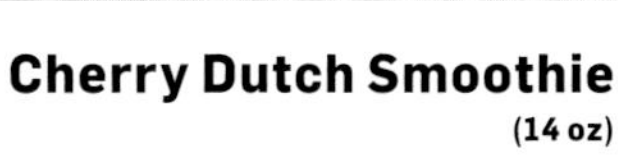

Wild Cherry Dutch Smoothie (14 oz)

300 calories
10 g fat (7 g saturated)
44 g sugars

CONDIMENT CATASTROPHE

Melted Cheese Dip

80 calories
6 g fat
(1 g saturated, 1 g trans)
580 mg sodium

It's a great mystery as to why this is different than the regular cheese sauce, but the hot stuff contains a shocking 2 grams of trans fat in just 2 ounces.

MEET YOUR MATCH

Sour Cream & Onion Pretzel
(1,180 mg sodium)
=
7 (1-ounce) bags of Lay's Classic potato chips

BAD BREED

Dutch Shakes

The worst of them pack up to 880 calories, and even the small vanilla shake contains 510 calories and 27 grams of fat. For a healthier sweet treat, try a Dutch Ice—the small Orange Crème is fat-free and just 190 calories.

Baja Fresh

D It's a surprise that Baja Fresh's menu has not yet collapsed under the weight of its own fatty fare. About a third of the items on the menu have more than 1,000 calories, and most are spiked with enough sodium to melt a polar ice cap. Fajitas, nachos, and burritos are all off-limits fare. First-rate tacos and the Baja Ensaladas are the only redeeming features of this otherwise troubling menu.

SURVIVAL STRATEGY
Unless you're comfortable stuffing 110 grams of fat into your arteries, avoid the nachos at all costs. In fact, avoid almost everything on this menu. The only safe options are the Baja tacos or a salad topped with salsa verde and served without the elephantine tortilla bowl.

Eat This

Chicken Baja Tacos

(2)

420 calories
10 g fat (2 g saturated)
460 mg sodium

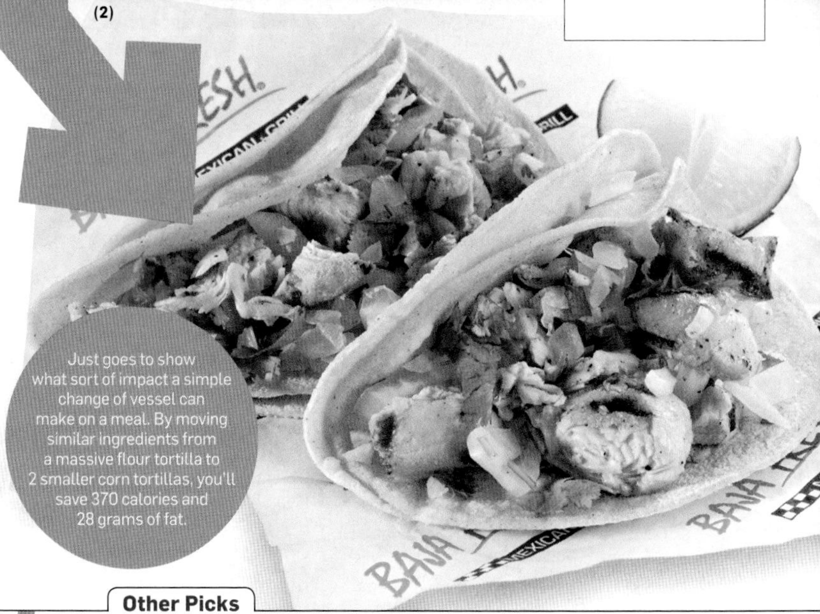

Just goes to show what sort of impact a simple change of vessel can make on a meal. By moving similar ingredients from a massive flour tortilla to 2 smaller corn tortillas, you'll save 370 calories and 28 grams of fat.

Other Picks

Charbroiled Chicken Salad
with fat-free salsa verde dressing

325 calories
7 g fat (2 g saturated)
1,580 mg sodium

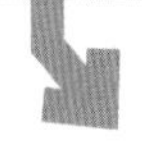

Veggie and Cheese Bare Burrito

580 calories
10 g fat (4 g saturated)
1,950 mg sodium

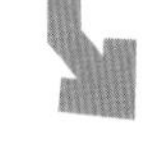

Corn Tortilla Chips
(1.5 oz side) and Guacamole (3 oz side)

320 calories
22 g fat (2 g saturated)
325 mg sodium

790 calories
38 g fat (15 g saturated, 1 g trans)
2,140 mg sodium

Not That!

Chicken Baja Burrito

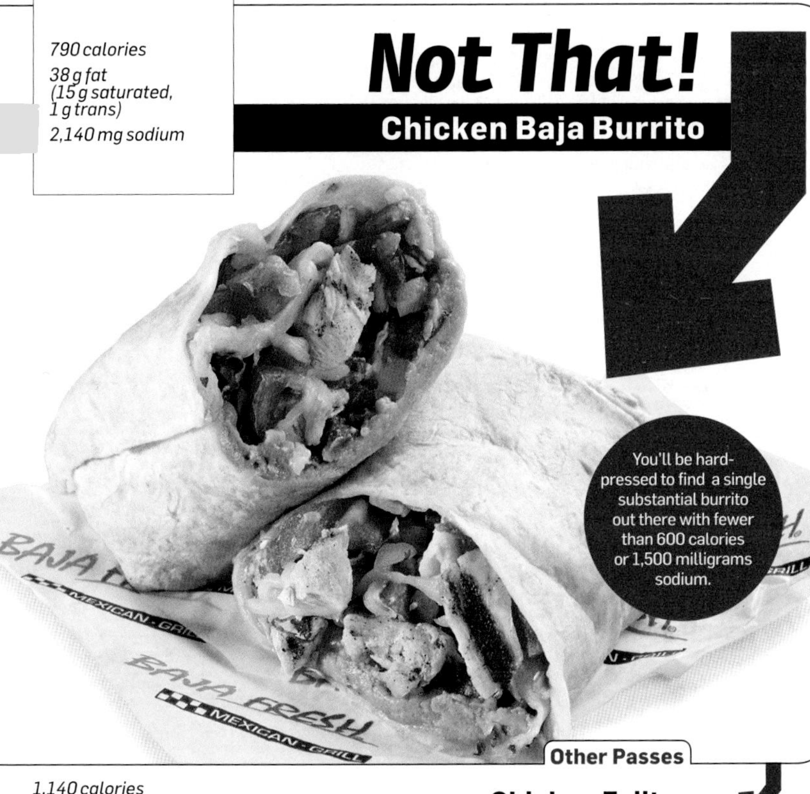

You'll be hard-pressed to find a single substantial burrito out there with fewer than 600 calories or 1,500 milligrams sodium.

Other Passes

1,140 calories
33 g fat (10 g saturated)
3,240 mg sodium

Chicken Fajitas
with flour tortillas

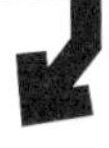

1,260 calories
78 g fat (37 g saturated)
2,310 mg sodium

Veggie Quesadilla

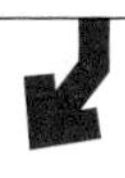

1,340 calories
83 g fat (8 g saturated, 2.5 g trans)
950 mg sodium

Chips and Guacamole

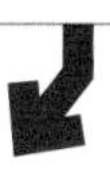

BAD BREED

Nachos

Since a mere 5 ounces of Baja's tortilla chips contain a whopping 740 calories, it's no surprise that a mountain of them smothered in melted cheese, guacamole, and sour cream will cost you big: at least 1,890 calories (for the plain cheese variety). Add meat and you'll cross the dreaded 2,000-calorie threshold. Unless you've got a crew of 6 to split 'em, nix the nachos.

HIDDEN DANGER

Tostada Salad with Chicken

Chicken salad isn't so bad—until you drown it in cheese and sour cream and serve it up in a deep-fried tortilla shell. (And that's without dressing!) Stick to a Baja Ensalada and save 830 calories.

1,140 calories
55 g fat (14 g saturated, 1 g trans)
2,370 mg sodium

Baskin-Robbins

D+

Baskin-Robbins did health-conscious consumers a solid by nixing their line of Premium Sundaes and Shakes. But the reality is that it would take more than just a little pruning to really clean up this menu; its soft serve is among the most caloric in the country, the smoothies and shakes contain a glut of added sugars, and anything that Baskin turns into a sundae winds up with more fat than a steakhouse buffet.

SURVIVAL STRATEGY
With choices like frozen yogurt, sherbet, and no-sugar-added ice cream, Baskin's lighter menu is the one bright spot in this otherwise darkly caloric place. Just be sure to ask for a sugar or cake cone—the waffle cone will swaddle your treat in an extra 160 calories.

Eat This

You're actually better off with this soft serve concoction than you are with a majority of Starbucks' blended Frappuccinos.
31 Baskin Robbins.

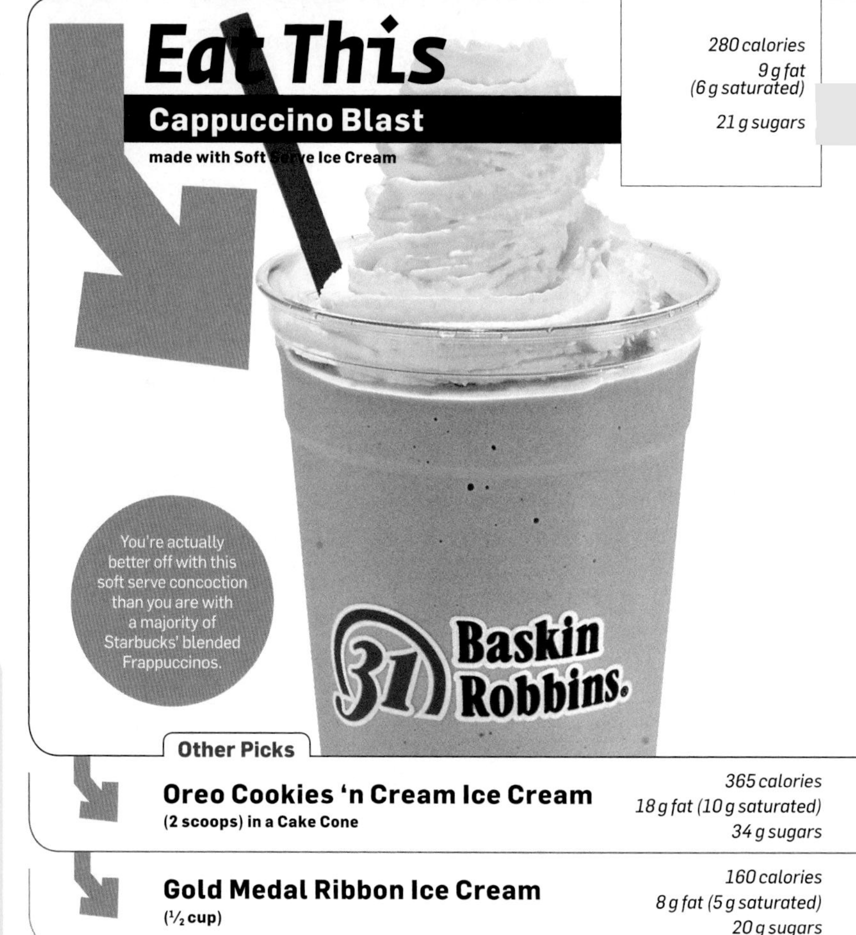

Cappuccino Blast

made with Soft Serve Ice Cream

280 calories
9 g fat (6 g saturated)
21 g sugars

Other Picks

Oreo Cookies 'n Cream Ice Cream
(2 scoops) in a Cake Cone
365 calories
18 g fat (10 g saturated)
34 g sugars

Gold Medal Ribbon Ice Cream
(½ cup)
160 calories
8 g fat (5 g saturated)
20 g sugars

Rainbow Sherbert
(½ cup)
100 calories
1.5 g fat (1 g saturated)
21 g sugars

670 calories
31 g fat (21 g saturated, 1 g trans)
73 g sugars

Not That!

Small Vanilla Shake

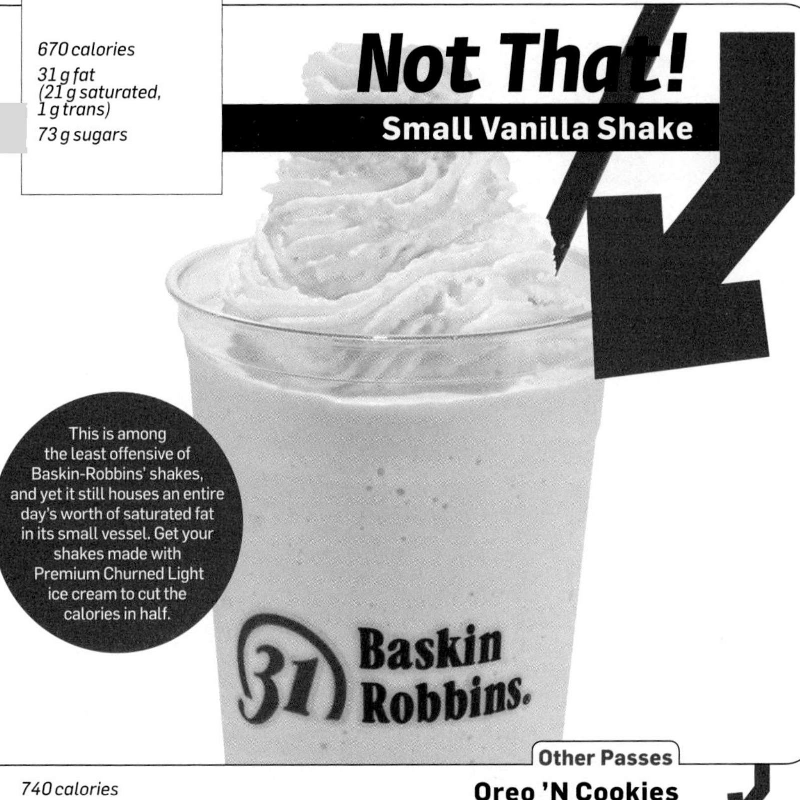

This is among the least offensive of Baskin-Robbins' shakes, and yet it still houses an entire day's worth of saturated fat in its small vessel. Get your shakes made with Premium Churned Light ice cream to cut the calories in half.

Other Passes

Oreo 'N Cookies Cappuccino Blast (medium)
740 calories
29 g fat (15 g saturated)
86 g sugars

Chocolate Mousse Royale Ice Cream (1/2 cup)
190 calories
11 g fat (8 g saturated)
19 g sugars

Strawberry Shortcake (1/2 cup)

170 calories
9 g fat (6 g saturated)
18 g sugars

BAD BREED

31° BELOW

These blended desserts all pack at least 600 calories—and most are closer to 1,000. In fact, the Fudge Brownie 31° Below contains 1,390 calories and 28 grams of saturated fat. That's 140% of your recommended daily allowance!

MENU DECODER

BRIGHT CHOICES: Baskin-Robbins' lower-calorie, low- or no-fat, and/or low-sugar options, such as Premium Churned Ice Cream. These are the most reliable items on the menu and, along with sherbets and frozen yogurts, really the only guarantee that you won't be overindulging when you go out for a simple scoop.

FOOD COURT

THE CRIME
Oreo Sundae
(1,290 calories)

THE PUNISHMENT
Mop the floor for 5 hours

Ben & Jerry's

C

What sets B&J's apart from the competition amounts to more than just an affinity for jam bands and green pastures. The shop also adheres to a lofty commitment to the quality and sources of its ingredients. All dairy is free from rBGH (recombinant bovine growth hormone) and the chocolate, vanilla, and coffee ingredients are all Fair Trade Certified. From a strictly nutritional standpoint, though, it's still just an ice cream shop.

SURVIVAL STRATEGY
With half of the calories of the ice cream, sorbet makes the healthiest choice on the menu. If you demand dairy, the frozen yogurt can still save you up to 100 calories per scoop.

Eat This

Strawberry Cheesecake Ice Cream

(1/2 cup)

210 calories
11 g fat (6 g saturated)
20 g sugars

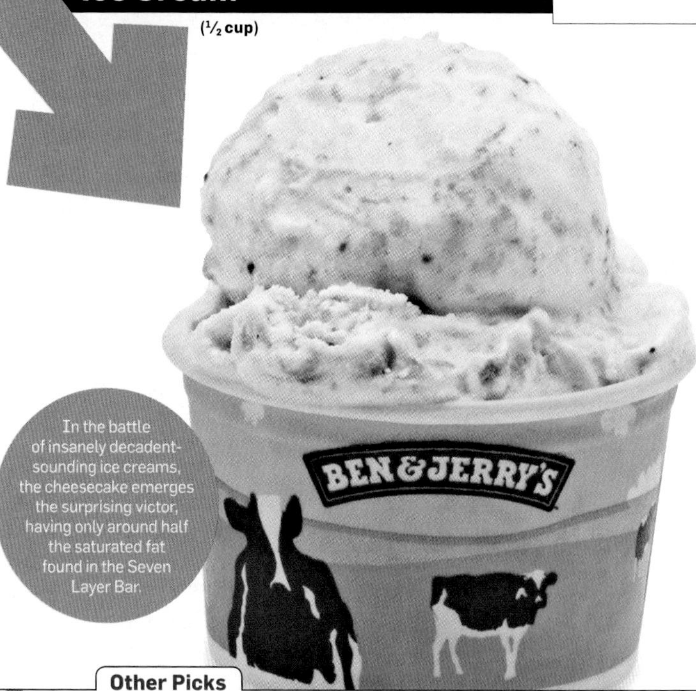

In the battle of insanely decadent-sounding ice creams, the cheesecake emerges the surprising victor, having only around half the saturated fat found in the Seven Layer Bar.

Other Picks

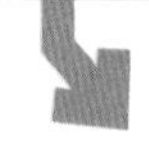

Chocolate Chip Cookie Dough Original Ice Cream
(1/2 cup)

220 calories
12 g fat (7 g saturated)
20 g sugars

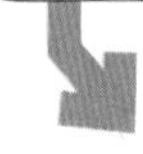

Half Baked Frozen Yogurt
(1/2 cup)

160 calories
2.5 g fat (1 g saturated)
20 g sugars

276 calories
17 g fat
(11 g saturated,
0.5 g trans)
20 g sugars

Not That!

Coconut Seven Layer Bar Ice Cream

(½ cup)

Every small scoop of this coconut calamity packs in more than half a day's worth of saturated fat. The trans fat and the 28 ingredients it takes to make this one flavor don't help improve matters, either.

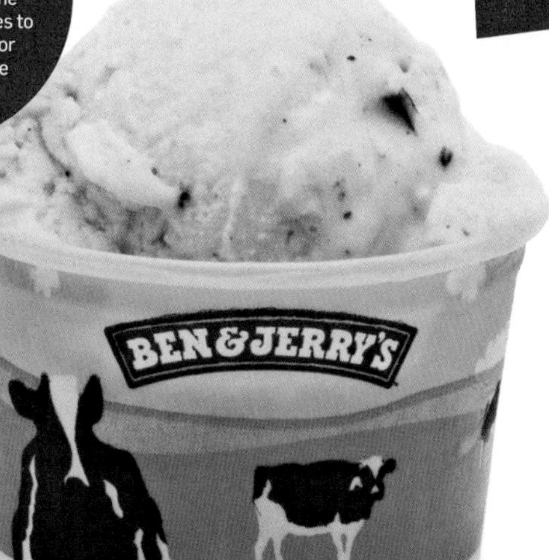

Other Passes

340 calories
24 g fat (12 g saturated)
24 g sugars

Peanut Butter Cup Original Ice Cream
(½ cup)

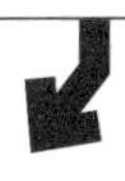

260 calories
20 g fat (8 g saturated)
24 g sugars

Butter Pecan Original Ice Cream
(½ cup)

ICE CREAM EQUATIONS

SORBET
Water + sugar + fruit puree =
100 calories per serving for any and all flavors

FROZEN YOGURT
Skim milk + water + sugar + flavorings (cookie dough, raspberry puree, and so on) =
130–160 calories per serving

NO SUGAR ADDED
[Ice cream]— sugar + artificial sweetener =
About 180 calories per serving

ICE CREAM
Cream + skim milk + sugar + ingredients =
152–276 calories per serving (from Orange and Cream and Coconut Seven Layer Bar, respectively)

MENU DECODER

GUAR GUM AND CARRAGEENAN: These two industrial thickening agents, found in nearly every pint of Ben & Jerry's, are used to give commercial ice cream a richer texture.

Blimpie

B In the past, we admonished Blimpie for its love of trans fat. Since then, the chain has quietly removed all the dangerous oils from its menu and earned itself a place of honor in our book. But that doesn't mean the menu is free from danger. Blimpie likes to splash oil on just about everything containing deli meat, and there are a handful of sinful subs that top the 1,000-calorie mark.

SURVIVAL STRATEGY
A ham Bluffin makes a decent breakfast, and the Grilled Chicken Teriyaki Sandwich is one of the best in the sandwich business. But skip the wraps and most of the hot sandwiches. And no matter which sandwich you choose, swap out mayo and oil for mustard or light dressing.

Eat This

Hot Pastrami
(6")

435 calories
16 g fat (7 g saturated)
1,354 mg sodium

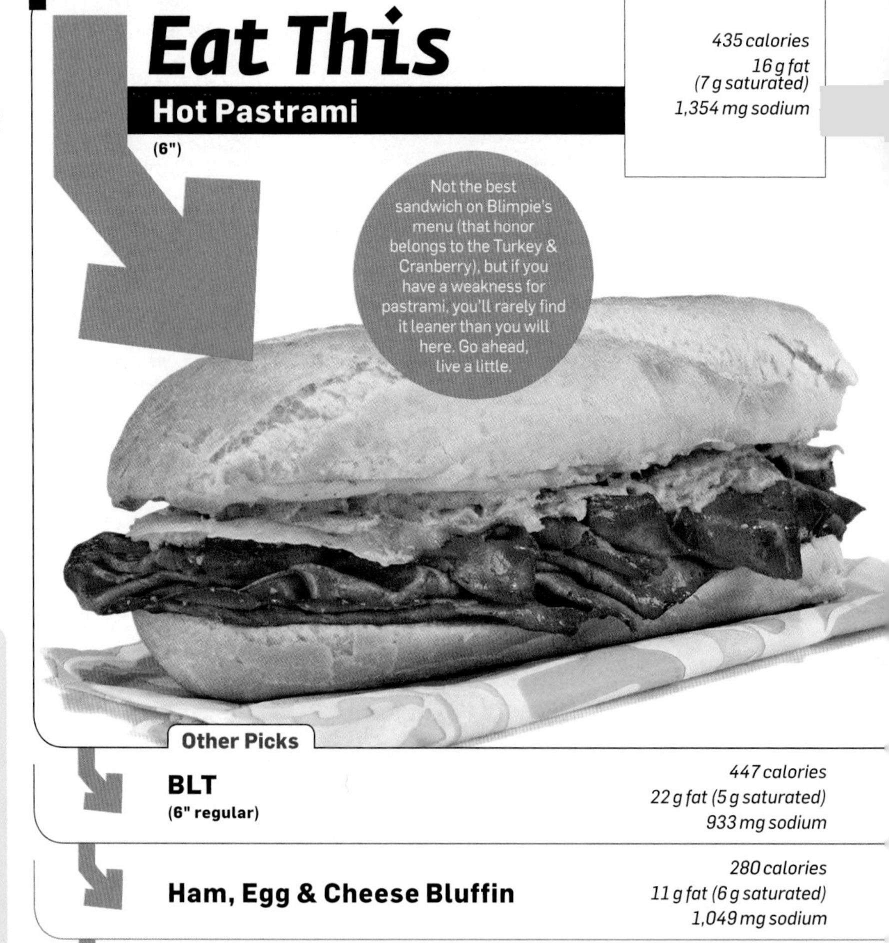

Not the best sandwich on Blimpie's menu (that honor belongs to the Turkey & Cranberry), but if you have a weakness for pastrami, you'll rarely find it leaner than you will here. Go ahead, live a little.

Other Picks

BLT
(6" regular)
447 calories
22 g fat (5 g saturated)
933 mg sodium

Ham, Egg & Cheese Bluffin
280 calories
11 g fat (6 g saturated)
1,049 mg sodium

Brownie
182 calories
7 g fat (3 g saturated)
115 mg sodium

607 calories
29 g fat
(9 g saturated)
1,586 mg sodium

Not That!

Chicken Caesar Wrap

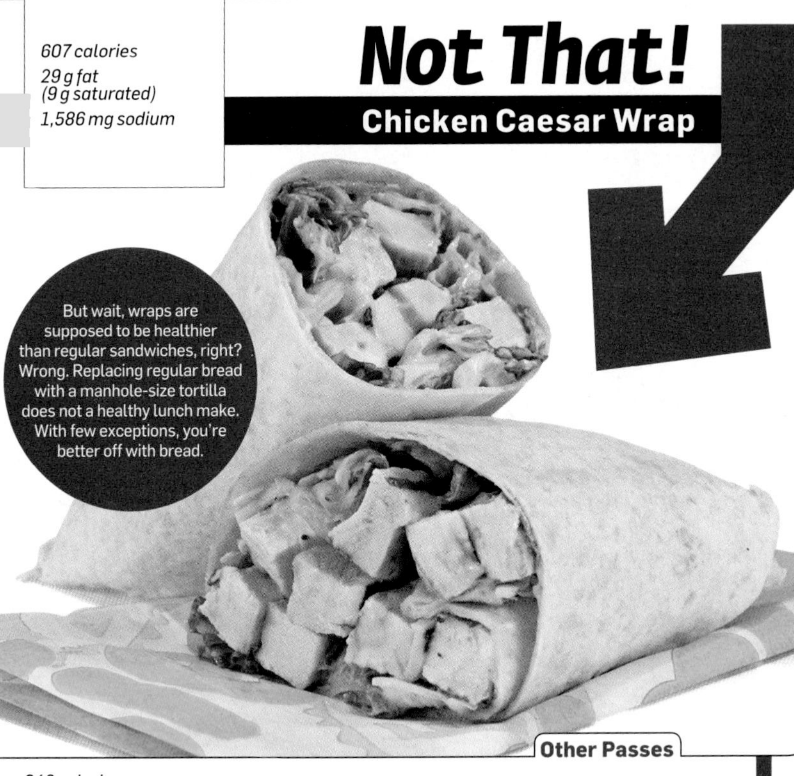

But wait, wraps are supposed to be healthier than regular sandwiches, right? Wrong. Replacing regular bread with a manhole-size tortilla does not a healthy lunch make. With few exceptions, you're better off with bread.

Other Passes

642 calories
34 g fat (10 g saturated)
1,648 mg sodium

Chicken Cheddar Bacon Ranch
(6" regular)

656 calories
34 g fat (16 g saturated)
2,202 mg sodium

Sausage, Egg & Cheese Burrito

327 calories
17 g fat (6 g saturated)
286 mg sodium

Sugar Cookie

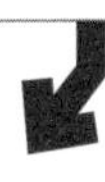

WEAPON OF MASS DESTRUCTION

Special Vegetarian
(12")

1,186 calories
60 g fat (19 g saturated)
3,532 mg sodium

This sandwich is so special, it even comes with its own defibrillator. Okay, so it doesn't, but maybe it should, considering that Blimpie manages to cram an entire day's worth of fat, saturated fat, and sodium onto a roll without the use of meat. Blimpie does, however, employ the use of multiple slices of cheese, plus crushed Doritos. (Seriously.) Just goes to disprove yet another prevalent food myth: Vegetarian food is always healthier for you. Clearly not.

GUILTY PLEASURE

Club Sandwich
(6")

386 calories
10 g fat (4 g saturated)
1,063 mg sodium

You don't generally think of a club sandwich as the healthiest item on a sub shop menu, but Blimpie's version is one of the best you'll find—and one of the leanest subs they offer.

Bob Evans

C- Bob offers up an array of healthy entrée and side options on the menu, but too much of the food here suffers from an overdose of dangerous trans fat. The Stacked & Stuffed Hotcakes, for instance, have between 6 and 9 grams per serving, and the apple pie packs a devastating 13 grams (nearly a full week's worth!) of the LDL cholesterol-spiking fat.

SURVIVAL STRATEGY

Remember this: If it sounds unhealthy (chicken fried steak, potpie, stuffed hotcakes), it is. Breakfast should consist of staples like oatmeal, eggs, fruit, and yogurt; for lunch and dinner, stick with grilled chicken or fish paired with one of the fruit and vegetable sides that avoid the fry treatment.

Eat This

Steak Tips

with Glazed Carrots and Green Beans

388 calories
20 g fat (6 g saturated)
1,428 mg sodium

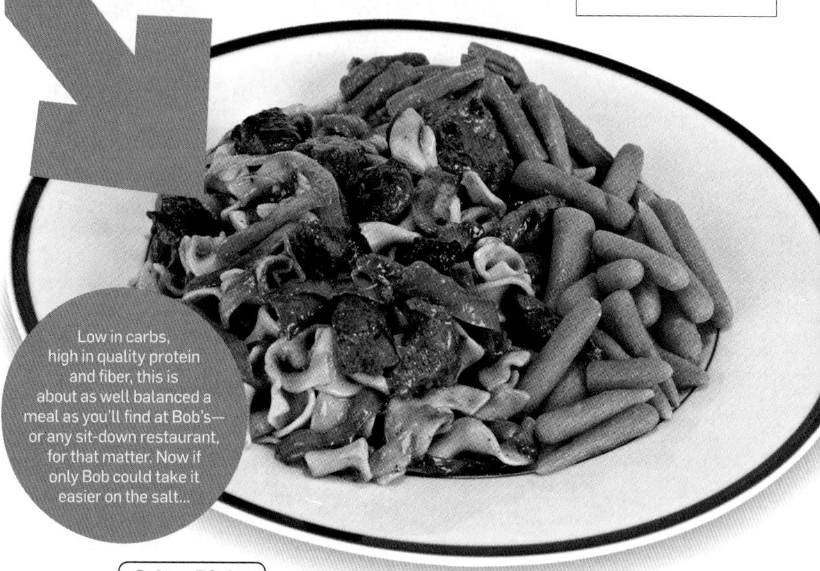

Low in carbs, high in quality protein and fiber, this is about as well balanced a meal as you'll find at Bob's—or any sit-down restaurant, for that matter. Now if only Bob could take it easier on the salt...

Other Picks

Bob-B-Q Pulled Pork Sandwich

599 calories
25 g fat (4 g saturated)
741 mg sodium

Savor Size Heritage Chef Salad
with vinegar & oil dressing

321 calories
21 g fat (9 g saturated)
923 mg sodium

Border Scramble Omelet
(made with Egg Lites)

441 calories
25 g fat (13 g saturated)
1,248 mg sodium

809 calories
48 g fat (20 g saturated, 3 g trans)
1,860 mg sodium

Not That!

Garden Vegetable Alfredo

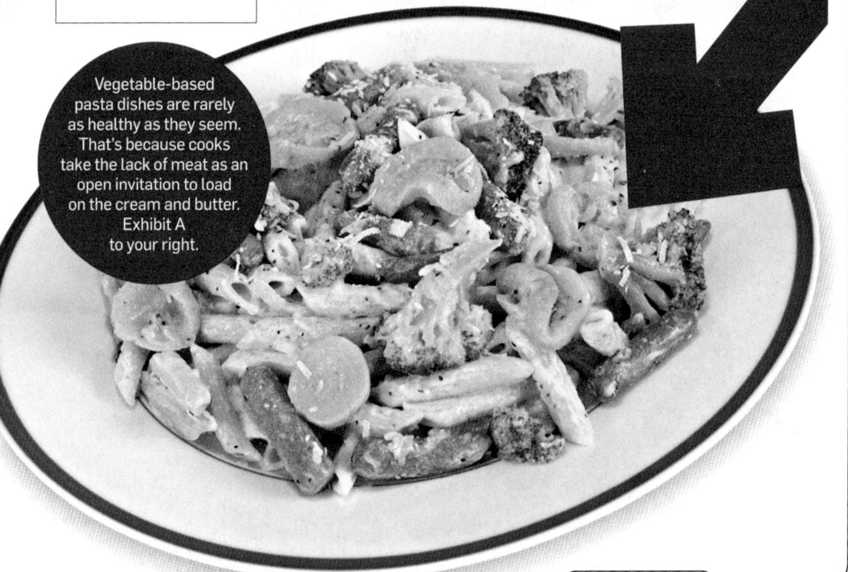

Vegetable-based pasta dishes are rarely as healthy as they seem. That's because cooks take the lack of meat as an open invitation to load on the cream and butter. Exhibit A to your right.

Other Passes

859 calories
32 g fat (9 g saturated)
1,176 mg sodium

Knife & Fork Bob-B-Q Pulled Pork Sandwich

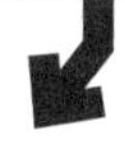

1,277 calories
100 g fat (23 g saturated)
3,008 mg sodium

Cranberry Pecan Chicken Salad
with avocado ranch dressing

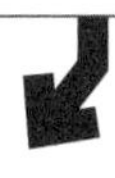

792 calories
50 g fat (18 g saturated, 4 g trans)
592 mg sodium

Blueberry Crepes
(2)

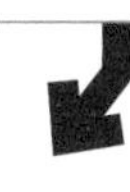

LITTLE TRICK

Don't skip the sausage—just be more selective about where it comes from. Pork and beef are the default sausages at big breakfast joints, but you can eliminate two-thirds of the fat if you ask the waiter to make yours turkey sausage, instead. And here's another boon: Bob's turkey links are a quarter bigger than the fattier stuff. That means more belly-filling mass at a fraction of the calories.

BAD BREED

Stacked & Stuffed Hotcakes

Thanks to the layers of vanilla cream cheese and the whipped cream and toppings (not to mention the sugary, calorie-laden hotcakes themselves), these sorry excuses for pancakes tip the scales at more than 1,000 calories.

Boston Market

Boston Market's menu has plenty of land mines—including healthy-sounding salads and sandwiches and nutritional disasters disguised as comfort foods, such as potpies and creamed spinach. Plus too many items have freakishly long, polluted ingredient lists. But those items are mostly offset by a host of lean, roasted meats and steamed vegetables. Choosing wisely here could mean the difference of 1,000 calories.

SURVIVAL STRATEGY
Pair roasted turkey, ham, white-meat chicken, or even sirloin with a vegetable side or two, and you've got a solid dinner. But avoid calorie-laden dark-meat chicken, meat loaf, potpie, and hot Carver Sandwiches.

Eat This

Beef Brisket, Green Beans, and Dill Potatoes

480 calories
27 g fat (4 g saturated)
560 mg sodium

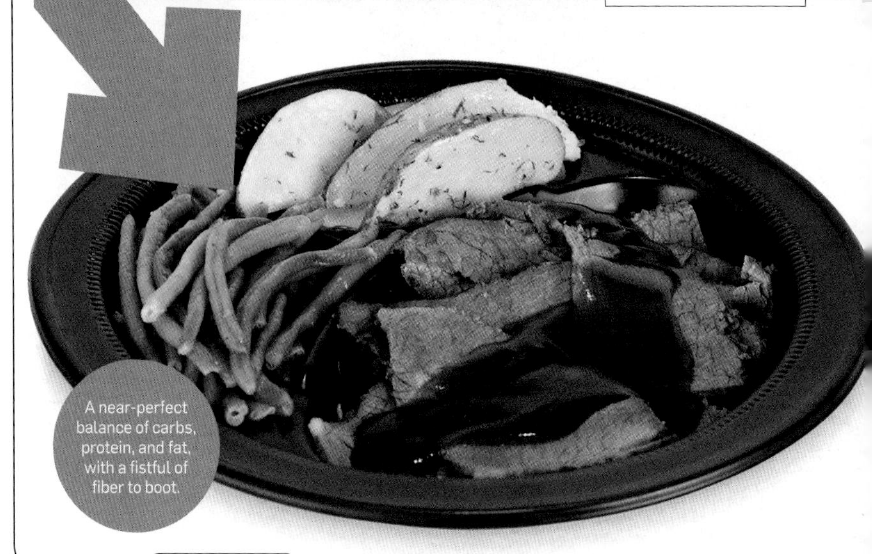

A near-perfect balance of carbs, protein, and fat, with a fistful of fiber to boot.

Other Picks

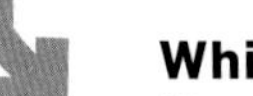

White Rotisserie Chicken (½, no skin) with Garden Fresh Cole Slaw
540 calories
24 g fat (5.5 g saturated)
1,170 mg sodium

Award Winning Roasted Sirloin
290 calories
15 g fat (6 g saturated)
440 mg sodium

Caesar Side Salad
170 calories
17 g fat (3.5 g saturated)
410 mg sodium

800 calories
41 g fat (7 g saturated, 5 g trans)
1,900 mg sodium

Not That!

Chicken Salad Sandwich

All research points to the fact that mayo-masked chicken salad is rarely as healthy as you'd think, but it's unfathomable how one sandwich could pack nearly 3 days' worth of trans fat.

3.5

The number of days' worth of heart-clobbering trans fat lurking in the Pastry Top Chicken Pot Pie.

HIDDEN DANGER

Sweet Potato Casserole

This one vegetable side dish can pack enough calories for an entire meal (and more sugar than 3 scoops of vanilla ice cream.) Blame it on 2 culprits: sugar and oil. You're better off sticking with a fresh fruit salad, some garlic spinach, or broccoli with garlic butter—or all 3.

460 calories
16 g fat
(4.5 g saturated)
39 g sugars

Other Passes

700 calories
26 g fat (8 g saturated, 5 g trans)
1,710 mg sodium

Boston Turkey Carver

480 calories
36 g fat (16 g saturated, 1.5 g trans)
1,030 mg sodium

Meatloaf

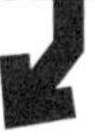

480 calories
40 g fat (8 g saturated, 1 g trans)
1,640 mg sodium

Market Chopped Side Salad

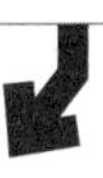

Burger King

C We got word from Burger King in October 2008 that they were finally removing the trans fat from their deep fryer. Excellent news, but the burgers are still sullied with the dangerous oils. Although the King holds the dubious distinction of being the unhealthiest of the Big Three burger joints, the trans fat transition and the introduction of healthy sides like Apple Fries signal that Burger King is finally trying to move in the right nutritional direction.

SURVIVAL STRATEGY
For breakfast, pick the Ham Omelet Sandwich. For lunch, match the regular hamburger, the Whopper Jr., or the Tendergrill Sandwich with Apple Fries and water, and you'll escape for about 500 calories.

Eat This

Whopper Jr.

(without mayo)

290 calories
12 g fat (4.5 g saturated)
500 mg sodium

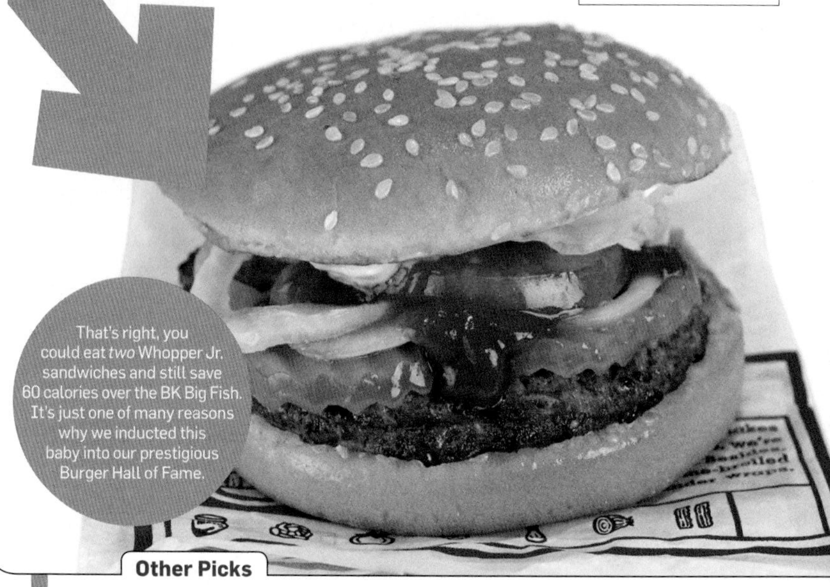

That's right, you could eat *two* Whopper Jr. sandwiches and still save 60 calories over the BK Big Fish. It's just one of many reasons why we inducted this baby into our prestigious Burger Hall of Fame.

Other Picks

Flame Broiled Double Cheeseburger

510 calories
29 g fat (14 g saturated, 1.5 g trans)
1,020 mg sodium

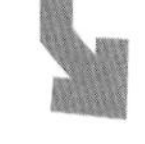

Onion Rings
(small)

310 calories
17 g fat (3 g saturated)
490 mg sodium

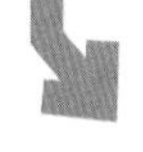

Croissan'wich Bacon, Egg & Cheese

350 calories
19 g fat (8 g saturated)
870 mg sodium

Not That!

BK Big Fish

650 calories
32 g fat (5 g saturated, 0.5 g trans)
1,540 mg sodium

Less of a fish, more of a whale. In fact, when it first belly flopped onto the scene, it was called the BK Whaler, until some mediocre marketing exec got harpooned.

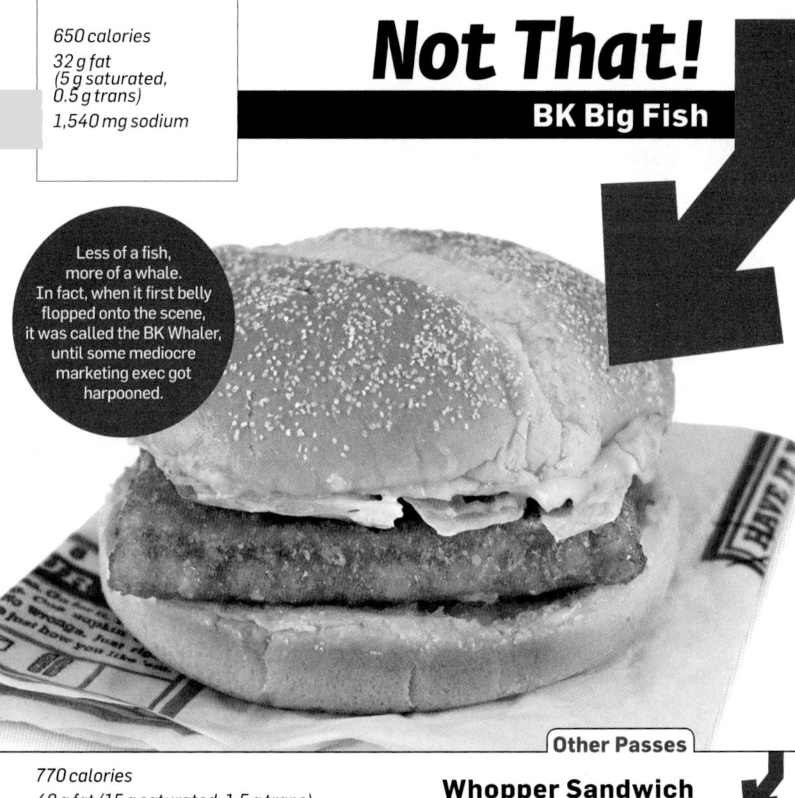

Other Passes

Whopper Sandwich with cheese

770 calories
48 g fat (15 g saturated, 1.5 g trans)
1,450 mg sodium

French Fries (small)

340 calories
17 g fat (3.5 g saturated)
590 mg sodium

Sausage, Egg & Cheese Biscuit

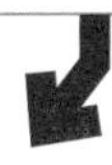

560 calories
37 g fat (19 g saturated, 1 g trans)
1,560 mg sodium

SMART SIDES

Your best bet at BK is an order of Apple Fries—fresh apples sliced to look like fries. But if you feel odd ordering from the kids' menu, stick with onion rings rather than French fries. They may not be healthy, but they'll save you a little in calories, sodium, and carbs.

LITTLE TRICK

Ask to 86 the mayo on your burger or sandwich. You'll save about 150 calories and 18 grams of fat.

GUILTY PLEASURE

Chicken Tenders (8 pieces)

360 calories
21 g fat (3.5 g saturated)
610 mg sodium

Even BK's largest serving of chicken tenders isn't half bad —it contains the same amount of calories as the relatively harmless Whopper Jr., plus it packs in 19 grams of protein. Pair them with ketchup, barbecue sauce, or sweet and sour sauce, rather than high-cal ranch or honey mustard.

California Pizza Kitchen

F Since CPK is unwilling to relinquish the nutritional numbers for their menu, we're forced to fail them, but our research found that they wouldn't fare much better than that, anyway. Among their many offenses: one of the most caloric salad menus in America; a disastrously fat-burdened Specialties lineup; and a few of the worst pasta dishes we've seen anywhere. Thankfully, the pizzas provide a surprisingly low-cal respite from the menu mayhem.

SURVIVAL STRATEGY
Either turn a healthier appetizer (like the chicken dumplings, crab cakes, or spring rolls) into an entrée, or stick with pizza—thin crust, preferably.

Eat This

Original Barbecue Chicken Pizza

(3 slices)

*525 calories**

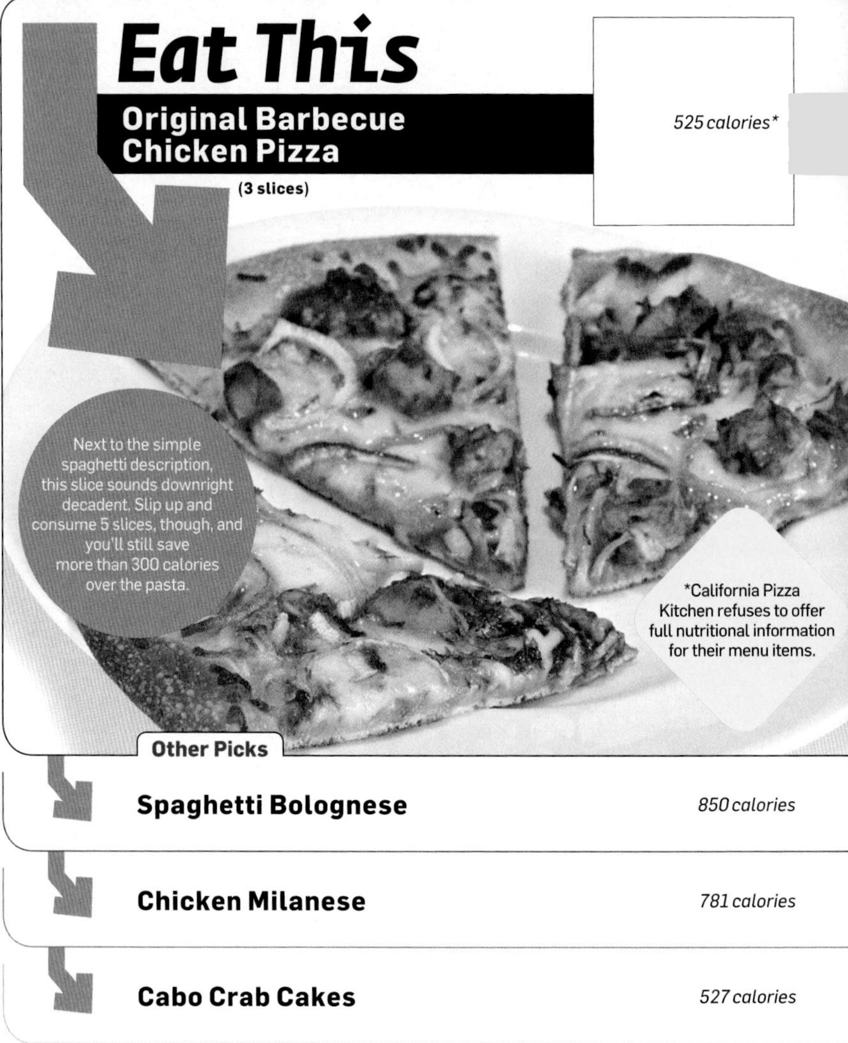

Next to the simple spaghetti description, this slice sounds downright decadent. Slip up and consume 5 slices, though, and you'll still save more than 300 calories over the pasta.

*California Pizza Kitchen refuses to offer full nutritional information for their menu items.

Other Picks

Spaghetti Bolognese *850 calories*

Chicken Milanese *781 calories*

Cabo Crab Cakes *527 calories*

Not That!

1,223 calories*

Tomato Basil Spaghettini

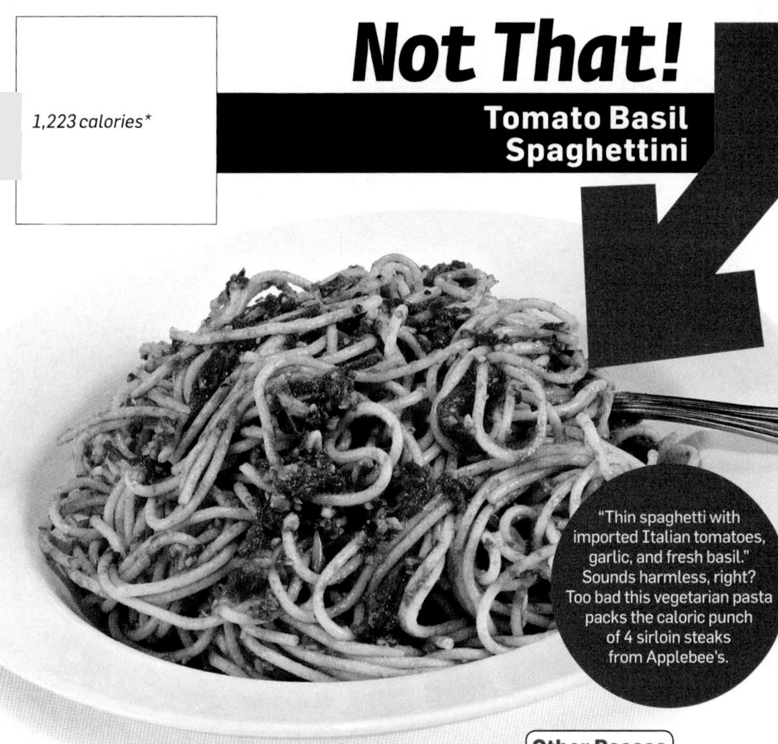

"Thin spaghetti with imported Italian tomatoes, garlic, and fresh basil." Sounds harmless, right? Too bad this vegetarian pasta packs the caloric punch of 4 sirloin steaks from Applebee's.

Other Passes

1,116 calories

Asparagus and Spinach Spaghettini

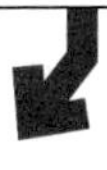

1,408 calories

Chicken Marsala

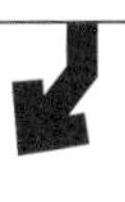

896 calories

Lettuce Wraps with Shrimp

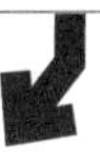

WEAPON OF MASS DESTRUCTION Thai Crunch Salad

2,115 calories

The lineup reads like a roster of nutritional superstars: shredded cabbage, julienne cucumbers, edamame, and grilled chicken breast. But together, these ingredients constitute America's worst salad, trouncing the runner-up—On the Border's greasy taco salad served in a giant fried tortilla bowl—by a staggering 400 calories.

GUILTY PLEASURE

Sticky Toffee Cake

311 calories

Sadly, desserts at CPK may be some of the healthiest dishes in the entire restaurant. The 530-calorie Tiramisu and 510-calorie Apple Crisp are both solid ways to satisfy a sweet tooth, but this new Toffee Cake deserves induction into our Dessert Hall of Fame. How do they serve salads so bad and desserts so good? Ah, the mysteries...

Carl's Jr.

D+

Most fast-food restaurants today are making at least some attempt to offset their bulging burgers and fried sides with healthier options. But Carl's Jr. is swimming against the nutritional current in nearly every way imaginable. The burgers are the worst in the fast-food industry, the breakfast menu has no entrée with fewer than 450 calories, and not a single side is spared a deep-fried fate.

SURVIVAL STRATEGY
Fast-food chains tend to group in clusters, so your first strategy should be to find another place to grab lunch. Failing that, settle on either the Charbroiled Chicken Salad with low-fat balsamic dressing or the Charbroiled BBQ Chicken Sandwich.

Eat This

Charbroiled BBQ Chicken Sandwich

380 calories
7 g fat (0.5 g saturated)
1,010 mg sodium

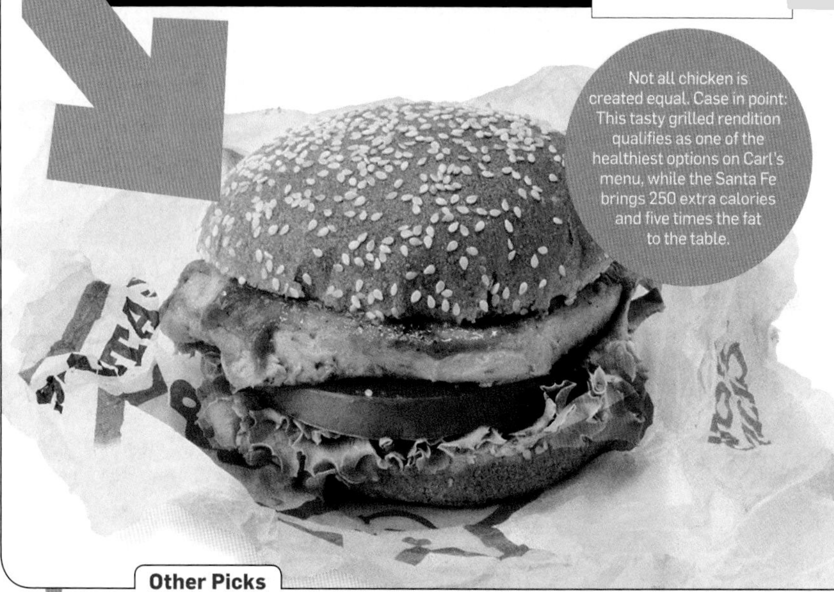

Not all chicken is created equal. Case in point: This tasty grilled rendition qualifies as one of the healthiest options on Carl's menu, while the Santa Fe brings 250 extra calories and five times the fat to the table.

Other Picks

Single Teriyaki Burger

610 calories
29 g fat (11 g saturated)
1,020 mg sodium

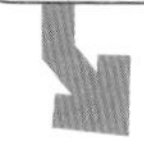

Sourdough Breakfast Sandwich

450 calories
21 g fat (8 g saturated)
1,470 mg sodium

Chicken Stars
(4 pieces)

210 calories
16 g fat (4 g saturated)
310 mg sodium

630 calories
35 g fat
(8 g saturated)
1,410 mg sodium

Not That!

Charbroiled Santa Fe Chicken Sandwich

Triple Whoppers are supposedly charbroiled, but that doesn't make them healthy. Here, the addition of cheese and a mayo-based sauce ups the fat ante by a factor of five.

Other Passes

890 calories
54 g fat (20 g saturated, 2 g trans)
2,040 mg sodium

The Original Six Dollar Burger

780 calories
41 g fat (15 g saturated, 1 g trans)
1,460 mg sodium

Breakfast Burger

460 calories
22 g fat (4.5 g saturated)
1,180 mg sodium

Natural Cut Fries **(medium)**

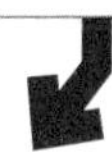

WEAPON OF MASS DESTRUCTION

Guacamole Bacon Six Dollar Burger

1,040 calories
70 g fat (25 g saturated, 2 g trans)
2,240 mg sodium

Paris Hilton, Padma Lakshmi, and Audrina Partridge have all shilled for Carl's infamous line of burgers, but don't let these rail-thin starlets give you the wrong idea: Few foods have the ability to make you fat quicker than a Six Dollar Burger. Add fries and a drink, and you'll need to make a 2½-hour date with a treadmill to work off the 1,700 calories.

GUILTY PLEASURE

Strawberry Swirl Cheesecake

290 calories
16 g fat (9 g saturated)
21 g sugars

There are 2 reasons why we find Carl's cheesecake irresistible: 1) It has 410 fewer calories than the strawberry shake, and 2) it stacks up remarkably well next to the slices dispensed elsewhere. (Uno Chicago Grill's has 920 calories and 64 grams of fat!)

Chevys Fresh Mex

D Don't let the made-fresh-daily shtick distract you from the massive portions that push many of Chevy's meals beyond the 1,000-calorie threshold. The taco trader earns its dismal grade by cramming a consistently dangerous amount of fat into its entrées; by having salt levels that make it difficult to find a meal with fewer than 2,000 milligrams of sodium; and by failing to offer complete nutritional disclosure.

SURVIVAL STRATEGY
Stick to the best items on the menu: the Homemade Tortilla Soup and the Santa Fe Chopped Salad. If you can't resist an entrée, order it without all the fixin's—tamalito, rice, sour cream, and cheese. That should knock more than 300 calories off your meal.

Eat This

Grilled Chicken Tacos

(no tamalito or rice)

779 calories
26 g fat
(7 g saturated)
2,101 mg sodium

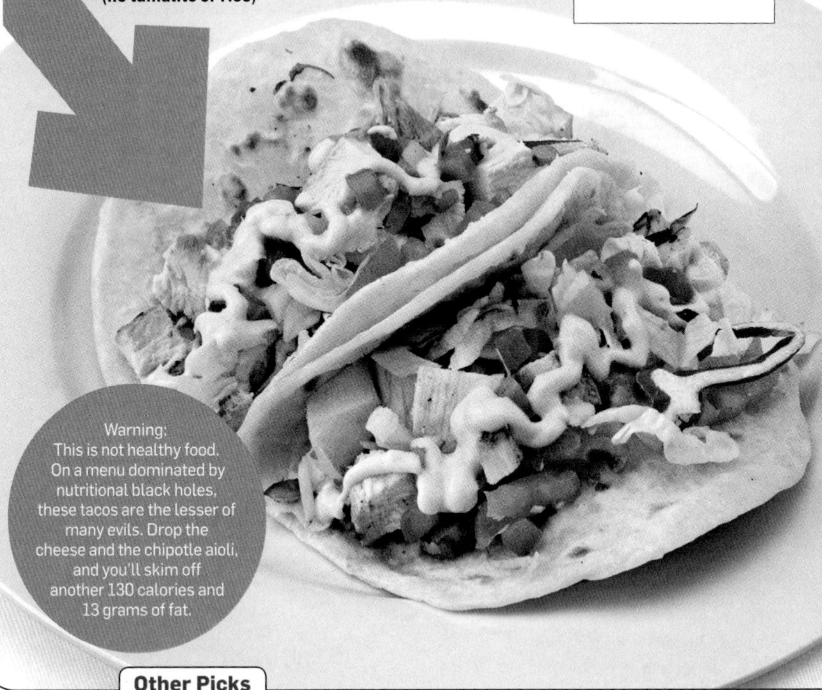

Warning:
This is not healthy food. On a menu dominated by nutritional black holes, these tacos are the lesser of many evils. Drop the cheese and the chipotle aioli, and you'll skim off another 130 calories and 13 grams of fat.

Other Picks

Santa Fe Chopped Salad
without cheese

471 calories
23 g fat (6 g saturated)
1,067 mg sodium

Black Beans
with cheese and pico de gallo

190 calories
2 g fat (1 g saturated)
930 mg sodium

1,551 calories
94 g fat
(37 g saturated)
2,480 mg sodium

Not That!

Tostada Salad with Chicken

Containing nearly a day's worth of calories and as much fat as 19 Twinkies, this bowl of leaves qualifies as one of the worst salads in America. (Only On the Border's Grande Taco Salad and CPK's Thai Crunch Salad are worse.)

4,993

The amount of sodium, in milligrams, in one order of Juicy Shrimp Fajitas with Tortillas. That's more than twice the amount you should consume daily.

HIDDEN DANGER

Fajita Fixings

A platter of sizzling meat and vegetables sounds like a pretty smart dinner choice, but as with all Tex-Mex cuisine, it's not the star of the plate that will get you in trouble—it's the long list of supporting actors. Combined, the rice, guac, sour cream, and tortillas bring the caloric equivalent of a Whopper to your dinner plate.

669 calories
27 g fat
(11 g saturated)
1531 mg sodium

Other Passes

1,040 calories
39 g fat (9 g saturated)
3,090 mg sodium

Grilled Salmon Tacos

275 calories
14 g fat (5 g saturated)
729 mg sodium

Refried Beans
without cheese or pico de gallo

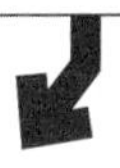

Chick-fil-A

A-

For those trying to cut down on calories, it's hard to beat Chick-fil-A. Between the breakfast and lunch menus, there are only two entrées that break the 500-calorie barrier. This means that it's hard to do too much harm—especially if you stick to the chicken. And unlike the typical fast-food chain, Chick-fil-A offers a list of sides that goes beyond breaded and fried potatoes and onions.

SURVIVAL STRATEGY

Instead of nuggets or strips, look to the Chargrilled Chicken Sandwiches, which average only 315 calories apiece. And sub in a healthy side—fruit or soup—for the standard fried fare. Just don't supplement your meal with a shake—none has fewer than 600 calories.

Eat This

Chick-fil-A Chargrilled Chicken Sandwich

270 calories
3 g fat (1 g saturated)
1,270 mg sodium

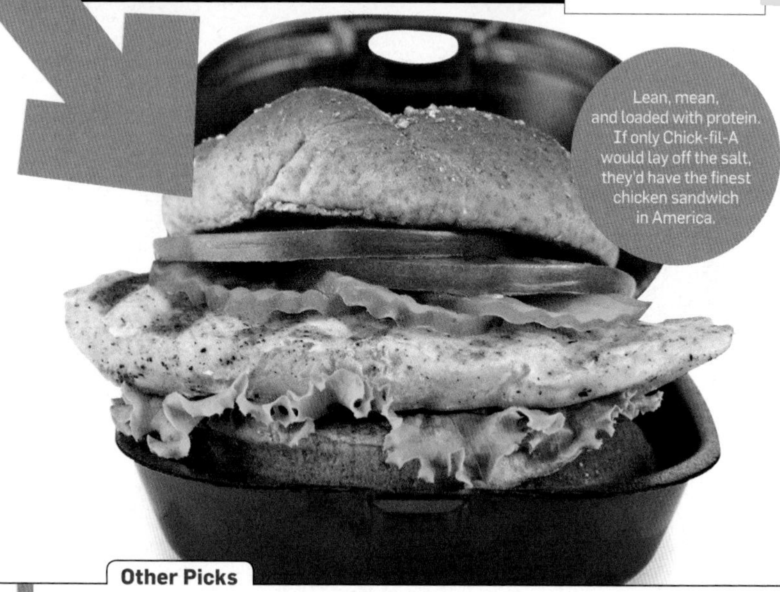

Lean, mean, and loaded with protein. If only Chick-fil-A would lay off the salt, they'd have the finest chicken sandwich in America.

Other Picks

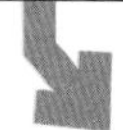

Chick-fil-A Chicken Sandwich

410 calories
16 g fat (3.5 g saturated)
1,300 mg sodium

Chicken Breakfast Burrito

420 calories
18 g fat (7 g saturated)
890 mg sodium

Fruit Cup
(medium)

70 calories
0 g fat
14 g sugars

600 calories
38 g fat (9 g saturated)
1,470 mg sodium

Not That!

Chick-fil-A Chick-n-Strips Salad

with blue cheese dressing

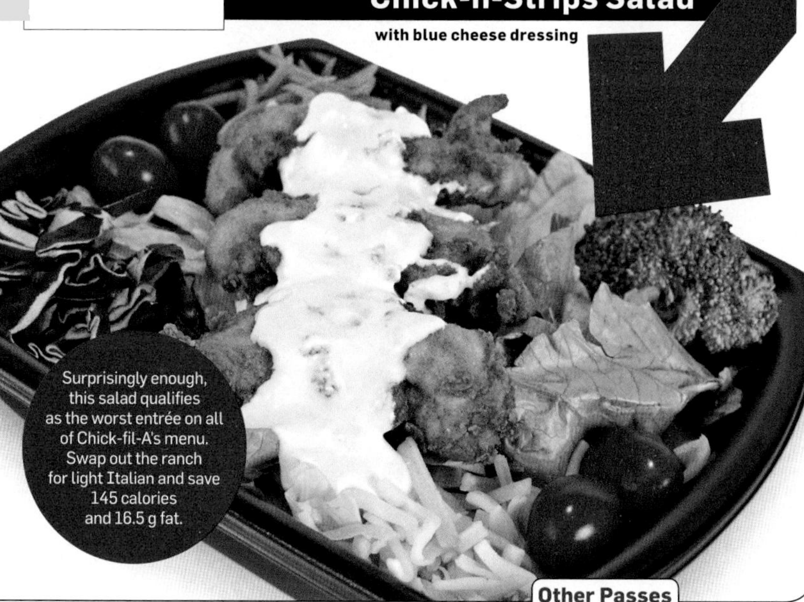

Surprisingly enough, this salad qualifies as the worst entrée on all of Chick-fil-A's menu. Swap out the ranch for light Italian and save 145 calories and 16.5 g fat.

Other Passes

480 calories
16 g fat (7 g saturated)
1,810 mg sodium

Chicken Caesar Cool Wrap

500 calories
20 g fat (7 g saturated)
1,260 mg sodium

Chicken, Egg & Cheese
on Sunflower Multigrain Bagel

270 calories
12 g fat (1.5 g saturated)
31 g sugars

Carrot and Raisin Salad

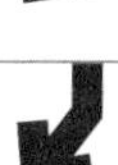

WEAPON OF MASS DESTRUCTION
Peach Milkshake

850 calories
21 g fat (13 g saturated)
144 g sugars

Does it seem odd that the single most caloric item on Chick-fil-A's menu invokes the spirit of fresh fruit? By name alone, this drink sounds almost like a smoothie, yet it packs in almost 200 calories more than Chick-fil-A's Vanilla Milkshake. The culprit is a massive sugar overload. You'd have to eat about a dozen real peaches to equal the sugar found in this one beverage.

GUILTY PLEASURE
Waffle Potato Fries

280 calories
15 g fat (3 g saturated)
100 mg sodium

As fries go, Chick-fil-A's are some of the best in the industry. They're relatively low in calories and fat, lightly dusted with salt, and—thanks to being fried in peanut oil—trans fat–free (as is the rest of their menu).

Chili's

D

From burgers to baby back ribs, Chili's serves up some of the country's saltiest, fattiest fare. Worst among the offenders are the burgers, fajitas, and appetizers, including the 2,130-calorie Onion String & Crispy Jalapeno Stack. The Guiltless Grill menu is Chili's attempt to offer healthier options, but with only 8 items and an average sodium content of 1,323 milligrams, it's a meager attempt at nutritional salvation.

SURVIVAL STRATEGY

There's not too much to choose from after you eliminate the ribs, burgers, fajitas, chicken, and salads. You're better off with a Classic Sirloin and steamed vegetables or broccoli. Or stick with the Chicken Fajita Pita with black beans and pico de gallo.

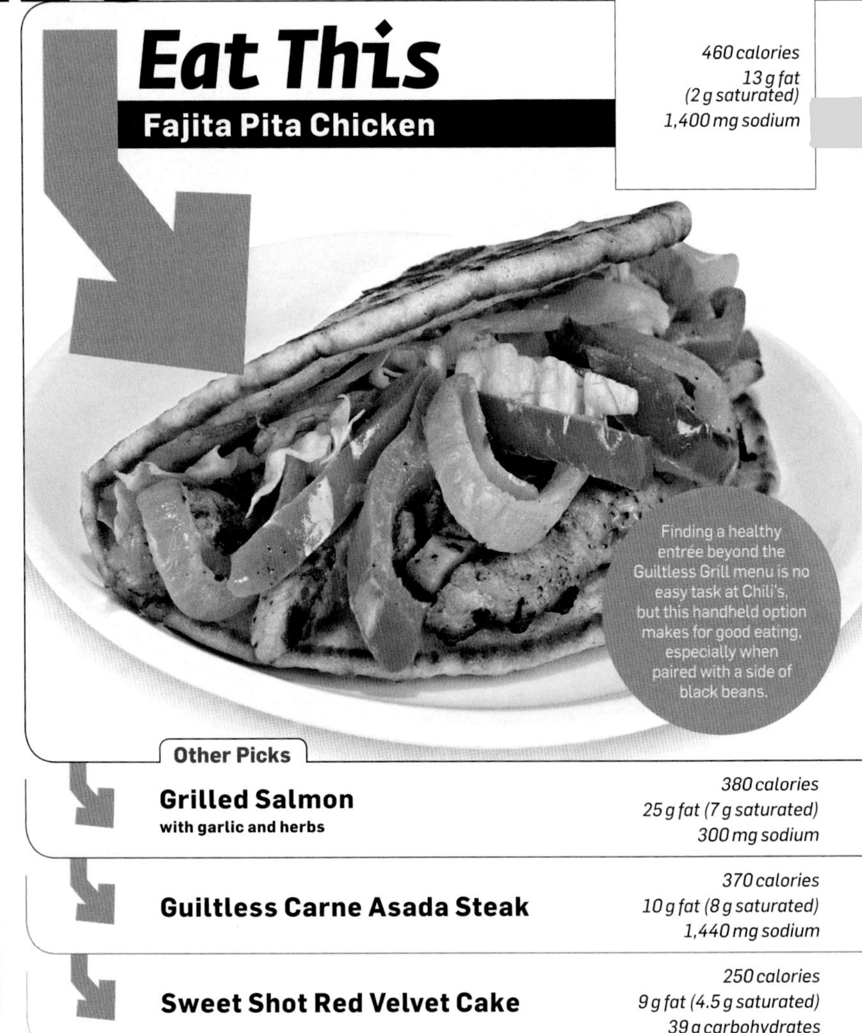

Eat This

Fajita Pita Chicken

460 calories
13 g fat (2 g saturated)
1,400 mg sodium

Finding a healthy entrée beyond the Guiltless Grill menu is no easy task at Chili's, but this handheld option makes for good eating, especially when paired with a side of black beans.

Other Picks

Grilled Salmon
with garlic and herbs
380 calories
25 g fat (7 g saturated)
300 mg sodium

Guiltless Carne Asada Steak
370 calories
10 g fat (8 g saturated)
1,440 mg sodium

Sweet Shot Red Velvet Cake
250 calories
9 g fat (4.5 g saturated)
39 g carbohydrates

1,170 calories
71 g fat
(11 g saturated)
2,910 mg sodium

Not That!

Chicken Ranch Sandwich

You're looking at nearly three times the calories, five times the fat, and twice the number of carbs as are in the Fajita Pita. This one's a no-brainer.

Other Passes

1,320 calories
76 g fat (38 g saturated)
3,650 mg sodium

Grilled Shrimp Alfredo

610 calories
11 g fat (2 g saturated)
1,790 mg sodium

Guiltless Black Bean Burger

1,140 calories
66 g fat (32 g saturated)
129 g carbohydrates

Chocolate Chip Paradise Pie

FOOD COURT

THE CRIME

Crispy Honey-Chipotle Chicken Crispers
(1,990 calories)

THE PUNISHMENT

Swim freestyle laps for 3 hours and 45 minutes

CONDIMENT CATASTROPHE

Citrus Balsamic Vinaigrette

250 calories
25 g fat (3.5 g saturated)
220 mg sodium

Balsamic is normally a safe bet, but Chili's rendition packs on more calories than both their ranch and blue cheese. Shave 160 calories with the tomato vinaigrette.

LITTLE TRICK

Ignore the preset menu options entirely. Instead, build a meal out of skewers of Spicy Lime & Garlic Shrimp and a few healthy sides (Chili's one really strong suit).

Chipotle

C+ There are only a few bad items at Chipotle, but unfortunately, with Chipotle's pared-down menu, they form the backbone of most meals. Without realizing it, the careless customer can easily construct a 1,000-calorie entrée. Add chips and the meal reaches towering heights. Still, Chipotle gets bonus points for using responsible, sustainable purveyors like Niman Ranch to fill up their fridges.

SURVIVAL STRATEGY
Chipotle assures us that they'll make anything a customer wants, as long as they have the ingredients. With fresh salsa, beans, lettuce, and grilled vegetables, you can do plenty of good. Skip the 13-inch tortillas, white rice, cheese, and sour cream and you'll do well.

Eat This

Crispy Steak Tacos

with black beans, tomato salsa, and lettuce

515 calories
13.5 g fat
(3.5 g saturated)
1,070 mg sodium

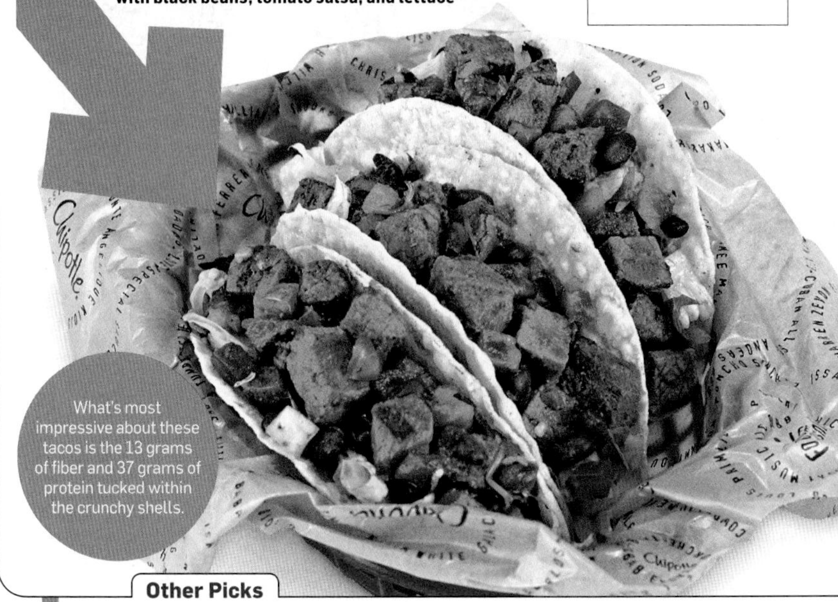

What's most impressive about these tacos is the 13 grams of fiber and 37 grams of protein tucked within the crunchy shells.

Other Picks

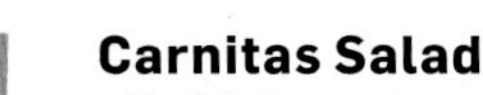

Carnitas Salad
with pinto beans, cheese, and green salsa

435 calories
17.5 g fat (8 g saturated)
1,335 mg sodium

Chicken Bowl
with black beans, cheese, lettuce, and tomato salsa

435 calories
16 g fat (7 g saturated)
1,270 mg sodium

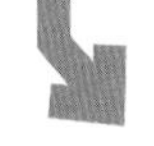

Guacamole
with crispy taco shells (3)

330 calories
19 g fat (3.5 g saturated)
220 mg sodium

1,035 calories
39.5 g fat (17.5 g saturated)
2,060 mg sodium

Not That!

Chicken Burrito

with rice, black beans, corn salsa, cheese, sour cream, and lettuce

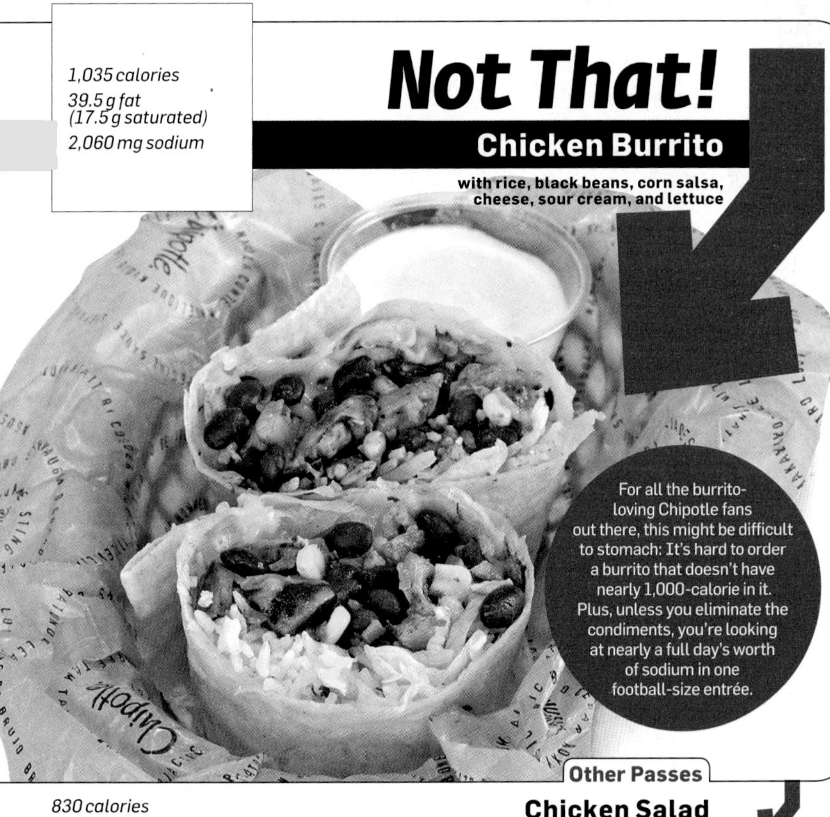

For all the burrito-loving Chipotle fans out there, this might be difficult to stomach: It's hard to order a burrito that doesn't have nearly 1,000-calorie in it. Plus, unless you eliminate the condiments, you're looking at nearly a full day's worth of sodium in one football-size entrée.

Other Passes

Chicken Salad

with black beans, cheese, guacamole, and chipotle vinaigrette

830 calories
53.5 g fat (13 g saturated)
1,695 mg sodium

Chicken Soft Tacos

with black beans, cheese, lettuce, and tomato salsa

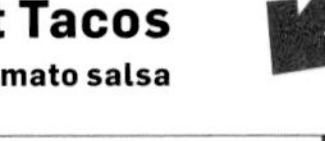

525 calories
18.5 g fat (8 g saturated)
1,470 mg sodium

Chips

with red salsa

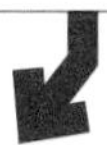

590 calories
28 g fat (3.5 g saturated)
930 mg sodium

STEALTH HEALTH FOOD
Cilantro

Found in several of Chipotle's sauces and dips (including the fresh tomato salsa, green tomatillo salsa, and guacamole), cilantro can help control blood sugar, fight bacteria, and cleanse your body of heavy metals.

HIDDEN DANGER

Chips

Made with kosher salt and fresh lime, Chipotle's guac-scoopers are hard to resist. But switch them out for 3 or 4 crunchy taco shells, and you'll save nearly 400 calories and 20 grams of fat.

570 calories
27 g fat
(3.5 g saturated)
420 mg sodium

LITTLE TRICK

Save 245 calories by using green salsa instead of the vinaigrette on your salads.

Cold Stone Creamery

C-

"Overindulge" is the silent message emanating from every menu board in every ice-cream shop in the country, and Cold Stone is no different. In fact, their largest size ice cream bears the spurious name "Gotta Have It." Small milk shakes weigh in at 1,000 calories, and troublesome toppings add up fast. On the other hand, Cold Stone offers a nice variety of sorbet, frozen yogurt, and Sinless Sans Fat ice cream.

SURVIVAL STRATEGY

Keep your intake to 300 calories by filling a 6-ounce Like It–size cup with one of the lighter scoops, and then sprinkle fresh fruit on top. Or opt for one of the creamery's 16-ounce real-fruit smoothies, which average only 290 calories apiece.

Eat This

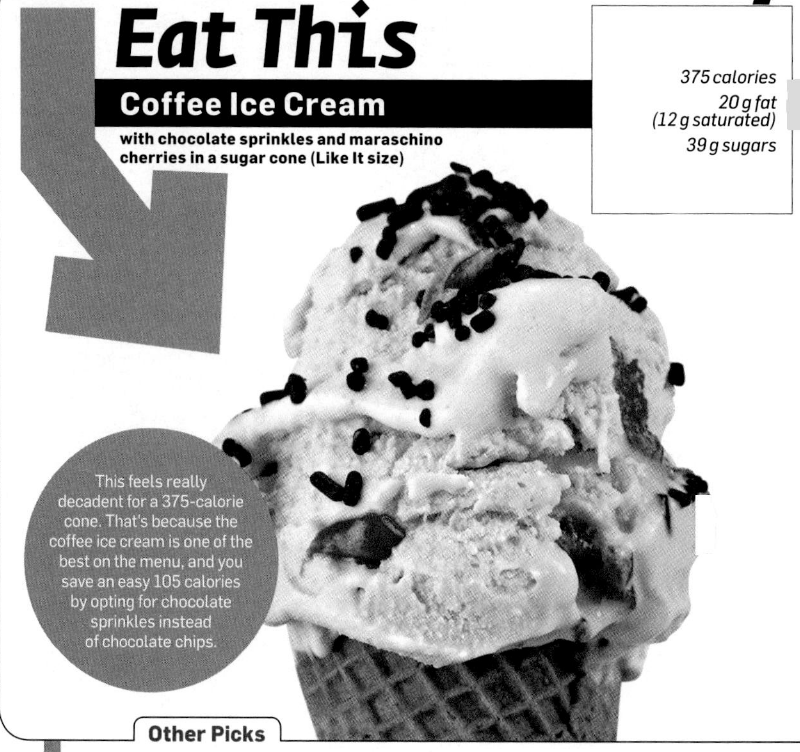

Coffee Ice Cream

with chocolate sprinkles and maraschino cherries in a sugar cone (Like It size)

375 calories
20 g fat (12 g saturated)
39 g sugars

This feels really decadent for a 375-calorie cone. That's because the coffee ice cream is one of the best on the menu, and you save an easy 105 calories by opting for chocolate sprinkles instead of chocolate chips.

Other Picks

Egg Nog Ice Cream
with blackberries (Like It size)

270 calories
15 g fat (10 g saturated)
23 g sugars

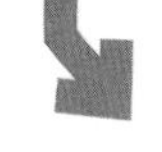

Sinless Sans Fat Sweet Cream
with York Peppermint Patties in a sugar cone (Like It size)

300 calories
2 g fat (1.5 g saturated)
30 g sugars

Strawberry Bananza Low-Cal Smoothie
(Like It size)

140 calories
1 g fat
24 g sugars

Not That!

Lotta Caramel Latte

(Like It size)

1,320 calories
62 g fat (39 g saturated, 1.5 g trans)
134 g sugars

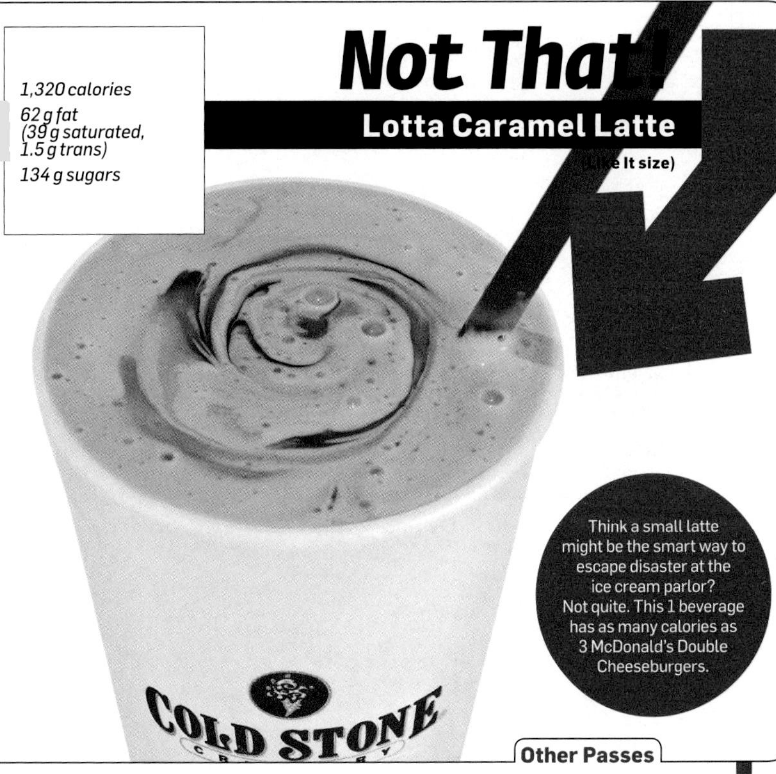

Think a small latte might be the smart way to escape disaster at the ice cream parlor? Not quite. This 1 beverage has as many calories as 3 McDonald's Double Cheeseburgers.

Other Passes

Cake Batter Ice Cream
with white chocolate chips (Like It size)

500 calories
28 g fat (20 g saturated, 0.5 g trans)
50 g sugars

French Vanilla Ice Cream
with cookie dough in a dipped waffle cone (Like It size)

830 calories
42 g fat (23.5 g saturated, 3.5 g trans)
90 g sugars

Savory Strawberry Shake
(Like It size)

1,000 calories
55 g fat (35 g saturated, 1.5 g trans)
98 g sugars

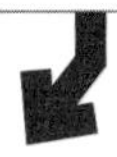

THE TOPPING TOTEM POLE

BLUEBERRIES
10 calories, 0 g fat, 2 g sugars

CHOCOLATE SPRINKLES
25 calories, 0 g fat, 6 g sugars

CHERRY PIE FILLING
50 calories, 0 g fat, 0 g sugars

KIT KAT CANDY BAR
110 calories, 5 g fat, 10 g sugars

COOKIE DOUGH
180 calories, 8 g fat, 26 g sugars

REESE'S PEANUT BUTTER CUP
190 calories, 11 g fat, 17 g sugars

PEANUTS
210 calories, 18 g fat, 0 g sugars

STEALTH HEALTH FOOD
Cinnamon

Ground cinnamon has been shown to be effective in bolstering insulin resistance, which means it may help prevent the sugar in your ice cream from passing through your stomach too quickly, suppressing the post–Cold Stone blood-sugar spike. Have some sprinkled atop your next cone or cup.

Così

B Answering the call for healthier options, Così recently unveiled the new Lighten Up! Menu, which relies on light dressings, low-fat mayo, and modest cheese servings to turn some of the more egregious menu items into some decent nosh. That's a step in the right direction, to be sure, but it does little to blunt the breakfast menu's oversize muffins or bagel sandwich belt-busters, not to mention the long lineup of deleterious desserts, including the 1,594-calorie Double Trouble Brownie Sundae.

SURVIVAL STRATEGY
Get cozy with Così's Lighten Up! Menu. Only 2 items top the 500-calorie mark: the Cosi Cobb Light Salad and the Chicken T.B.M. Light.

Eat This

Shanghai Chicken Salad

305 calories
13 g fat
824 mg sodium

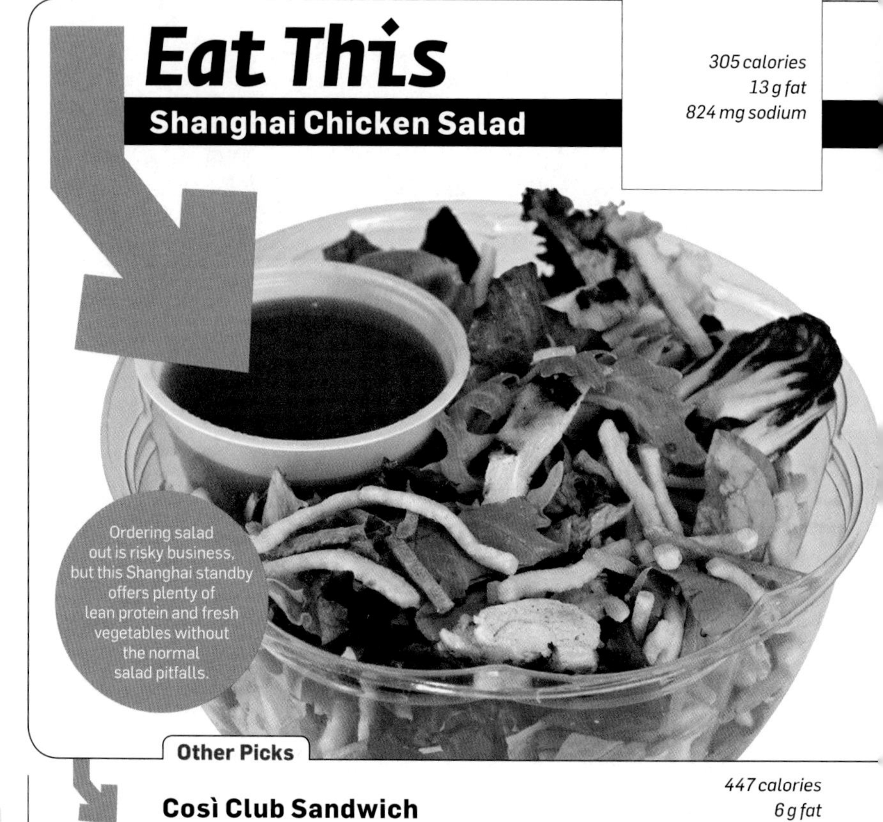

Ordering salad out is risky business, but this Shanghai standby offers plenty of lean protein and fresh vegetables without the normal salad pitfalls.

Other Picks

Così Club Sandwich
447 calories
6 g fat
677 mg sodium

Meatball Aurora
558 calories
25 g fat
1,158 mg sodium

Chocolate Croissant
324 calories
17 g fat
41 g carbohydrates

708 calories
55 g fat
1,328 mg sodium

Not That!

Cosi Cobb Salad

Learn to Lighten Up! On sandwiches and salads that include Così Vinaigrette, this little phrase will switch you to fat-free vinaigrette. Easiest 300-calorie savings ever.

Other Passes

722 calories
40 g fat
845 mg sodium

Grilled Chicken T.B.M.

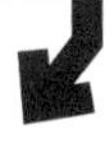

747 calories
42 g fat
2,210 mg sodium

Italiano

500 calories
25 g fat
61 g carbohydrates

Carrot Muffin

WEAPON OF MASS DESTRUCTION
Etruscan Whole Grain Bread
(2 slices)

470 calories
4 g fat
92 g carbohydrates

Can you imagine making a sandwich between two Dunkin' Donuts Chocolate Frosted Donuts? That's exactly what you're doing (calorically, at least) everytime you order a sandwich made on Etruscan, the worst bread we've ever seen.

GUILTY PLEASURE

Bacon Turkey Cheddar Melt

572 calories
24 g fat
1,101 mg sodium

The words "bacon," "Cheddar," and "melt" are usually harbingers for dietary disaster—especially at Così, where most melts are more than 600 calories—but with 45 grams of protein, this sandwich defies expectations. Add an unsweetened ice tea for a decent lunch that feels like a splurge.

Dairy Queen

D+

Dairy Queen has a taste for excess that rivals that of other fast-food failures such as Carl's Jr. and Hardee's. But unlike Carl's, DQ offers a whole slew of abominable ice cream creations to pair with its calorie-riddled savory bites. Here's a look at one hypothetical meal: a Mushroom Swiss Burger with regular onion rings and a small Snickers Blizzard—a shocking 1,650-calorie meal with 78 grams of fat.

SURVIVAL STRATEGY
Your best offense is a solid defense: Skip elaborate burgers, fried sides, and specialty ice cream concoctions. Order a Grilled Chicken Sandwich or an Original Burger, and if you must have a treat, stick to soft serve cone or a small sundae.

Eat This

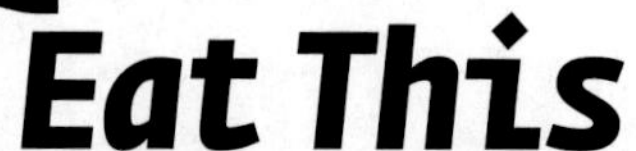

All-Beef Chili Cheese Dog

430 calories
22 g fat (10 g saturated)
1,010 mg sodium

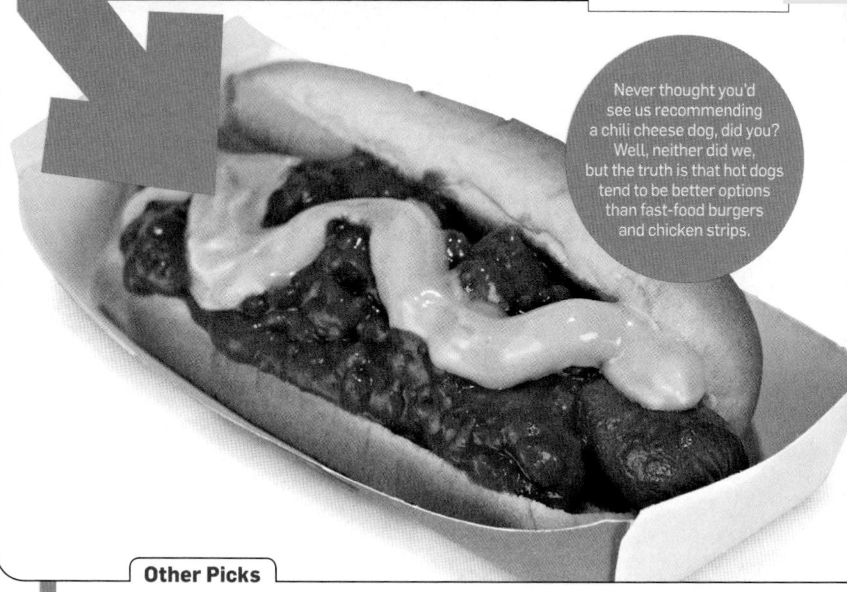

Never thought you'd see us recommending a chili cheese dog, did you? Well, neither did we, but the truth is that hot dogs tend to be better options than fast-food burgers and chicken strips.

Other Picks

DQ Original Cheeseburger

400 calories
18 g fat (9 g saturated, 0.5 g trans)
920 mg sodium

Pancake Platter with bacon

400 calories
13 g fat (3.5 g saturated)
1,030 mg sodium

Hot Fudge Sundae (small)

300 calories
10 g fat (7 g saturated)
37 g sugars

1,360 calories
63 g fat (11 g saturated, 1 g trans)
2,910 mg sodium

Not That!

Chicken Strip Basket with Country Gravy

(4 pieces)

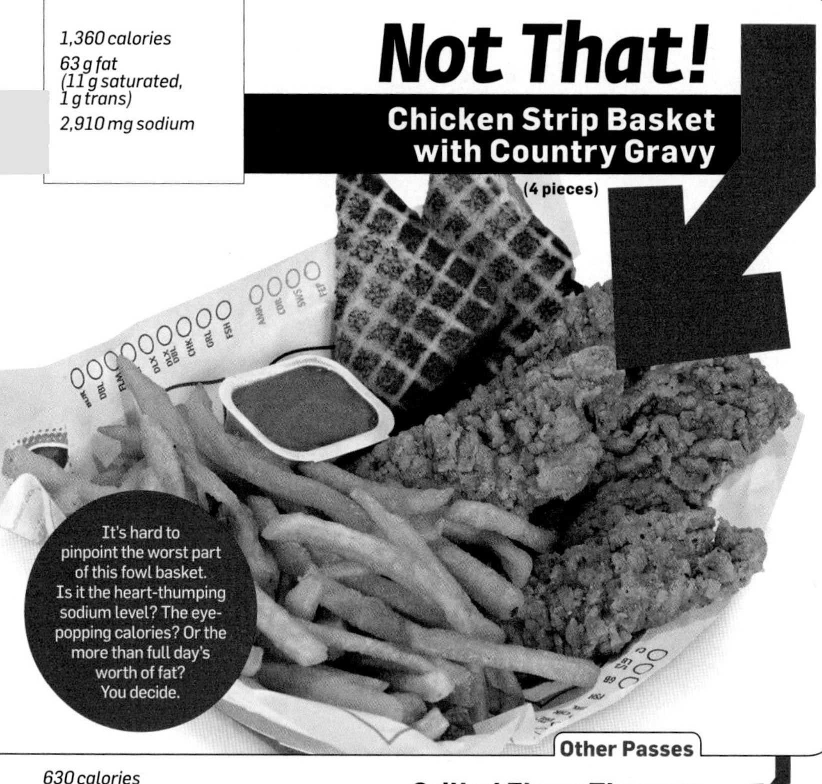

It's hard to pinpoint the worst part of this fowl basket. Is it the heart-thumping sodium level? The eye-popping calories? Or the more than full day's worth of fat? You decide.

1,216

The average number of calories in one of Dairy Queen's Basket Meals.

HIDDEN DANGER

Iron Grilled Veggie Quesadilla Basket

Don't let the phrase "grilled veggie" fool you—this gut bomb has more calories and fat than 90% of DQ's burgers and cheeseburgers.

1,020 calories
49 g fat (19 g saturated)
2,470 mg sodium

Other Passes

630 calories
36 g fat (9 g saturated)
1,580 mg sodium

Grilled FlameThrower Chicken Sandwich

750 calories
49 g fat (17 g saturated, 2.5 g trans)
1,470 mg sodium

Ultimate Hash Browns with Bacon

710 calories
27 g fat (14 g saturated, 3 g trans)
76 g sugars

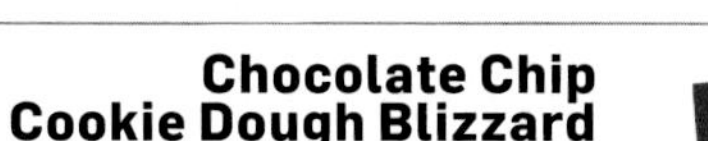

Chocolate Chip Cookie Dough Blizzard (small)

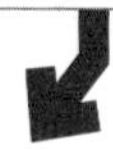

FOOD COURT

THE CRIME
6-Piece Chicken Strip Basket with Country Gravy
(1,640 calories)

THE PUNISHMENT
Lift weights for 7½ hours

Denny's

C-

Too bad the adult menu at Denny's doesn't adhere to the same standard as the kids' menu, which is loaded with low-calorie entrées and sides. The famous Slam breakfasts all top 800 calories, and the burgers are even worse. But Denny's does have an array of reliable sides and six dinner entrées with fewer than 500 calories, including the 340-calorie sirloin and shrimp dinner.

SURVIVAL STRATEGY

Look for the Fit Fare menu, which gathers together all the best options on the menu. Outside of that, stick to the sirloin, grilled chicken, or soups. For breakfast, order a Veggie Cheese Omelette or create your own meal from à la carte options such as fruit, oatmeal, toast, and eggs.

Eat This

Buffalo Wings

(9)

300 calories
21 g fat
(5 g saturated)
1,940 mg sodium

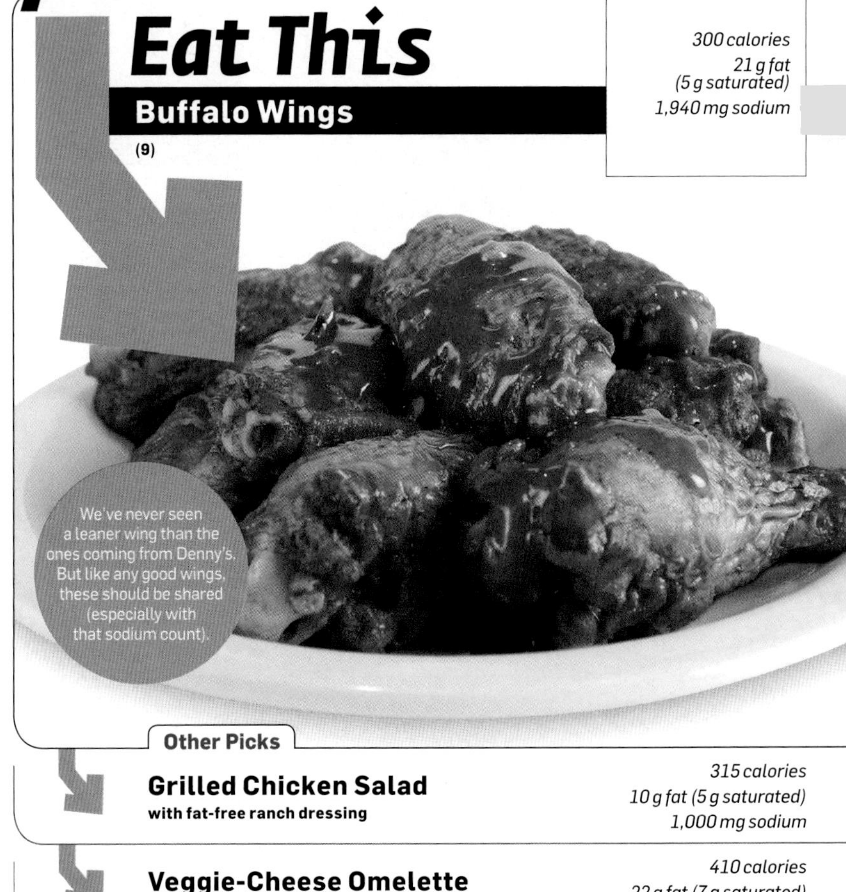

We've never seen a leaner wing than the ones coming from Denny's. But like any good wings, these should be shared (especially with that sodium count).

Other Picks

Grilled Chicken Salad
with fat-free ranch dressing

315 calories
10 g fat (5 g saturated)
1,000 mg sodium

Veggie-Cheese Omelette
made with Egg Beaters

410 calories
22 g fat (7 g saturated)
1,100 mg sodium

Cheesecake
no sugar added

290 calories
23 g fat (14 g saturated)
2 g sugars

Not That!

Buffalo Chicken Strips

(5)

730 calories
32 g fat
(0 g saturated)
2,940 mg sodium

Another example of how 2 seemingly similar items can be worlds apart in terms of nutrition. We've seen worse strips, to be sure, but when you can have a basket of wings for fewer than half the calories, why would you choose these?

WEAPON OF MASS DESTRUCTION
Potachos

1,460 calories
110 g fat (53 g saturated, 1.5 g trans)
2,700 mg sodium

This freakish Frankenfood turns two of the most troublesome appetizers—potato skins and nachos—into one of the worst starters in America. Divide them by 4 and each person will still be taking in more than a dozen bacon strips' worth of saturated fat.

Other Passes

Grilled Chicken Sandwich
with honey mustard dressing

970 calories
58 g fat (10 g saturated)
2,070 mg sodium

Heartland Scramble

1,150 calories
66 g fat (20 g saturated, 0.5 g trans)
2,800 mg sodium

French Silk Pie

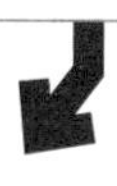

770 calories
57 g fat (30 g saturated, 1.5 g trans)
38 g sugars

SMART SIDES

Denny's side options range from 10 calories (tomato slices) to 520 calories (onion rings), so your choices here can make or break your dinner. The best combo is mixed veggies and cottage cheese, which will limit your calorie intake and offer both protein and fiber, which sure beats the blood-sugar spiking effects of a basket of fries or a scoop of mashed potatoes would. Shrimp skewers and cinnamon apples also do the trick.

Domino's Pizza

B The Bad News Pies on Domino's menu are the same as those at any other pizza purveyor: Think oversize crusts, fatty meats, and greasy shag carpets of cheese. But Domino's Crunchy Thin Crust cheese pizza is one of the lowest-calorie pies in America, which makes it a sound foundation for a decent dinner. Just avoid the breadsticks and Domino's appalling line of pasta bread bowls and oven-baked sandwiches.

SURVIVAL STRATEGY
Domino's thin crust has fewer calories than any other national pizza chain's. Show your apprecia-tion by making it your go-to order. Want toppings? Stick to ham and pineapple or just veggies.

Eat This

Ham, Mushroom, Green Pepper, and Onion Pizza

(2 slices; large, thin crust)

396 calories
20 g fat (7 g saturated)
820 mg sodium

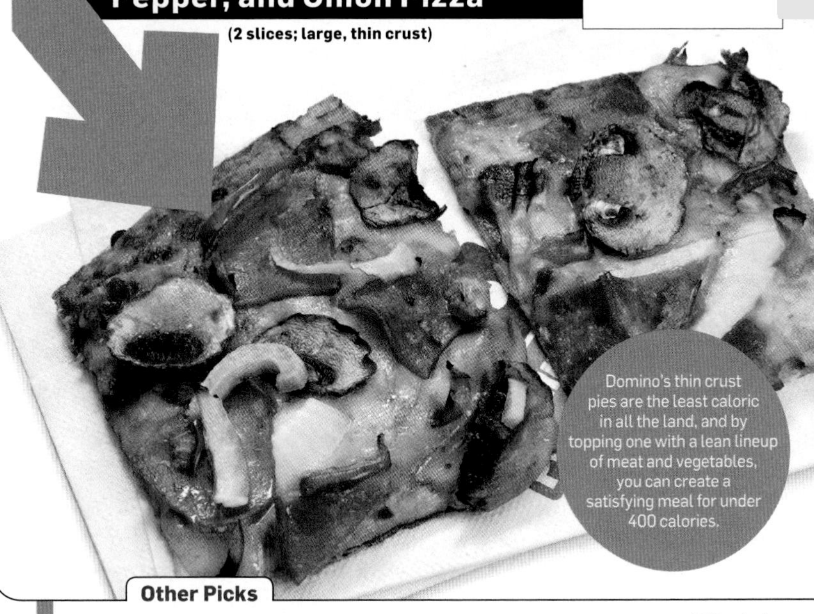

Domino's thin crust pies are the least caloric in all the land, and by topping one with a lean lineup of meat and vegetables, you can create a satisfying meal for under 400 calories.

Other Picks

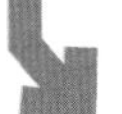

Deluxe Feast Pizza
(2 slices; medium, hand-tossed crust)

452 calories
19 g fat (7 g saturated)
1,010 mg sodium

Buffalo Chicken Kickers
(6 pieces)

300 calories
13.5 g fat (1.5 g saturated)
840 mg sodium

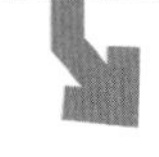

Garden Fresh Salad
with light Italian dressing (1/2 salad)

90 calories
5 g fat (2.5 g saturated)
860 mg sodium

594 calories
25 g fat (9 g saturated)
1,360 mg sodium

Not That!

Pepperoni Pizza

(2 slices; large, hand-tossed crust)

Pepperoni slices are like miniature disks of obesity. With a few exceptions, keep them off your pizza.

Other Passes

620 calories
35 g fat (12 g saturated)
1,250 mg sodium

Cali Chicken Bacon Ranch Pizza
(2 slices; medium, hand-tossed crust)

690 calories
42 g fat (10.5 g saturated)
1,230 mg sodium

Barbeque Buffalo Wings
(6 pieces)

355 calories
28.5 g fat (5.5 g saturated)
890 mg sodium

Grilled Chicken Caesar Salad
with croutons and creamy Caesar dressing (1/2 salad)

STEALTH HEALTH FOOD
Anchovies

The much maligned anchovy is one of the greatest source of lean protein and omega-3s in the animal kingdom. Can't stomach the thought of them on your pizza? Order them with onions and jalapeños, which will pair well with their intense flavor.

BAD BREEDS
Oven-Baked Sandwiches

Bet you never thought we'd tell you it's better to eat pizza than sandwiches—well, that's the case at Domino's. Their leanest oven-baked sandwich clocks in at a whopping 690 calories (the worst, the Chicken Bacon Ranch, contains 890 calories), and all contain 1 gram of trans fat.

61

The number of ingredients in Domino's Cheesy Bread.

Dunkin' Donuts

B- The Dunkin' camp has made major improvements in recent years. The doughnut king cast out the trans fat in 2007, and they've been pushing the menu toward healthier options ever since—including the DDSmart Menu, which emphasizes the menu's nutritional champions and introduces the low-fat and protein-packed flatbread sandwiches. Now there's no excuse to settle for bagels, muffins, or doughnuts, which are as bad as ever.

SURVIVAL STRATEGY
Use the DDSmart Menu as a starting point, then stick to the sandwiches served on flatbread or English muffins. If you must order doughnuts, always opt for yeast donuts over their cakey counterparts.

Eat This

Bacon, Egg, and Cheese

on an english muffin

360 calories
16 g fat (6 g saturated)
920 mg sodium
35 g carbohydrates

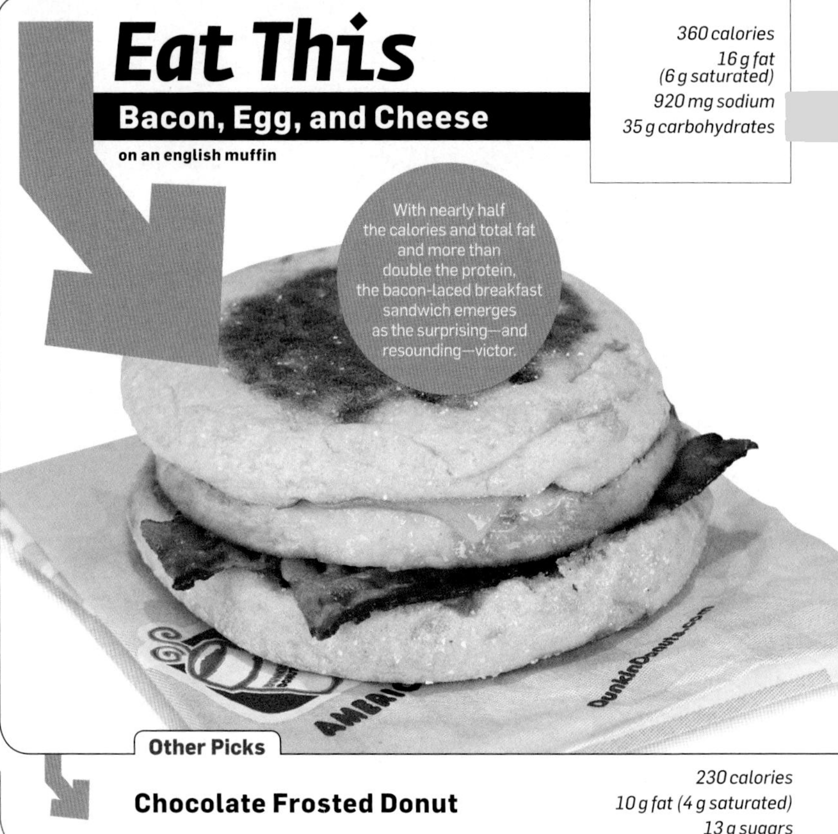

With nearly half the calories and total fat and more than double the protein, the bacon-laced breakfast sandwich emerges as the surprising—and resounding—victor.

Other Picks

Chocolate Frosted Donut
230 calories
10 g fat (4 g saturated)
13 g sugars

Turkey, Cheddar & Bacon Flatbread
420 calories
17 g fat (7 g saturated)
1,270 mg sodium

Cappuccino (small)
80 calories
4 g fat (2.5 g saturated)
7 g sugars

650 calories
29 g fat (5 g saturated)
520 mg sodium
91 g carbohydrates

Not That!

Pumpkin Muffin

Despite the healthy-sounding names—banana-walnut, blueberry, cran-orange—muffins are little more than glorified cake. Case in point: This one has more sugar than 3 ice cream sandwiches.

Other Passes

460 calories
14 g fat (8 g saturated)
49 g sugars

Apple Crumb Donut

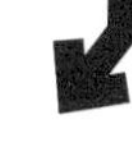

770 calories
30 g fat (7 g saturated)
1,560 mg sodium

Tuna Melt Sandwich

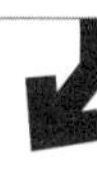

230 calories
11 g fat (9 g saturated)
24 g sugars

Dunkaccino (small)

WEAPON OF MASS DESTRUCTION
Vanilla Bean Coolatta (large)

860 calories
11 g fat (7 g saturated)
172 g sugars

This ranks up there among the very worst of the liquid-calorie offenders. Sip this and you'll be slurping up 6 Snickers bars' worth of sugar through a straw.

BAD BREEDS

Cake Donuts

Cake doughnuts are made without yeast, so they end up as dense as the most decadent pastries and levy a significantly heftier caloric toll than yeast doughnuts. A glazed cake doughnut, for example, has 100 more calories than a regular glazed does.

536

The average number of calories in a muffin from Dunkin' Donuts.

Five Guys

C

Without much more than burgers, hot dogs, and French fries on the menu, it's difficult to find anything nutritionally redeeming about Five Guys. The only option geared toward health-conscious consumers is the Veggie Sandwich. The burgers range from 480 to 920 calories, so how you order can make a big difference to your waistline. Keep your burgers small, choose your topping wisely, and skip the fries.

SURVIVAL STRATEGY

The regular hamburger is actually a double, so order a Little Hamburger and load up on the vegetation. And if you must indulge somewhere, don't do it with the fries—the smallest order will set you back 620 calories.

Eat This

Little Cheeseburger

with lettuce, tomato, and onion

573 calories
32 g fat (15 g saturated)
677 mg sodium

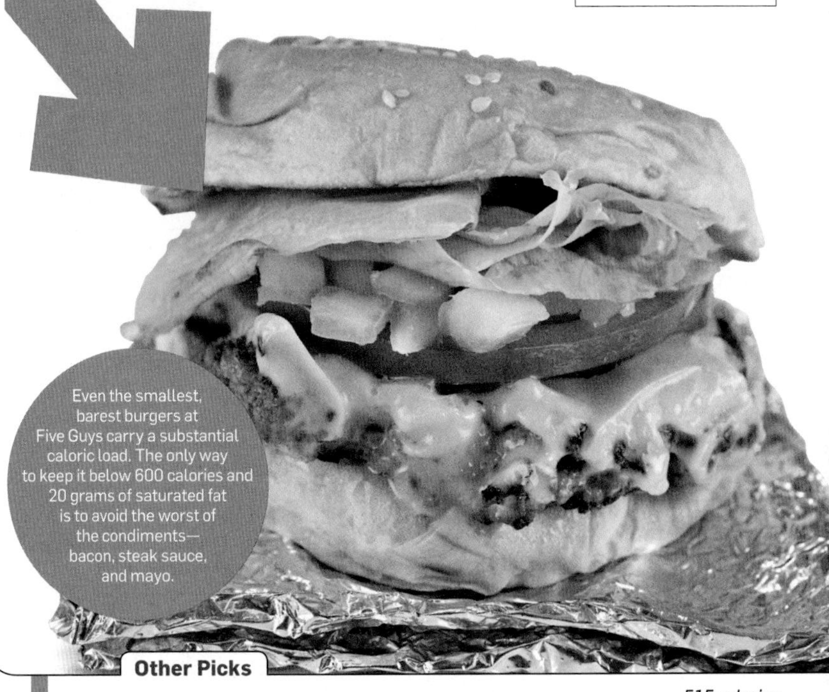

Even the smallest, barest burgers at Five Guys carry a substantial caloric load. The only way to keep it below 600 calories and 20 grams of saturated fat is to avoid the worst of the condiments—bacon, steak sauce, and mayo.

Other Picks

Little Hamburger
with mushrooms, grilled onions, and A1 Steak Sauce

515 calories
26 g fat (11.5 g saturated)
761 mg sodium

BLT
4 slices of bacon, lettuce, tomato, and mustard

434 calories
23 g fat (9 g saturated)
915 mg sodium

615 calories
41 g fat
(19 g saturated)
1,440 mg sodium

Not That!

Cheese Dog

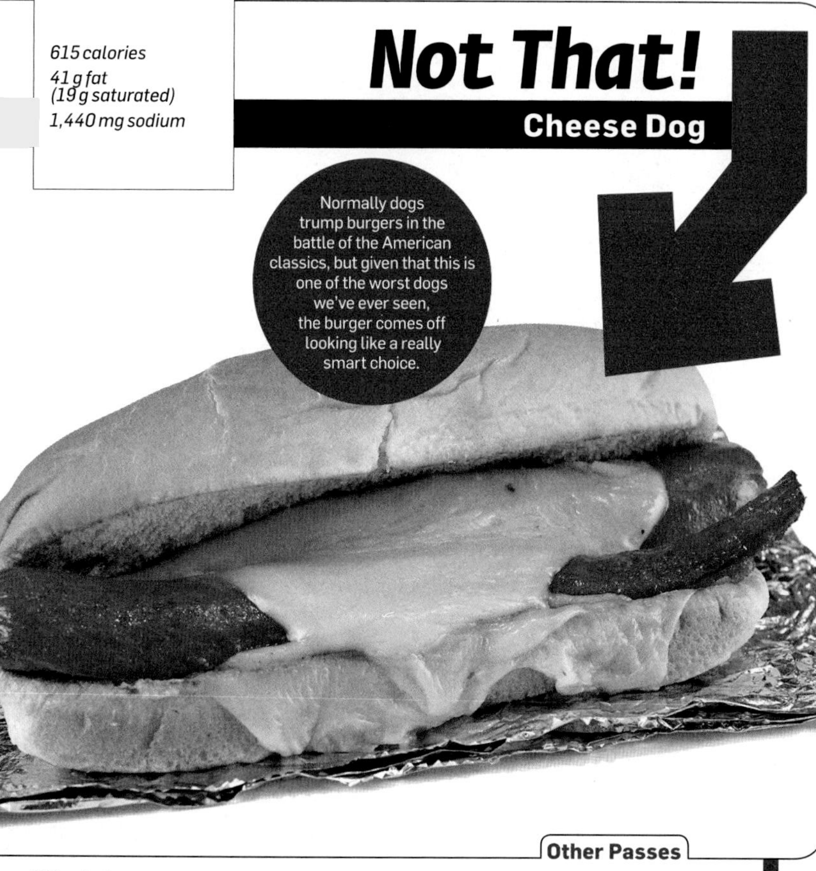

Normally dogs trump burgers in the battle of the American classics, but given that this is one of the worst dogs we've ever seen, the burger comes off looking like a really smart choice.

Other Passes

Cheeseburger with ketchup

855 calories
55 g fat (26.5 g saturated)
1,240 mg sodium

Hamburger

700 calories
43 g fat (19.5 g saturated)
430 mg sodium

SAUCE SELECTOR
(per Tbsp)

MUSTARD
0 calories, 0 g fat,
55 mg sodium

KETCHUP
15 calories, 0 g fat,
190 mg sodium

A1 STEAK SAUCE
15 calories, 0 g fat,
280 mg sodium

BBQ SAUCE
60 calories, 0 g fat,
400 mg sodium

MAYONNAISE
100 calories,
11 g fat (2 g saturated),
75 mg sodium

GUILTY PLEASURE

Little Bacon Burger

560 calories
33 g fat (14.5 g saturated)
640 mg sodium

Sometimes you just want bacon on your burger. For those moments, turn to this reasonable rendition.

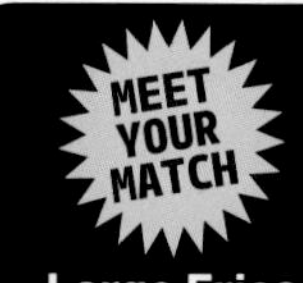

Large Fries
(1,464 calories)
=
42 chicken wings
from Denny's

Hardee's

C- A 1997 purchase by CKE Restaurants put Hardee's under the same parent company as Carl's Jr., and the adopted brothers are slowly coming to look like identical twins. Hardee's penchant for oversize eats plays out most potently in the line of Monster Thick-burgers. But while the Hardee's menu tips toward the heavy side, it also serves up a few more modest choices, which helps it earn a slightly less dismal grade than its big brother.

SURVIVAL STRATEGY
Choose a breakfast sandwich topped with ham or jelly, and avoid anything served in a bowl or on a platter. For lunch, stick to single-patty burgers or go for the roast beef or BBQ Chicken Sandwich.

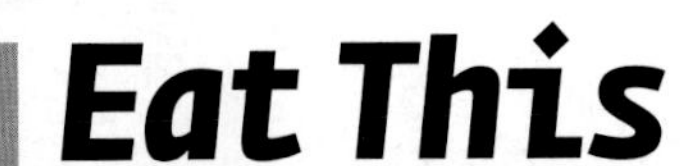

Eat This

Double Cheeseburger

510 calories
26 g fat
(5 g saturated)
1,120 mg sodium

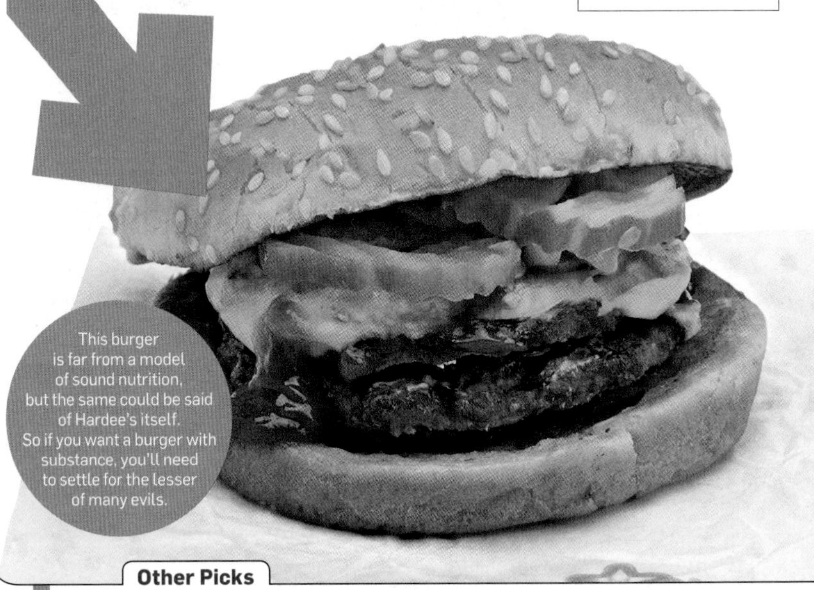

This burger is far from a model of sound nutrition, but the same could be said of Hardee's itself. So if you want a burger with substance, you'll need to settle for the lesser of many evils.

Other Picks

BBQ Chicken Sandwich
320 calories
6 g fat (1 g saturated)
1,200 mg sodium

Frisco Breakfast Sandwich
420 calories
20 g fat (7 g saturated)
1,340 mg sodium

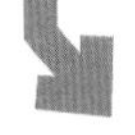

Mashed Potatoes
90 calories
15 g fat (2 g saturated)
410 mg sodium

910 calories
64 g fat
(21 g saturated)
1,560 mg sodium

Not That!

Original Thickburger

(1/3 lb)

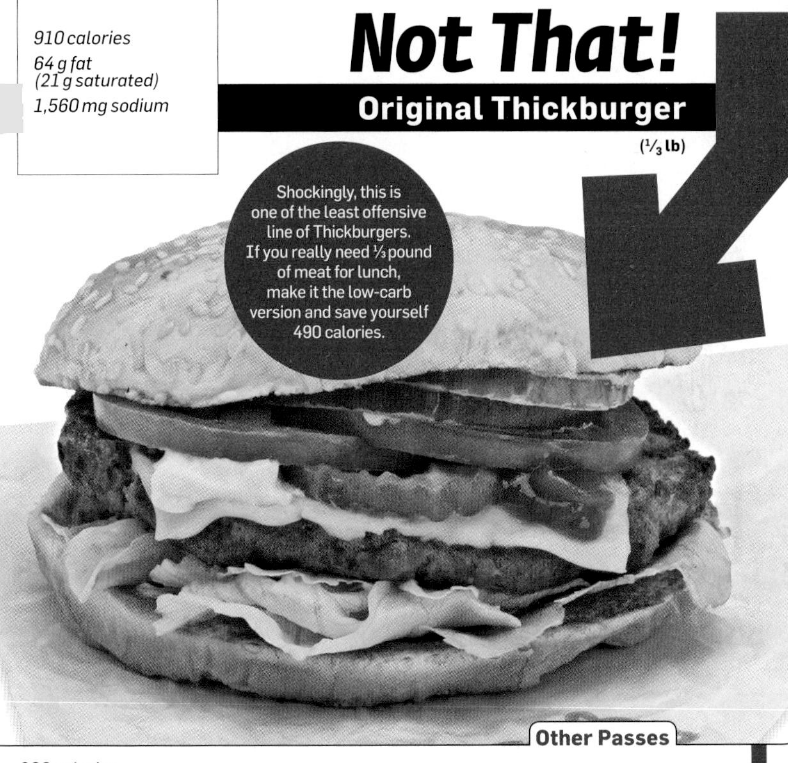

Shockingly, this is one of the least offensive line of Thickburgers. If you really need ⅓ pound of meat for lunch, make it the low-carb version and save yourself 490 calories.

Other Passes

800 calories
37 g fat (6 g saturated)
1,890 mg sodium

Big Chicken Fillet Sandwich

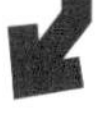

620 calories
50 g fat (21 g saturated)
1,380 mg sodium

Low-Carb Breakfast Bowl

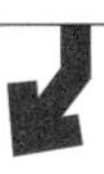

430 calories
19 g fat (4 g saturated)
960 mg sodium

Natural-Cut French Fries
(medium)

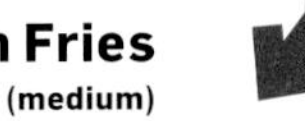

WEAPON OF MASS DESTRUCTION
Monster Thickburger
(2/3 lb)

1,420 calories
108 g fat
(43 g saturated)
2,770 mg sodium

The burger industry feels more like a nuclear arms race, with fast-food joints and sit-down restaurants constantly trying to one-up each other with their diet-destroying arsenals. If that's the case, then this absurdly oversize behemoth is the fast-food equivalent of the A-bomb, ready to lay waste to any shred of health consciousness that gets in its path.

STEALTH HEALTH FOOD
Cole slaw

170 calories
10 g fat (2 g saturated)
140 mg sodium

Okay, it would be better if it weren't robed in mayo, but cabbage contains a big dose of sulforaphane, a chemical shown to boost your body's production of enzymes that fend off cancer. So it earns your occasional affection.

IHOP

F

We knew IHOP was up to no good when it refused to reveal its nutritional information back when we first asked in 2007. But we were shocked when a New York City law forced them to post calorie counts: 1,000-calorie crepes, 1,200-calorie breakfast combos, and 1,700-calorie burgers. The F is for its closed-door policy, but IHOP might not score much better even if we ran the numbers.

SURVIVAL STRATEGY

You'll have a hard time finding a regular breakfast with fewer than 700 calories and a lunch or dinner with fewer than 1,000 calories. Your only safe bet is to stick to the IHOP for Me menu, where you'll find the nutritional content for a small selection of healthier items.

Eat This

Belgian Waffle

with Cool Strawberry and Grilled Ham

*650 calories**

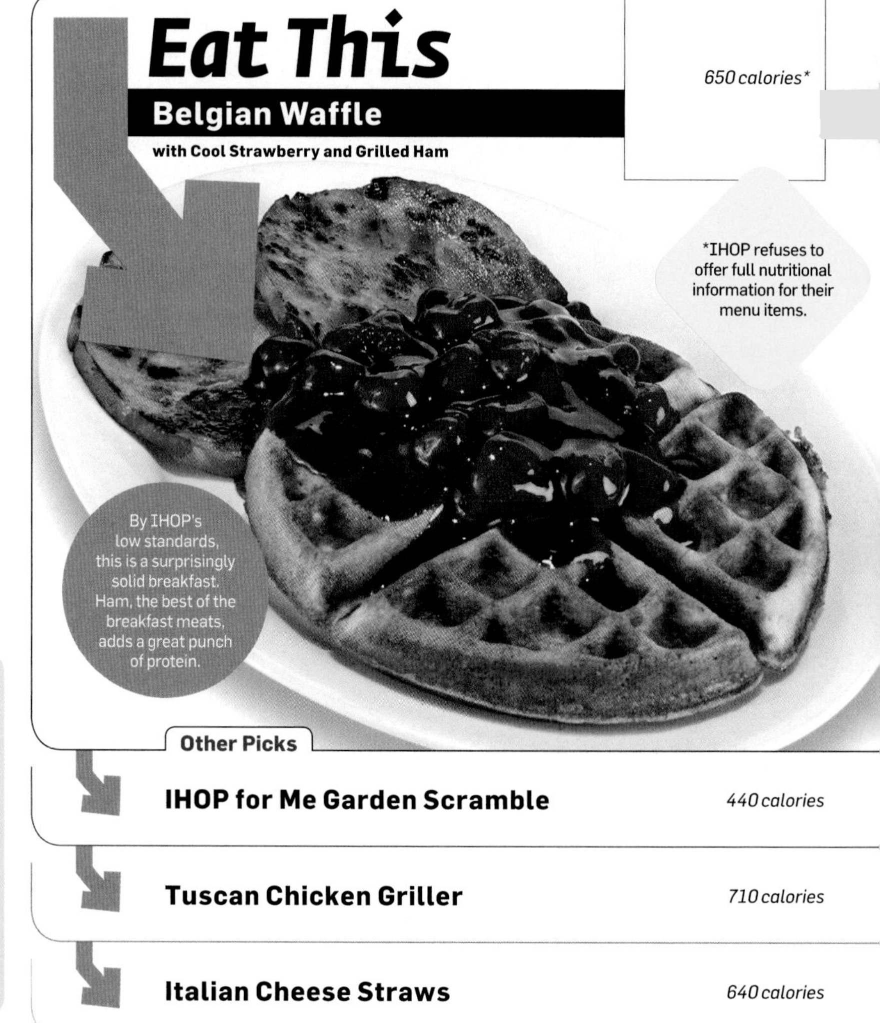

By IHOP's low standards, this is a surprisingly solid breakfast. Ham, the best of the breakfast meats, adds a great punch of protein.

*IHOP refuses to offer full nutritional information for their menu items.

Other Picks

IHOP for Me Garden Scramble	*440 calories*
Tuscan Chicken Griller	*710 calories*
Italian Cheese Straws	*640 calories*

*870 calories**

Not That!

Harvest Grain 'N Nut

with Warm Blueberry Compote

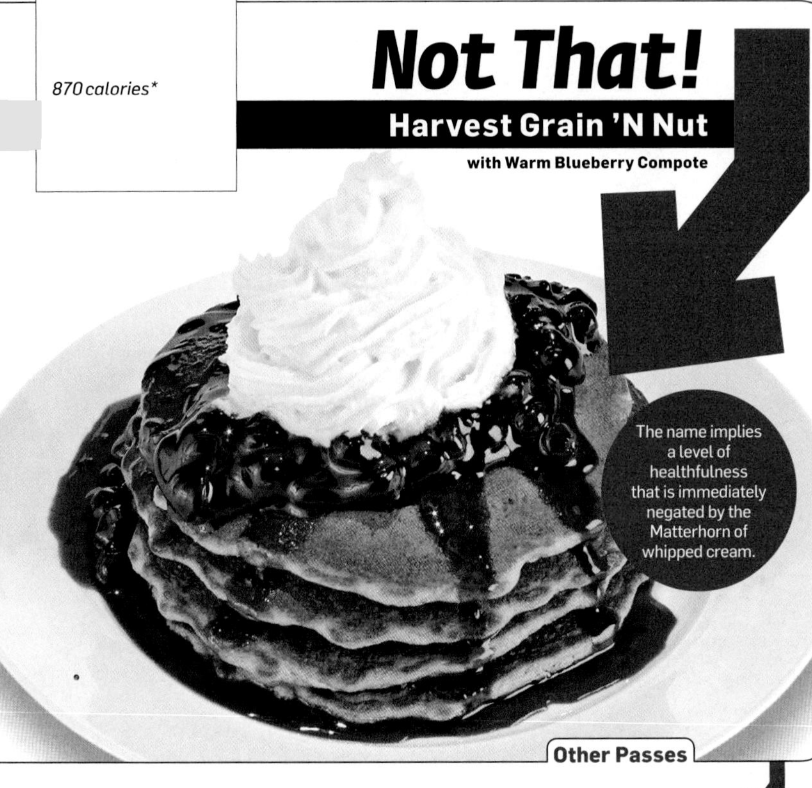

The name implies a level of healthfulness that is immediately negated by the Matterhorn of whipped cream.

Other Passes

1,210 calories **Spinach and Mushroom Omelette**

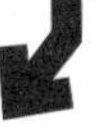

1,600 calories **Chicken, Spinach, and Apple Salad**

940 calories **Onion Rings**

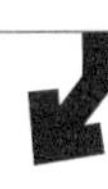

WEAPON OF MASS DESTRUCTION

Crispy Chicken Strips

1,850 calories

There's nary a menu in America that doesn't offer up this popular dish, but IHOP's rendition qualifies as one of the world's worst chicken dishes.

GUILTY PLEASURE

Crispy Banana Caramel Cheesecake

530 calories

The most decadent-sounding item on the entire IHOP menu just happens to have 700 fewer calories than the *average* entrée-size salad here. In fact, you might be better off going straight to dessert.

BAD BREED

Omelets

We've never seen a line of egg dishes as thoroughly appalling as the bomblets offered up by this pancake pusher. The "lightest" of the bunch, the Garden Omelette, packs 1,150 calories.

In-N-Out Burger

C+ In-N-Out has the most pared down menu in America. Wander in and you'll find nothing more than burgers, fries, shakes, and sodas. While that's certainly nothing to build a healthy diet on, In-N-Out earns points for offering plenty of calorie-saving menu tweaks, like the Protein-Style Burger, which replaces the bun with lettuce and saves you 150 calories.

SURVIVAL STRATEGY

A single cheeseburger and a glass of iced tea or H_2O make for a reasonable lunch, while the formidable Double-Double should be reserved for an occasional splurge (especially if you use a few of the calorie-lowering secret menu options). But flirt with the fries or the milk shake at your own peril.

Eat This

Double-Double

with grilled onion, ketchup, and mustard

590 calories
32 g fat (17 g saturated)
1,520 mg sodium

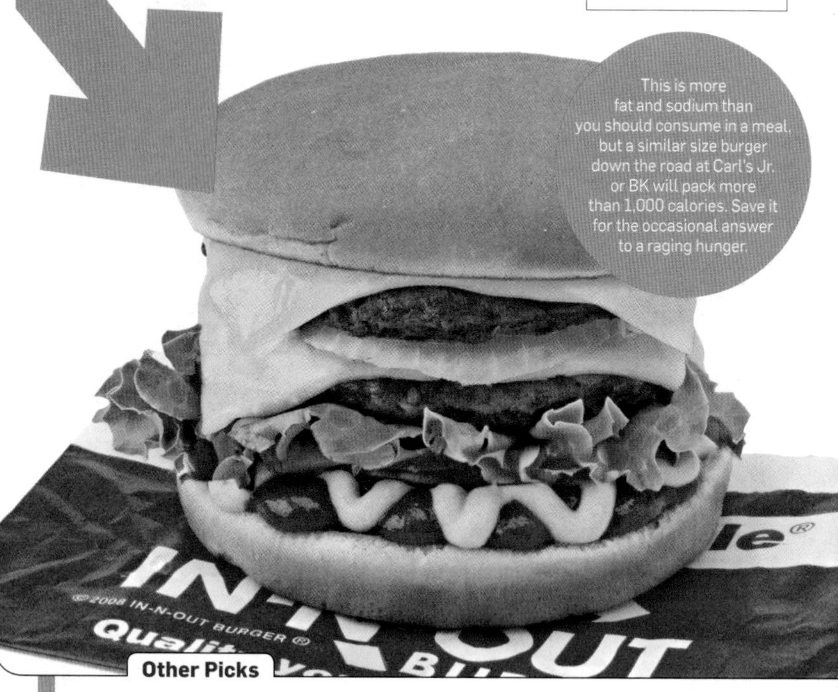

This is more fat and sodium than you should consume in a meal, but a similar size burger down the road at Carl's Jr. or BK will pack more than 1,000 calories. Save it for the occasional answer to a raging hunger.

Other Picks

Hamburger

with grilled onion, ketchup, and mustard

310 calories
10 g fat (4 g saturated)
730 mg sodium

Tea-Ade

(half lemonade, half iced tea, 16 oz)

90 calories
0 g fat
19 g sugars

880 calories
45 g fat (15 g saturated)
1,245 mg sodium

Not That!

Cheeseburger with Fries

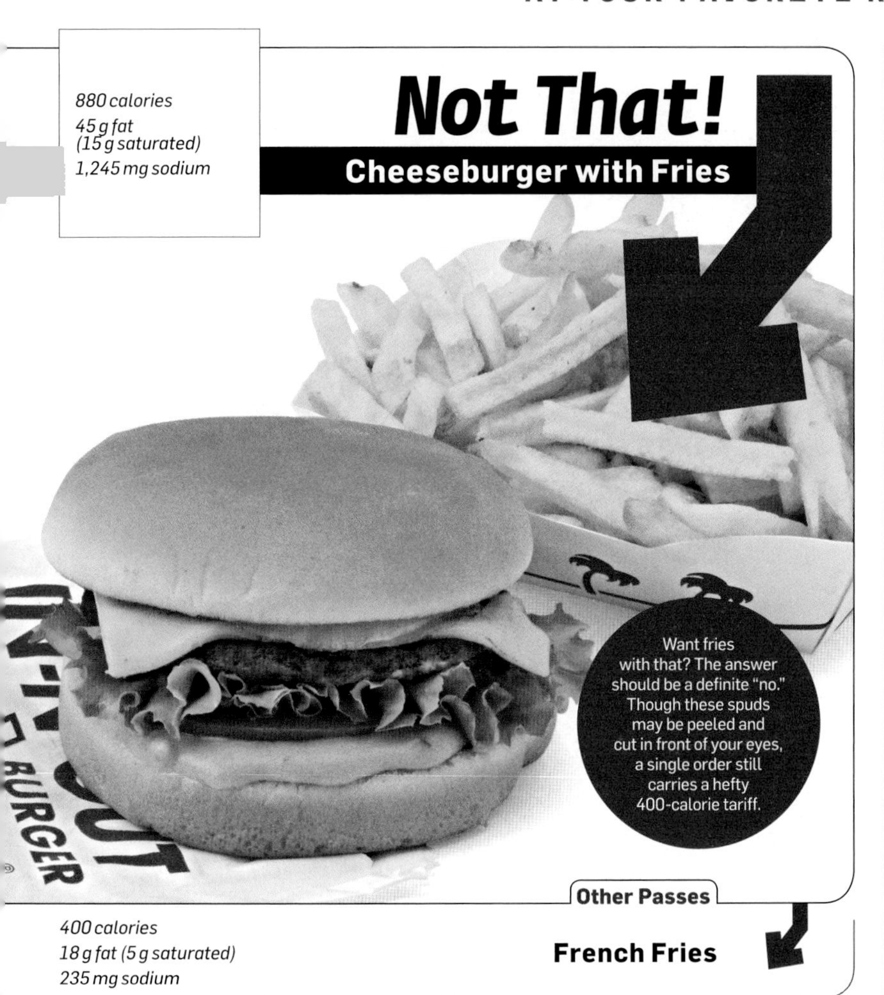

Want fries with that? The answer should be a definite "no." Though these spuds may be peeled and cut in front of your eyes, a single order still carries a hefty 400-calorie tariff.

Other Passes

400 calories
18 g fat (5 g saturated)
235 mg sodium

French Fries

198 calories
0 g fat
54 g sugars

Coca-Cola Classic (16 oz)

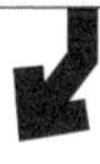

(SECRET) MENU DECODER

These are the most popular of In-N-Outs many off-menu items.

- **FLYING DUTCHMAN:** Beef patty (or patties) with double cheese served with no vegetables or bun.
- **VEGGIE BURGER:** All the veggie toppings on a bun, without meat or cheese.
- **A X B:** As many beef patties (A) with as many cheese slices (B) as you want.
- **ANIMAL STYLE:** Mustard-slathered patty, topped with grilled onions, plus extra pickles and secret sauce. Also offered on fries.
- **PROTEIN STYLE:** A regular burger wrapped in lettuce, instead of on a bun.
- **WELL-DONE FRIES:** Fries cooked for an extra minute for extra crispiness.

Jack in the Box

D+ This menu has plenty of suitable options, but where it fails, it fails in dangerous ways. At least half a dozen burgers surpass the horrifying 900-calorie mark, and everything that touches Jack's fryer emerges with a soggy load of trans fat. Until Jack follows the lead set by nearly every other restaurant in America and disposes of the trans fat, consumers need to be very careful about investing any cash (or calories) at this West Coast joint.

SURVIVAL STRATEGY

Keep your burger small, or order a Whole Grain Chicken Fajita Pita with a fruit cup on the side. For breakfast, order any Breakfast Jack without sausage. Whatever you do, don't touch the fried foods.

Eat This

Bacon Breakfast Jack

300 calories
14 g fat
(5 g saturated)
730 mg sodium

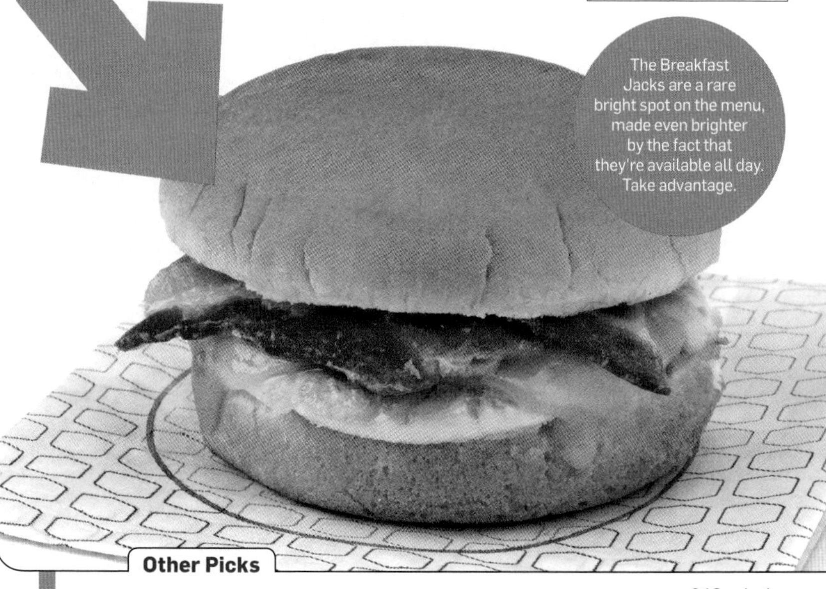

The Breakfast Jacks are a rare bright spot on the menu, made even brighter by the fact that they're available all day. Take advantage.

Other Picks

Hamburger Deluxe

340 calories
18 g fat (16 g saturated, 1 g trans)
550 mg sodium

Southwest Chicken Salad
with grilled chicken strips and low-fat balsamic vinaigrette

345 calories
13.5 g fat (5 g saturated)
1,300 mg sodium

Chocolate Overload Cake

300 calories
7 g fat (1.5 g saturated)
34 g sugars

580 calories
39 g fat
(13 g saturated, 4 g trans)
770 mg sodium

Not That!

Sausage Croissant

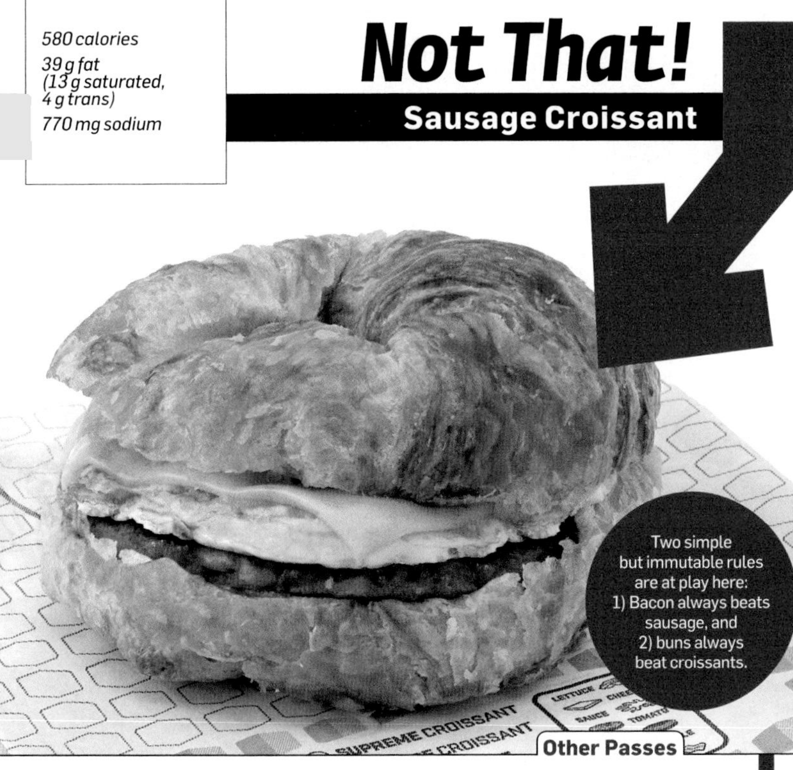

Two simple but immutable rules are at play here: 1) Bacon always beats sausage, and 2) buns always beat croissants.

Other Passes

950 calories
60 g fat (19 g saturated, 2 g trans)
1,920 mg sodium

Sirloin Cheeseburger

740 calories
53 g fat (14 g saturated, 4 g trans)
1,750 mg sodium

Chicken Club Salad
with crispy chicken strips and bacon ranch dressing

750 calories
36 g fat (24 g saturated, 1.5 g trans)
84 g sugars

Chocolate Ice Cream Shake
(16 oz)

WEAPON OF MASS DESTRUCTION
Bacon and Cheddar Wedges

13 g trans fat

While the rest of the restaurant world sheds their partially hydrogenated ways, Jack clings stubbornly to the use of cholesterol-spiking fats in all but 10 food items on their menu. These wedges, containing nearly seven times the amount of trans fat the American Heart Association deems safe for daily consumption, are the worst on the menu and the worst in the country.

GUILTY PLEASURE

Regular Beef Taco

160 calories
8 g fat
(3 g saturated, 1 g trans)
270 mg sodium

Many a late-night munchie-driven diner has professed a love for the ultracheap tacos at Jack's. We're here to tell you that if you end up with 1 or 2 of these instead of a burger, a chicken sandwich, or anything from the fryer, you've done yourself a favor.

Jamba Juice

A-

There's no doubt that smoothies can be part of a healthy diet, but there's an erroneous halo of health that seems to hang over all things smoothie-related. Make this your rule: If it includes added sugar, it ceases to be a smoothie. Jamba Juice makes more than a few faux-fruit blends, but their menu has a ton of real-deal smoothies, as well. Just as exciting is Jamba's new line of satisfying, low-calorie eats.

SURVIVAL STRATEGY
For a perfectly guilt-free treat, opt for a Jamba Light or an All Fruit Smoothie in a 16-ounce cup. And unless you're looking to put on weight for your latest movie role, don't touch the Peanut Butter Moo'd or any of the other Creamy Treats.

Eat This

Fresh Banana Oatmeal

(oatmeal, bananas, brown sugar crumble)

370 calories
5 g fat
(1 g saturated)
41 g sugars

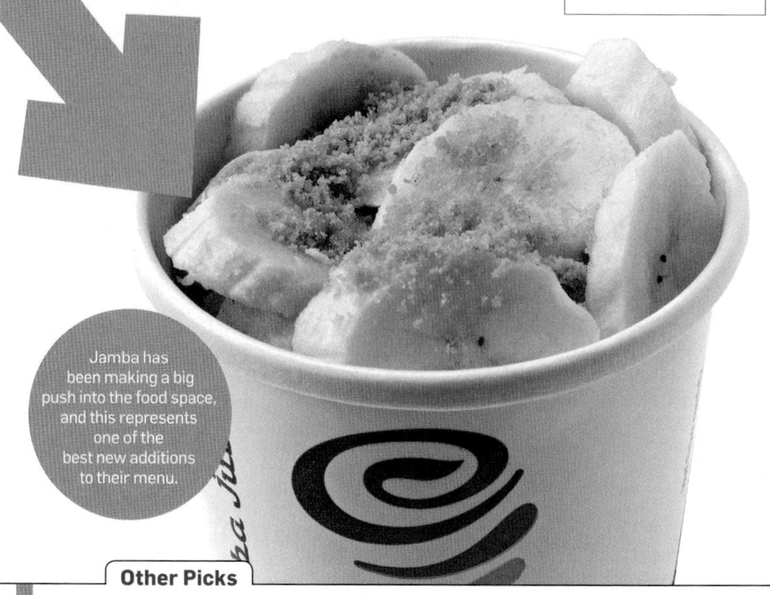

Jamba has been making a big push into the food space, and this represents one of the best new additions to their menu.

Other Picks

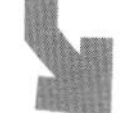

Strawberry Nirvana
(24 oz)

290 calories
1 g fat
54 g sugars

Peach Perfection
(24 oz)

340 calories
0.5 g fat
67 g sugars

Omega-3 Oatmeal Cookie

150 calories
6 g fat (1.5 g saturated)
15 g sugars

590 calories
18 g fat (3 g saturated)
55 g sugars

Not That!

Ideal Meal Chunky Strawberry

(16 oz)

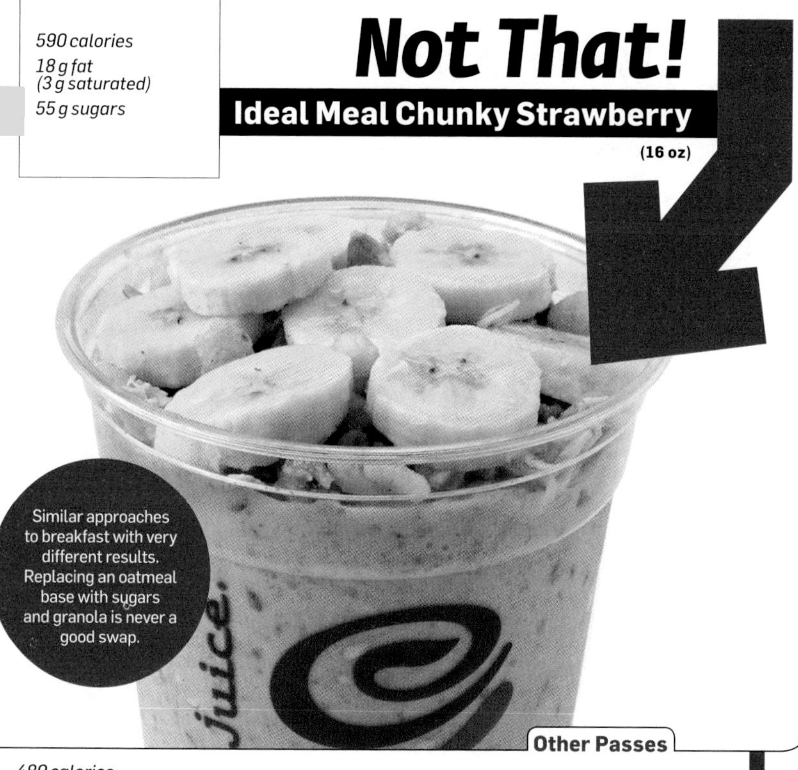

Similar approaches to breakfast with very different results. Replacing an oatmeal base with sugars and granola is never a good swap.

Other Passes

480 calories
1.5 g fat
105 g sugars

Strawberry Surf Rider
(24 oz)

450 calories
1 g fat
95 g sugars

Pomegranate Heart Happy
(24 oz)

310 calories
9 g fat (2 g saturated)
31 g sugars

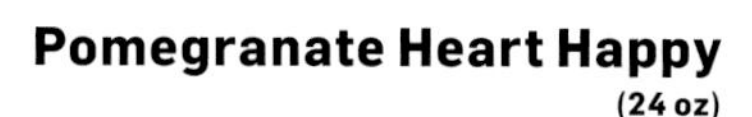

Reduced-Fat Cranberry Orange Loaf

STEALTH HEALTH FOOD

MediterraneYUM California Flatbread

250 calories
8 g fat (2.5 g saturated)
620 mg sodium

Jamba's new flatbreads all hover around 300 calories, which is just enough to turn a small smoothie into a great full meal. Plus, unlike so many flatbreads, these are actually healthy. They rely on flaxseed and olive oil to provide a tidy dose of healthy fats.

BAD BREED

Jamba Classics

Call us old-fashioned, but we just can't get behind a beverage that is made from anything but fruit. That's just what you'll find in Jamba's "classic" options, though—milk shakes in disguise.

9

Percentage of Americans who eat their daily recommended servings of fruits and vegetables.

KFC

B+ Hold on a second! KFC gets a B+? Surprisingly enough, KFC has more than a few things going for it. The menu's crispy bird bits are offset by skinless chicken pieces, low-calorie sandwich options, and a host of sides that come from beyond the fryer. Plus, they recently introduced grilled chicken to the menu, which shows that they're determined to cast aside the Kentucky fried nutritional demons of their past.

SURVIVAL STRATEGY
Go the skinless route, the new grilled route, or pal up with a Chicken Stacker or a Toasted Sandwich. Then adorn your plate with one of the Colonel's healthy sides. If you want fried chicken, make sure you order the strips.

Eat This

KFC Grilled Chicken Breast

and Drumstick and Mashed Potatoes with Gravy

380 calories
12.5 g fat (3 g saturated)
1,190 mg sodium

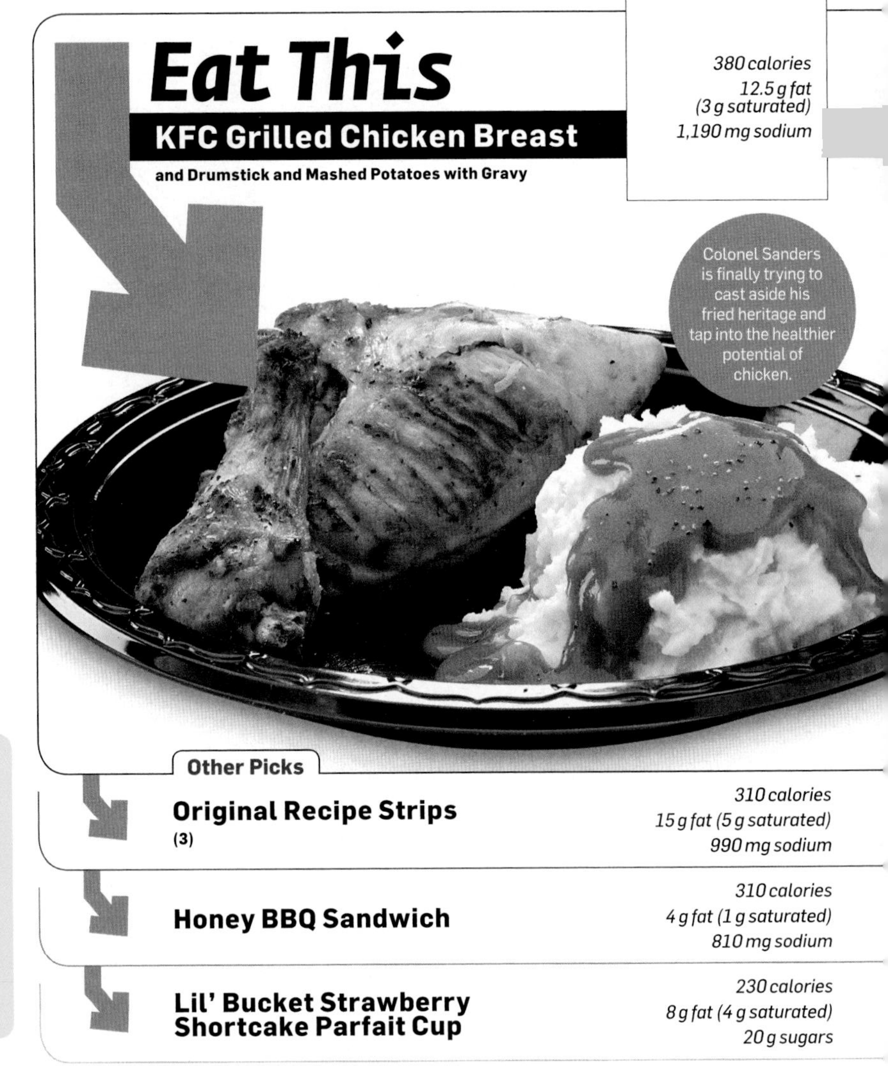

Colonel Sanders is finally trying to cast aside his fried heritage and tap into the healthier potential of chicken.

Other Picks

Original Recipe Strips (3)
310 calories
15 g fat (5 g saturated)
990 mg sodium

Honey BBQ Sandwich
310 calories
4 g fat (1 g saturated)
810 mg sodium

Lil' Bucket Strawberry Shortcake Parfait Cup
230 calories
8 g fat (4 g saturated)
20 g sugars

490 calories
31 g fat
(7 g saturated)
1,080 mg sodium

Not That!

Extra Crispy Chicken Breast

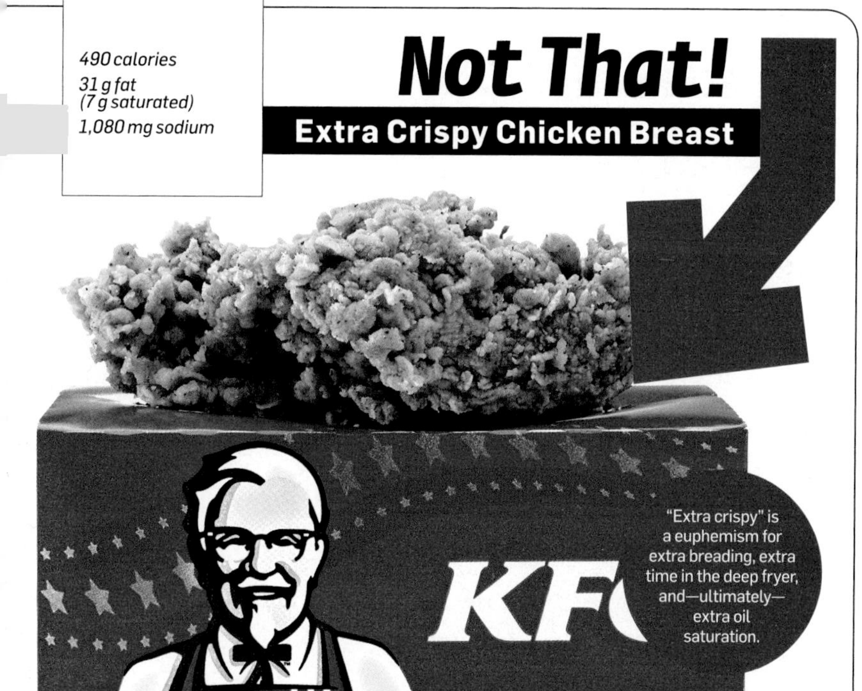

"Extra crispy" is a euphemism for extra breading, extra time in the deep fryer, and—ultimately—extra oil saturation.

Other Passes

400 calories
26 g fat (4.5 g saturated)
1,160 mg sodium

Popcorn Chicken (individual)

580 calories
30 g fat (7 g saturated)
1,250 mg sodium

Crispy Twister with Crispy Strip

390 calories
14 g fat (8 g saturated)
47 g sugars

Lil' Bucket Lemon Crème Parfait Cup

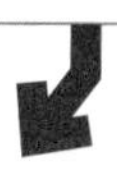

WEAPON OF MASS DESTRUCTION
KFC Famous Bowls—Rice and Gravy

790 calories
28 g fat (7 g saturated, 1 g trans)
2,690 mg sodium
106 g carbohydrates

With more sodium than you should consume in a day, this bowl is the single worst item on the KFC menu. Whether it's Taco Bell's Border Bowls or P.F. Chang's Lunch Bowls, foods served up in deep plastic shells are usually nutritional nightmares.

SMART SIDES

One of the best items on KFC's menu? Surprise: It's mashed potatoes and gravy, at just 130 calories and 4.5 grams of fat. In fact, sides are the best part of KFC's menu.

YOUR BEST BETS:
Green Beans: 25 calories, 0 g fat
Corn on the Cob, 3-inch: 70 calories, 0.5 g fat
KFC Mean Greens: 30 calories, 0 g fat
House Side Salad with Light Italian Dressing: 45 calories, 0 g fat
Three-Bean Salad: 70 calories, 0 g fat

Krispy Kreme

C-

While Dunkin' Donuts expands its menu to include more legitimate options, Krispy Kreme is stuck in the carb-heavy world of glazed, powdered, and jelly-filled doughnuts. Their one expansion move was to introduce Chillers, frozen beverages that can pack more than 1,000 calories into a 20-ounce cup. The good news is that Krispy Kreme has finally cut trans fat from its doughnuts. The bad news is that a single doughnut can still carry half a day's saturated fat.

SURVIVAL STRATEGY

To stay under 500 calories, you'll need to cap your sweet tooth at one filled or specialty doughnut or, worst-case scenario, two original glazed doughnuts.

Eat This

Sugar Doughnut

200 calories
12 g fat (6 g saturated)
10 g sugars

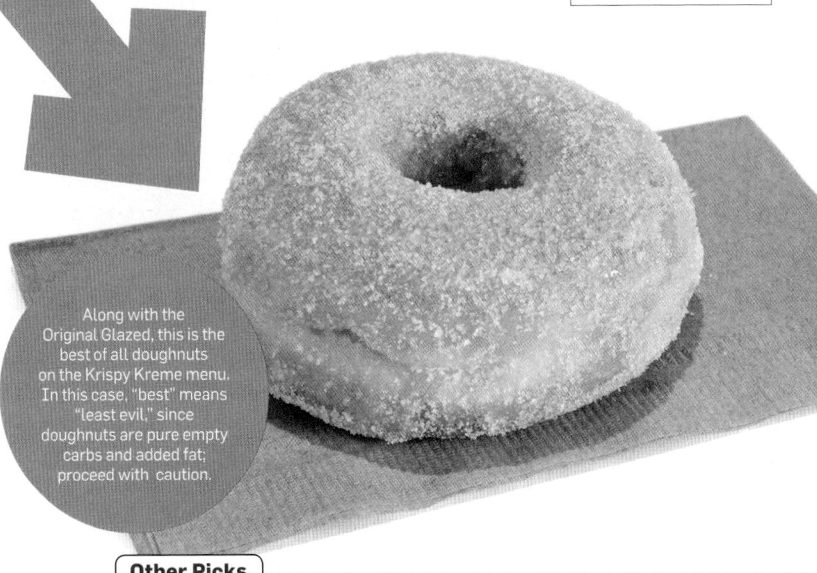

Along with the Original Glazed, this is the best of all doughnuts on the Krispy Kreme menu. In this case, "best" means "least evil," since doughnuts are pure empty carbs and added fat; proceed with caution.

Other Picks

Original Glazed Doughnut
200 calories
12 g fat (6 g saturated)
10 g sugars

Very Berry Chiller (12 oz)
170 calories
0 g fat
43 g sugars

Glazed Cruller
240 calories
14 g fat (7 g saturated)
14 g sugars

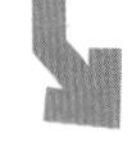

290 calories
14 g fat (6 g saturated)
19 g sugars

Not That!

Powdered Cake Doughnut

Both of these are classic sugar doughnuts, but in otherwise equal matchups, cake doughnuts will always lose out to yeast doughnuts. Make this mistake twice a week and you'll be looking at nearly 3 pounds of extra fat by the end of the year.

Other Passes

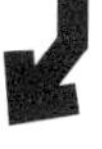

Glazed Blueberry Cake Doughnut

330 calories
17 g fat (4 g saturated)
28 g sugars

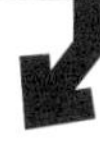

Berries & Kreme Chiller (12 oz)

620 calories
28 g fat (24 g saturated)
71 g sugars

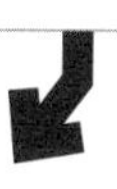

Glazed Kreme Filled

340 calories
20 g fat (10 g saturated)
23 g sugars

WEAPON OF MASS DESTRUCTION

Lotta Latte Chiller (20 oz)

1,050 calories
40 g fat (36 g saturated)
97 g sugars

All the "Kreme" Chillers come in above 600 calories, but this one ranks up there among the worst drinks on the planet. Most appalling of all is that 90% of the fat in this drink is saturated, conspiring to deliver nearly 2 full day's worth of the stuff to you through a straw. Save 500 calories or more by opting for a fruity chiller instead.

GUILTY PLEASURE

Original Glazed Doughnut Holes (4)

200 calories
11 g fat (5 g saturated)
15 g sugars

An order of these doughnut holes is one of the menu items lowest in calories, fat, saturated fat, and sugars. Plus, being able to pop 4 pieces into your mouth may help you feel more satisfied than just eating 1 doughnut would.

Long John Silver's

C-

Blame a stubborn reliance on partially hydrogenated oils for the sheen of trans fat that coats nearly everything that emerges from Long John's kitchen. The fish mogul has the healthy sides—Vegetable Medley, Corn Cobbettes—in place. But for now, it's not safe to eat fried food at a place where a snack-size box of Breaded Clam Strips means 7 grams of trans fat for your bloodstream.

SURVIVAL STRATEGY

The only fish that avoid the trans fat oils are those that are grilled or baked. Pair one of those options with a healthy side. If you need some extra flavor, choose cocktail sauce or malt vinegar instead of tartar sauce.

Eat This

Shrimp Scampi

110 calories
5 g fat (1 g saturated)
610 mg sodium

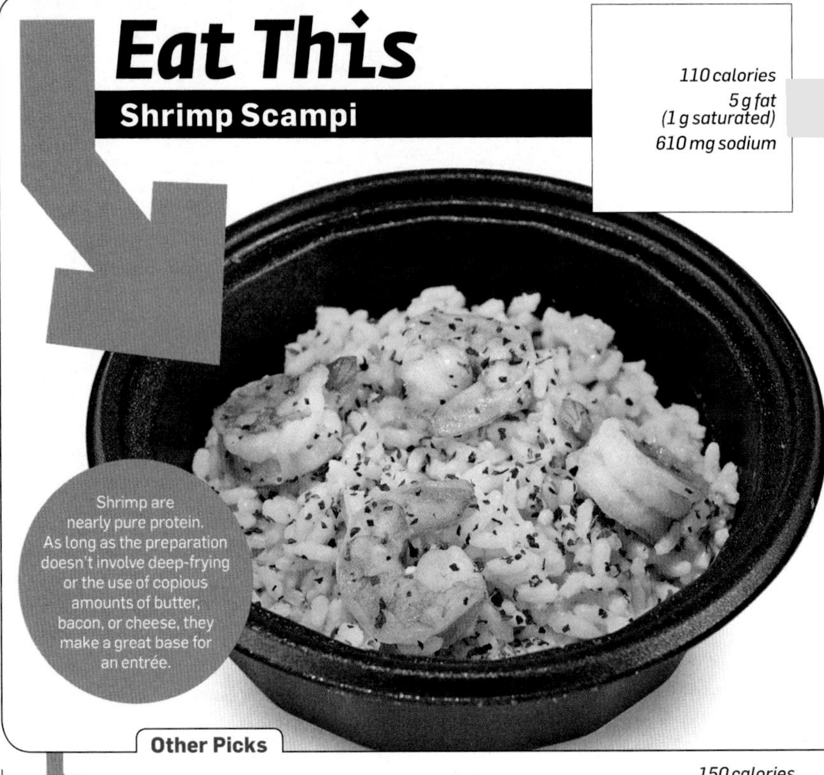

Shrimp are nearly pure protein. As long as the preparation doesn't involve deep-frying or the use of copious amounts of butter, bacon, or cheese, they make a great base for an entrée.

Other Picks

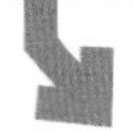

Grilled Pacific Salmon
150 calories
5 g fat (1 g saturated)
440 mg sodium

Lobster Stuffed Crab Cake
170 calories
9 g fat (2 g saturated)
390 mg sodium

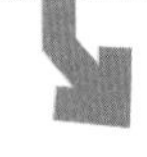

Corn Cobbette
(without butter oil)
90 calories
3 g fat (0.5 g saturated)
0 mg sodium

270 calories
16 g fat (4 g saturated, 4.5 g trans)
570 mg sodium

Not That!

Popcorn Shrimp

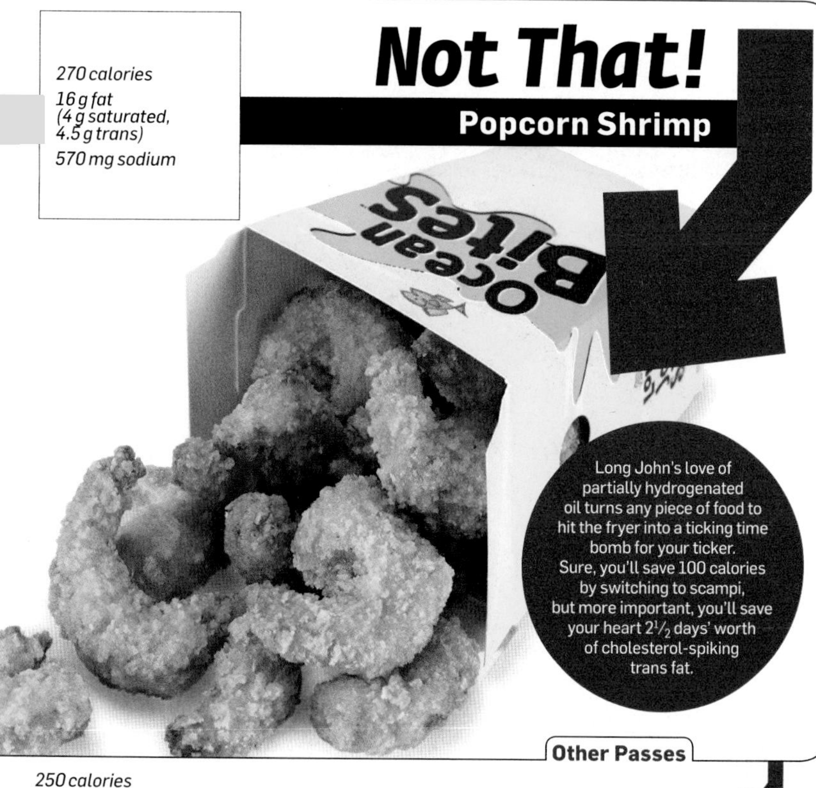

Long John's love of partially hydrogenated oil turns any piece of food to hit the fryer into a ticking time bomb for your ticker. Sure, you'll save 100 calories by switching to scampi, but more important, you'll save your heart 2½ days' worth of cholesterol-spiking trans fat.

Other Passes

Alaskan Flounder

250 calories
11 g fat (2.5 g saturated, 3 g trans)
910 mg sodium

Breaded Clam Strips
(1 snack box)

320 calories
19 g fat (4.5 g saturated, 7 g trans)
1,190 mg sodium

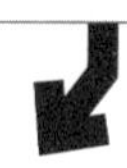

Cole Slaw

200 calories
15 g fat (2.5 g saturated)
340 mg sodium

3.6

The amount of trans fat, in grams, in the average fish sandwich or fish fillet at LJS.

MENU DECODER

- **CRUMBLIES:** Crunchy bits of batter thrown in with your fish—at a cost of 170 calories and 4 grams of trans fat a pop.
- **FRESHSIDE GRILLE:** LJS's new (much-needed!) healthier menu section.

CONDIMENT CATASTROPHE

Tartar Sauce

100 calories
9 g fat (1.5 g saturated)
250 mg sodium

There are worse sauces out there, but at LJS, you need all the help you can get. Cocktail sauce has one-quarter of the calories and no fat.

McDonald's

B+ The world-famous burger baron has come a long way since the publication of *Fast Food Nation*—at least nutritionally speaking. The trans fat is mostly gone, the number of calorie bombs reduced, and there are more healthy options, such as salads and yogurt parfaits, than ever. Still, too many of the breakfast and lunch items still top the 500-calorie mark, and the dessert menu is a total mess.

SURVIVAL STRATEGY
At breakfast, look no farther than the Egg McMuffin—it remains one of the best ways to start your day in the fast-food world. Grilled chicken and Snack Wraps make for a sound lunch. Splurge on a Big Mac or Quarter Pounder, but only if you skip the fries and soda.

Eat This

Big N' Tasty

460 calories
24 g fat (8 g saturated, 1.5 g trans)
720 mg sodium

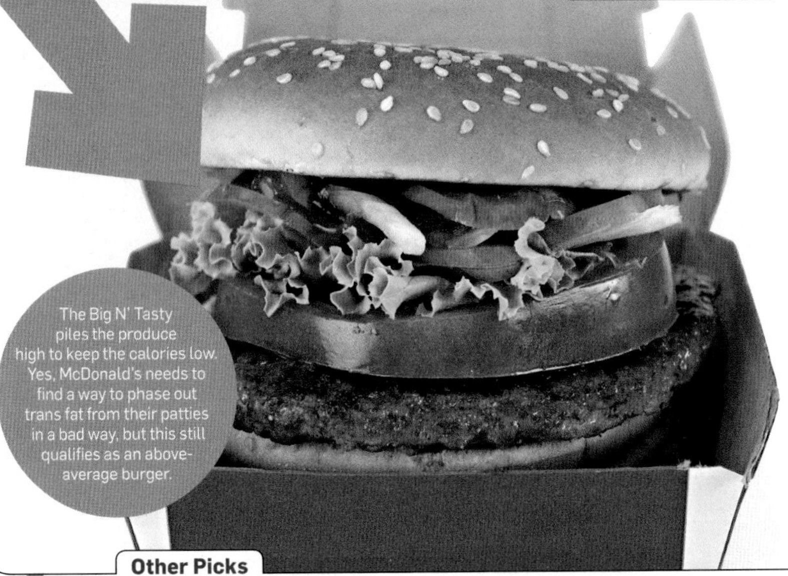

The Big N' Tasty piles the produce high to keep the calories low. Yes, McDonald's needs to find a way to phase out trans fat from their patties in a bad way, but this still qualifies as an above-average burger.

Other Picks

Filet-O-Fish

380 calories
18 g fat (3.5 g saturated)
640 mg sodium

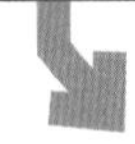

Honey Mustard Snack Wrap **(grilled)**

260 calories
9 g fat (3.5 g saturated)
800 mg sodium

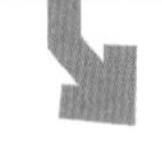

Sausage Patty with Scrambled Eggs **(2)**

340 calories
26 g fat (9 g saturated)
520 mg sodium

Not That!

Chicken Selects Premium Breast Strips

(5) with Creamy Ranch Sauce

860 calories
22 g fat
(9.5 g saturated)
2,000 mg sodium

Outside of eating a Double Quarter Pounder, there's no worse way to direct your dollars at the Golden Arches.

Other Passes

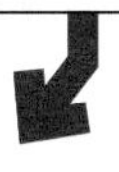

Premium Crispy Chicken Classic Sandwich

530 calories
20 g fat (3.5 g saturated)
1,150 mg sodium

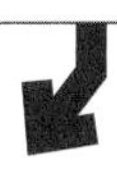

Southern Style Crispy Chicken Sandwich

400 calories
17 g fat (3 g saturated)
1,030 mg sodium

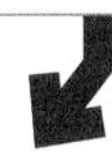

McSkillet Burrito with Sausage

610 calories
36 g fat (14 g saturated, 0.5 g trans)
1,390 mg sodium

WEAPON OF MASS DESTRUCTION

Chocolate Triple Thick Shake
(32 oz)

1,160 calories
27 g fat
(16 g saturated, 2 g trans)
168 g sugars

With as many calories as 20 doughnut holes and as much sugar as 14 bowls of Froot Loops, this thick shake will make you thick, too.

SMART SIDES

Fruit 'n Yogurt Parfait

160 calories
2 g fat
21 g sugars

Consider this a guilt-free way to indulge your sweet tooth on the go. Or sub it in for French fries with your next meal. The swap will save you 220 calories and 17 grams of fat.

FOOD COURT

THE CRIME
Large Deluxe Breakfast
(1,370 calories)

THE PUNISHMENT
Wash and wax cars for 4 hours
(fund-raiser, anyone?)

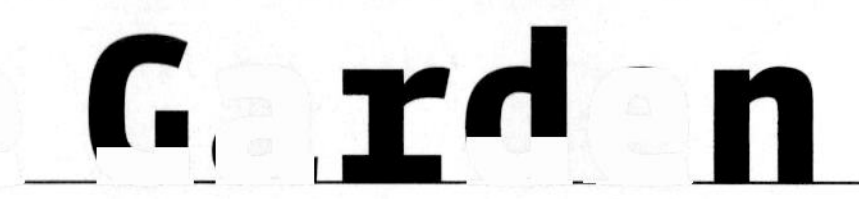

Olive Garden

D+

We initially gave the Garden an F for failing to disclose their nutritional content, and we really appreciate the effort they've made to increase their transparency since then. But when a typical entrée packs an average of 905 calories (and that's before you factor in appetizers, sides, drinks, and desserts), it's not time to celebrate just yet.

SURVIVAL STRATEGY

Most pasta dishes are packed with at least a day's worth of sodium and more than 1,000 calories, so choose either the Linguine alla Marinara or the Ravioli di Portobello; they're both reasonable options. As for chicken and seafood, stick with the Herb-Grilled Salmon, Parmesan Crusted Tilapia, or Shrimp and Asparagus Risotto.

Eat This

Parmesan Crusted Tilapia

590 calories
25 g fat (10 g saturated)
910 mg sodium

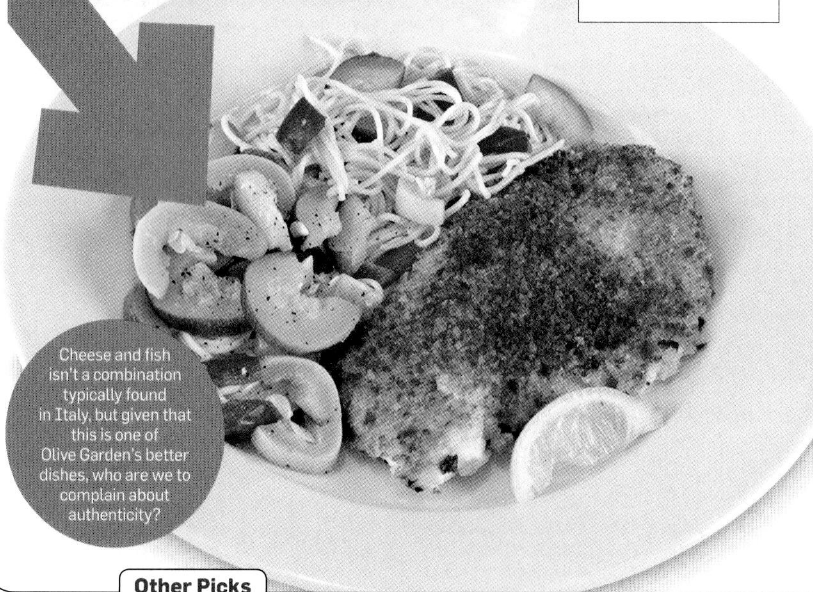

Cheese and fish isn't a combination typically found in Italy, but given that this is one of Olive Garden's better dishes, who are we to complain about authenticity?

Other Picks

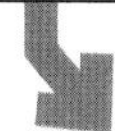

Linguine alla Marinara

430 calories
6 g fat (1 g saturated)
900 mg sodium

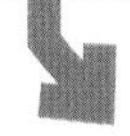

Venetian Apricot Chicken

380 calories
4 g fat (1.5 g saturated)
1,420 mg sodium

Mussels di Napoli
(1/2 order)

90 calories
4 g fat (2 g saturated)
900 mg sodium

900 calories
41 g fat (17 g saturated)
3,490 mg sodium

Not That!

Grilled Shrimp Caprese

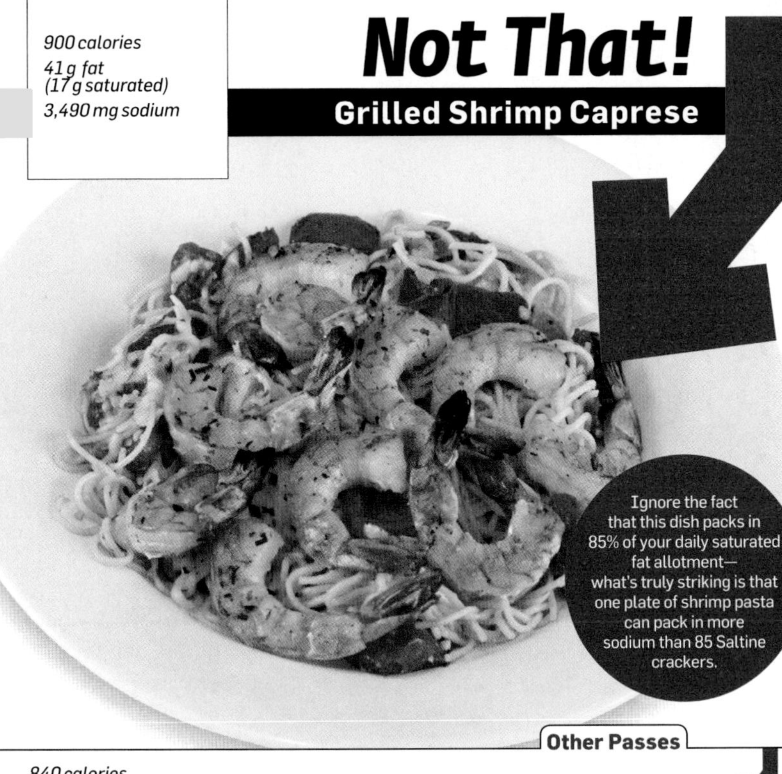

Ignore the fact that this dish packs in 85% of your daily saturated fat allotment—what's truly striking is that one plate of shrimp pasta can pack in more sodium than 85 Saltine crackers.

Other Passes

Capellini Pomodoro
840 calories
17 g fat (3 g saturated)
1,250 mg sodium

Chicken & Gnocchi Veronese
1,030 calories
58 g fat (26 g saturated)
2,580 mg sodium

Calamari (1/2 order)
445 calories
27 g fat (2.5 g saturated)
1,165 mg sodium

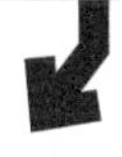

GUILTY PLEASURE

Pork Filettino
640 calories
19 g fat (3 g saturated)
840 mg sodium

Despite popular perception, pork is a great source of lean protein. Plus, this dish has the second-lowest sodium content of any entrée on Olive Garden's menu—probably because it's marinated in olive oil and rosemary for flavor, rather than slathered in a salty sauce. To top it all off, this one entrée offers a truly impressive 14 grams of fiber.

CONDIMENT CATASTROPHE

Alfredo Dipping Sauce
380 calories
35 g fat (22 g saturated)

Even in its best form, "dipping sauce" usually serves as a euphemism for "fat bath," but this Alfredo rendition makes ranch dressing look like wheatgrass. With more than a day's worth of saturated fat in a tiny tub, this qualifies as the most calorie-dense condiment we've ever seen. Dip your breadsticks in marinara, instead, and save 310 calories and more than 30 grams of fat.

On the Border

D-

On the Border is a subsidiary of Brinker International, the same parent company that owns Chili's and has a hand in Romano's Macaroni Grill. It should come as no surprise, then, that its food is potentially as detrimental as its corporate brothers' foods are. The massive menu suffers from appetizers with 120 grams of fat, salads with a full day's worth of sodium, and fish taco entrées with up to 2,350 calories. Don't come hungry.

SURVIVAL STRATEGY

The Border Smart Menu highlights 5 items with fewer than 600 calories and 25 grams of fat each. Those aren't great numbers, considering that the dishes average 1,600 milligrams of sodium apiece, but that's all you have to work with here.

Eat This

Grilled Fajita Chicken Tacos

570 calories
9 g fat
(2 g saturated)
1,910 mg sodium

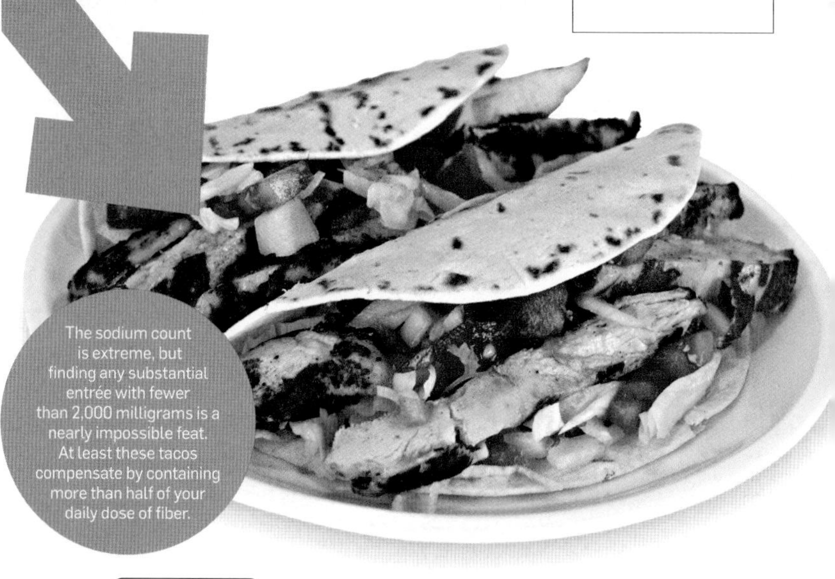

The sodium count is extreme, but finding any substantial entrée with fewer than 2,000 milligrams is a nearly impossible feat. At least these tacos compensate by containing more than half of your daily dose of fiber.

Other Picks

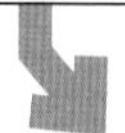

Pico Shrimp Tacos
with black beans and grilled vegetables

490 calories
5 g fat (1 g saturated)
1,650 mg sodium

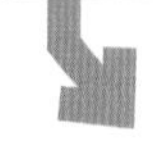

Beef Enchiladas
(2) with Chile Con Carne

420 calories
22 g fat (7 g saturated)
1,140 mg sodium

Chicken Tortilla Soup
(cup) and house salad with Fat-Free Mango-Citrus Vinaigrette

575 calories
30 g fat (10.5 g saturated)
1,290 mg sodium

1,340 calories
73 g fat (14 g saturated)
2,700 mg sodium

Not That!

Southwest Chicken Tacos

with Creamy Red Chile Sauce

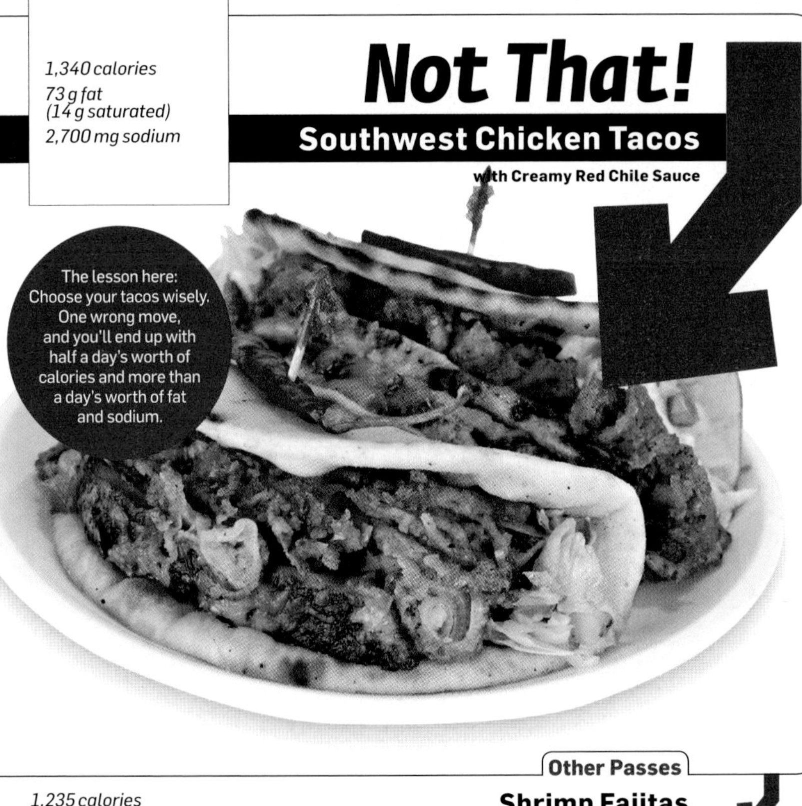

The lesson here: Choose your tacos wisely. One wrong move, and you'll end up with half a day's worth of calories and more than a day's worth of fat and sodium.

Other Passes

1,235 calories
81.5 g fat (21.5 g saturated)
3,555 mg sodium

Shrimp Fajitas
with Classic Veggies, Tequila Lime Chile Sauce, and condiments

1,120 calories
43 g fat (19 g saturated)
2,580 mg sodium

Classic Beef Burrito
with Chili Con Carne

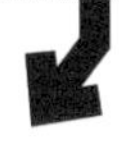

1,700 calories
124 g fat (37.5 g saturated)
2,620 mg sodium

Grande Taco Salad
with Seasoned Ground Beef and Chipotle Honey Mustard Dressing

STEALTH HEALTH FOOD
Guacamole

170 calories
14 g fat (3 g saturated)
500 mg sodium

Guacamole might be the single healthiest item on this Mexican menu. The avocados that form its base are loaded with a cholesterol-lowering fat called oleic acid. Want to enjoy the benefits without increasing your calories? Ask to have your tacos prepared without cheese, and then scoop on the guac, instead. Same rich, creamy effect, just with tons of nutrition.

LITTLE TRICK

The real trouble at Mexican restaurants is found in the condiments and sides. Ask to substitute grilled vegetables for the Mexican rice. You'll save up to 220 calories and 660 milligrams of sodium. Strip away another few hundred calories by banning cheese and sour cream from your plate.

Outback Steakhouse

F

You wouldn't order a meal if the restaurant refused to tell you the price, would you? Fat, calories, and sodium are all just as much a part of the overall cost of a meal as the dollar value. That's why we flunk Outback, along with the rest of the nutritional holdouts. You don't show up for the test, you can't make the grade.

SURVIVAL STRATEGY

Curb your desire to order the 14-ounce rib eye (1,190 calories) by starting with the protein-rich Seared Ahi Tuna. Then move on to one of the leaner cuts of beef: the petite fillet or the prime rib. Assuming you skip the bread and house salad (590 calories) and choose steamed vegetables as your side, you might have a shot at escaping dinner for less than 1,000 calories.

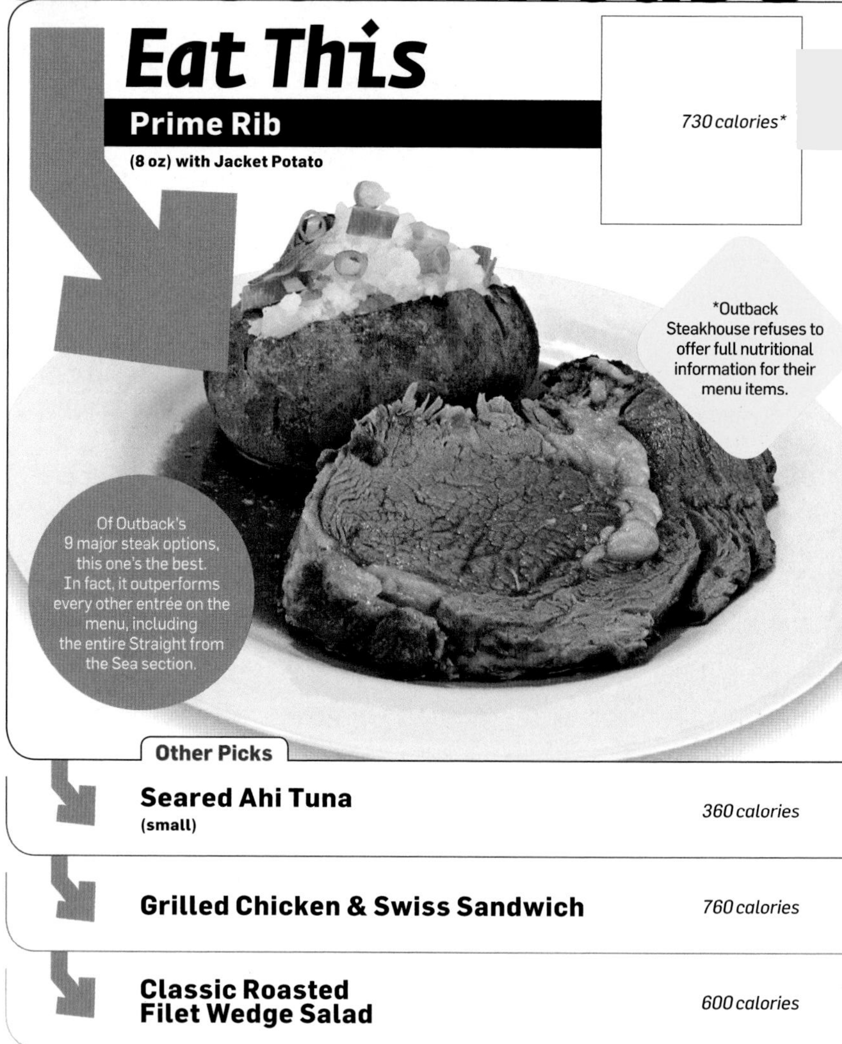

Eat This

Prime Rib

(8 oz) with Jacket Potato

*730 calories**

*Outback Steakhouse refuses to offer full nutritional information for their menu items.

Of Outback's 9 major steak options, this one's the best. In fact, it outperforms every other entrée on the menu, including the entire Straight from the Sea section.

Other Picks

Seared Ahi Tuna **(small)** — *360 calories*

Grilled Chicken & Swiss Sandwich — *760 calories*

Classic Roasted Filet Wedge Salad — *600 calories*

Not That!

1,330 calories*

Victoria's Filet

(9 oz) with Sweet Potato

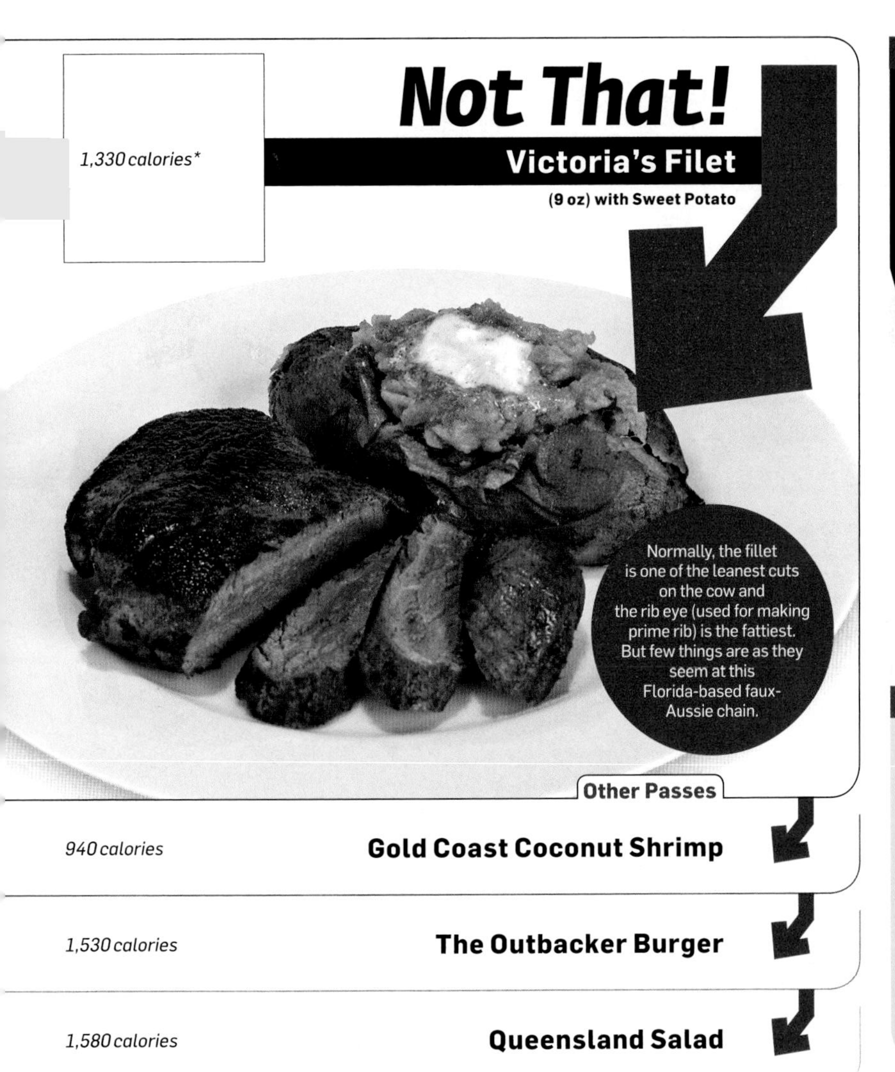

Normally, the fillet is one of the leanest cuts on the cow and the rib eye (used for making prime rib) is the fattiest. But few things are as they seem at this Florida-based faux-Aussie chain.

Other Passes

940 calories — **Gold Coast Coconut Shrimp**

1,530 calories — **The Outbacker Burger**

1,580 calories — **Queensland Salad**

HIDDEN DANGER

Sweet Potato

Normally, the fiber and vitamin A in sweet potatoes make them a smarter choice than regular potatoes, but not so here. We're not sure how Outback managed to create this spud missle (2 guesses: butter and oil), but we do know that a regular dressed baked potato will save you a shocking 410 calories.

600 calories*

GUILTY PLEASURE

Pinot Noir

100 calories

Need something to wash down the lean prime rib? Few things are better for your palate, or your ticker, than a glass of pinot. While the bold berry flavor pairs up perfectly with red meat, it's the extra dose of heart-healthy reservatol found in the pinot grape that makes this such a classic steak-house match.

Panda Express

C Oddly enough, it's not the wok-fried meat or the viscous sauces that do this menu the most harm—it's the more than 400 calories of rice and noodles that form the foundation of each meal. Scrape these starches from the plate, and Panda Express starts to look a lot healthier. Only one entrée item has more than 500 calories, and there's hardly a trans fat on the menu. Gut-bloating problems arise when multiple entrées and sides start piling up on one plate, though, so bring your self-restraint.

SURVIVAL STRATEGY
Avoid these entrées: Orange Chicken, Sweet & Sour Chicken, Beijing Beef, and anything with pork. Then swap in Mixed Veggies for the scoop of rice.

Eat This

Mongolian Beef

200 calories
9 g fat
(2 g saturated)
830 mg sodium

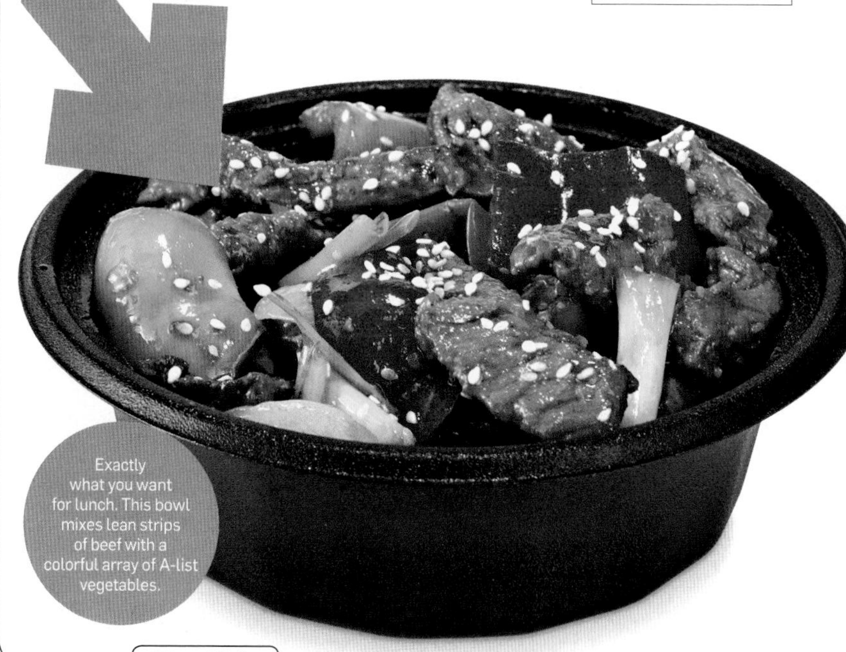

Exactly what you want for lunch. This bowl mixes lean strips of beef with a colorful array of A-list vegetables.

Other Picks

Pineapple Chicken

230 calories
10 g fat (2 g saturated)
710 mg sodium

Mixed Veggies (entrée)

100 calories
6 g fat (1 g saturated)
220 mg sodium

660 calories
41 g fat (7 g saturated)
860 mg sodium

Not That!

Beijing Beef

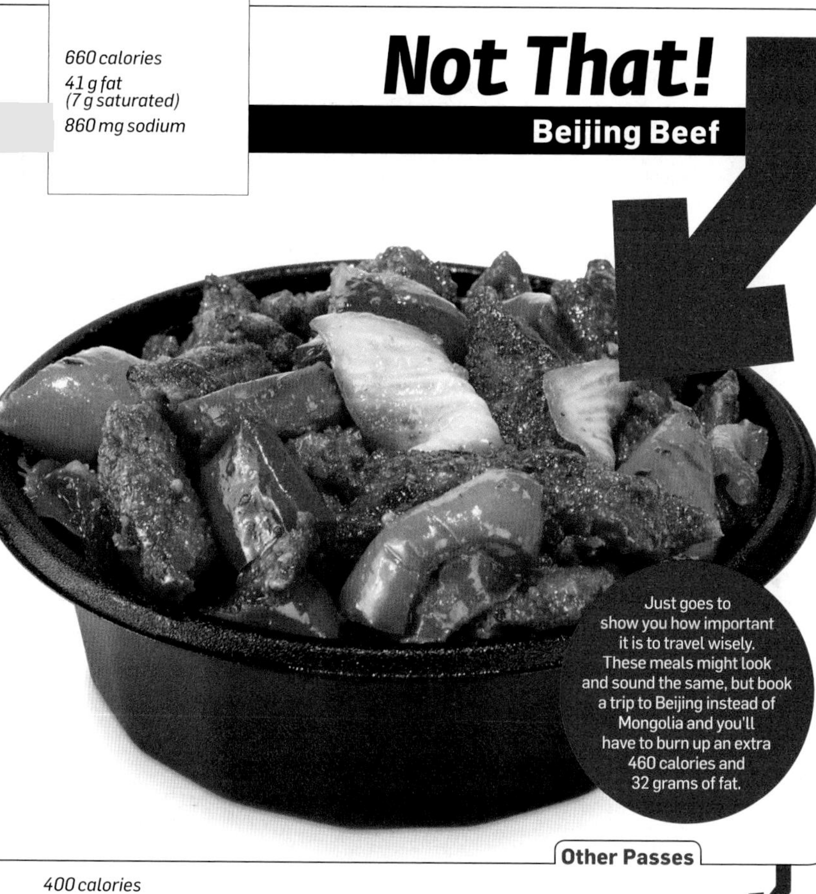

Just goes to show you how important it is to travel wisely. These meals might look and sound the same, but book a trip to Beijing instead of Mongolia and you'll have to burn up an extra 460 calories and 32 grams of fat.

Other Passes

Orange Chicken

400 calories
20 g fat (3.5 g saturated)
640 mg sodium

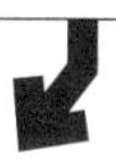

Eggplant and Tofu

310 calories
24 g fat (3 g saturated)
680 mg sodium

GUILTY PLEASURE

Fortune Cookie

32 calories
2 g fat
3 g sugars

The postmeal fortune cookie is a long-standing tradition in Chinese-America cuisine, so it's fortunate that it has only a few more calories than you'd find in a single Hershey Kiss. Plus, a few calories are a small price to pay for knowing the future.

BAD BREEDS

Rice & Noodle

Panda Express's Chow Mein and Steamed and Fried Rice are all higher in calories and carbs than almost any entrée on the menu.

STEALTH HEALTH FOOD

Tangy Shrimp

140 calories
4.5 g fat (1 g saturated)
660 mg sodium

Here's what you need to know about shrimp: Each one is constructed almost entirely from pure protein and is loaded with vitamins and minerals. They contain bone-strengthening vitamin D, joint-protecting selenium, and mood-enhancing tryptophan.

Panera Bread

B-

Artisan they may be, but some of the sandwiches push into quadruple digits, and a long list of brownies, pastries, and cookies almost qualifies Panera as a dessert shop. Breakfast, limited to carb-driven confections and fatty sandwiches and souffles, doesn't improve matters. But the healthy selection of soups and salads, plus the much-needed half sandwich option, really does. (Oh, and free Wi-Fi doesn't hurt, either.)

SURVIVAL STRATEGY

For breakfast, choose between the Egg & Cheese breakfast sandwich and 310-calorie granola parfait. Skip the stand-alone sandwich lunch. Instead, pair soup and a salad, or order the soup and half-sandwich combo.

Eat This

Half Asiago Roast Beef with Black Bean Soup

You Pick Two Combo

450 calories
17 g fat (6 g saturated)
1,510 mg sodium

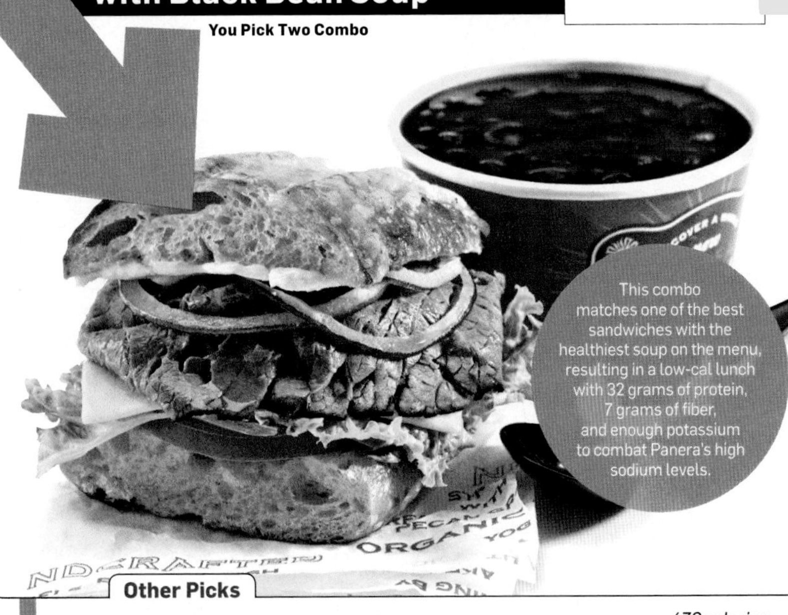

This combo matches one of the best sandwiches with the healthiest soup on the menu, resulting in a low-cal lunch with 32 grams of protein, 7 grams of fiber, and enough potassium to combat Panera's high sodium levels.

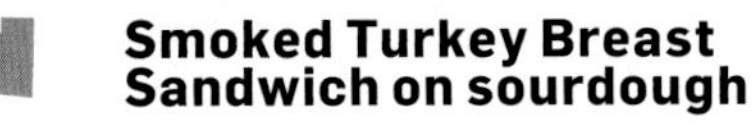

Other Picks

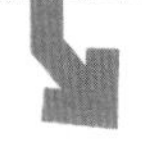

Smoked Turkey Breast Sandwich on sourdough

470 calories
17 g fat (2.5 g saturated)
1,680 mg sodium

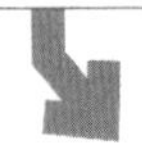

Egg & Cheese Grilled Breakfast Sandwich

380 calories
14 g fat (6 g saturated)
620 mg sodium

Caffe Latte

110 calories
4.5 g fat (3 g saturated)
11 g sugars

810 calories
59 g fat (12 g saturated)
1,870 mg sodium

Not That!

Half Sierra Turkey with Half Greek Salad

You Pick Two Combo

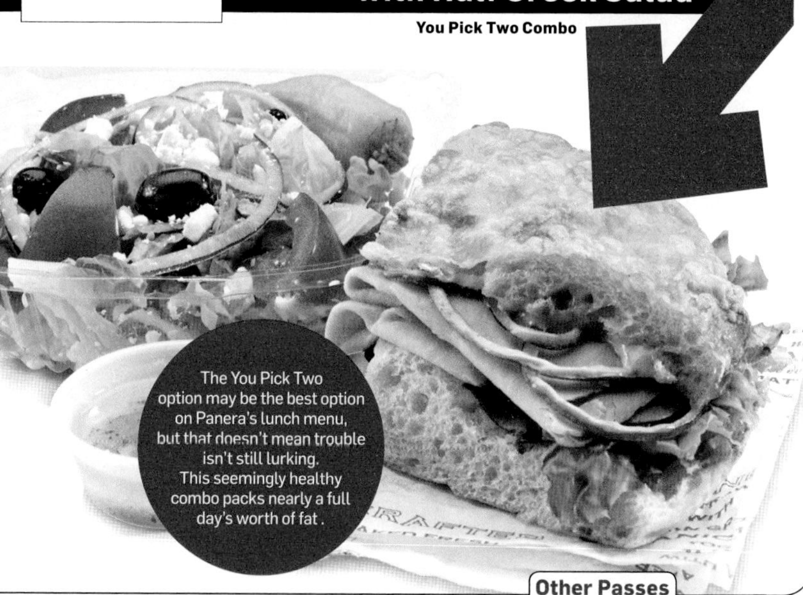

The You Pick Two option may be the best option on Panera's lunch menu, but that doesn't mean trouble isn't still lurking. This seemingly healthy combo packs nearly a full day's worth of fat.

Other Passes

1,070 calories
55 g fat (15 g saturated, 1 g trans)
2,570 mg sodium

Chipotle Chicken Sandwich on artisan French bread

490 calories
13.5 g fat (6 g saturated)
620 mg sodium

Whole Grain Bagel with reduced-fat veggie cream cheese
(2 oz)

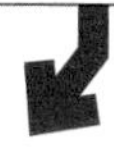

380 calories
17 g fat (11 g saturated)
41 g sugars

Caffe Mocha

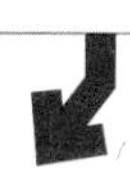

GUILTY PLEASURE

Petite Chocolate Duet with Walnuts Cookie

110 calories
6 g fat (3 g saturated)
9 g sugars

Enter exhibit A: a properly proportioned cookie. Note how it doesn't have belt-busting levels of fat and sugar. But it does have walnuts, arguably the world's healthiest nut—and the only nut loaded with omega-3 fats. Just be sure you ask for your cookie "petite." Otherwise you'll get stuck with the 450-calorie version.

BAD BREEDS

Signature Sandwiches

Sadly, not one of Panera's delicious signature sandwiches contains fewer than 700 calories and 30 grams of fat. The worst by far is the 1,070-calorie Chipotle Chicken. Stick with a lower-cal café sandwich, or get half a sandwich with a cup of soup.

LITTLE TRICK

Swap mayo and fatty spreads for light ranch—it'll save 100 calories or more on your next sandwich.

Papa John's

C

Give Papa John's credit for being the only pizza franchise to offer a whole wheat crust, thus providing a viable, fiber-rich option to pizza lovers the country over. Combine that with an innovative list of healthy toppings—including the surprisingly lean Spinach Alfredo—and you start to see hope for Papa John's devotees. The chain loses big points for its line of treacherous dipping sauces, its belly-building bread sticks, and its 400-calorie-a-slice pan-crust pizza, though.

SURVIVAL STRATEGY

There are only 2 crust options to consider: thin and wheat. Ask for light cheese, and cover it with anything other than sausage, pepperoni, or bacon.

Eat This

The Works

(2 slices, 12" original crust)

460 calories
16 g fat (7 g saturated)
1,240 mg sodium

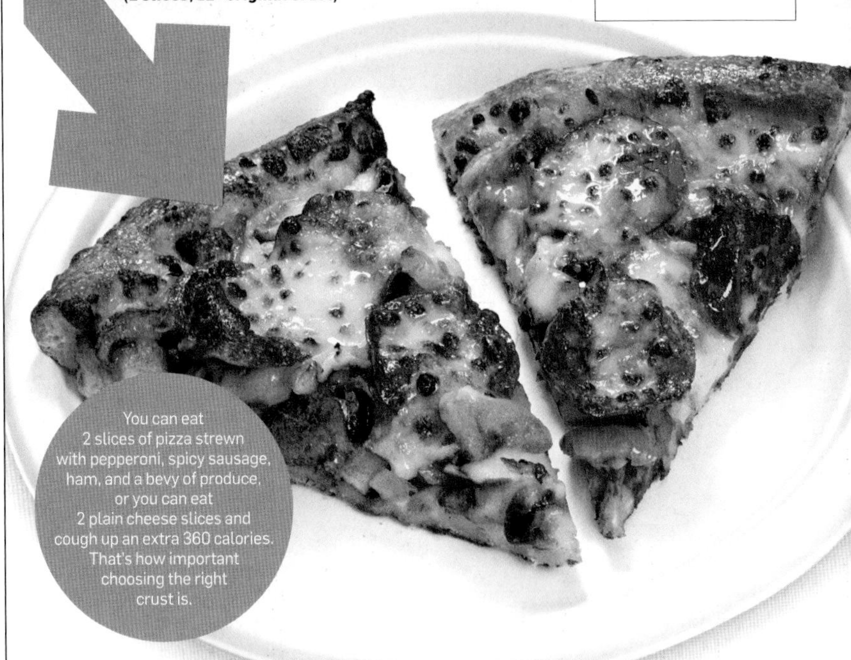

You can eat 2 slices of pizza strewn with pepperoni, spicy sausage, ham, and a bevy of produce, or you can eat 2 plain cheese slices and cough up an extra 360 calories. That's how important choosing the right crust is.

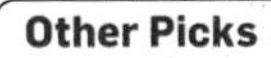

Other Picks

Spinach Alfredo Pizza

(2 slices, thin crust)

440 calories
26 g fat (9 g saturated)
840 mg sodium

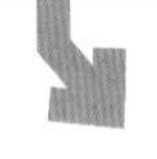

BBQ Wings

(2)

160 calories
12 g fat (3 g saturated)
560 mg sodium

820 calories
46 g fat (14 g saturated)
1,500 mg sodium

Not That!

Cheese Pizza

(2 slices, pan crust)

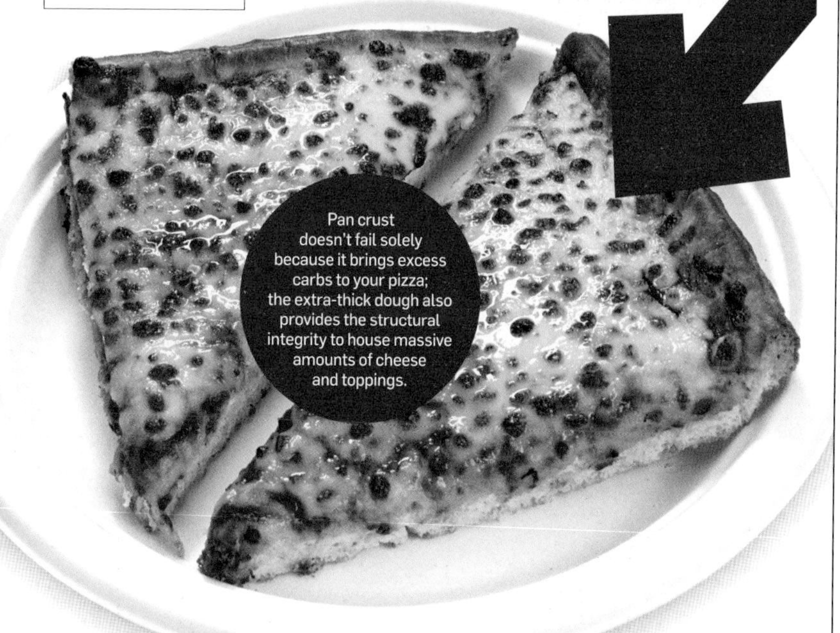

Pan crust doesn't fail solely because it brings excess carbs to your pizza; the extra-thick dough also provides the structural integrity to house massive amounts of cheese and toppings.

Other Passes

560 calories
26 g fat (7 g saturated)
1,500 mg sodium

Hawaiian BBQ Chicken Pizza
(2 slices, thin crust)

330 calories
10 g fat (1.5 g saturated)
720 mg sodium

Garlic Parmesan Breadsticks
(2)

SMART SIDES

Pizza Sauce
(1 oz)

20 calories
230 mg sodium

Pizza sauce, aka marinara, is made from cooked tomatoes, which just so happen to be the world's best source of lycopene—an antioxidant that battles cancer and helps your skin repair itself after a day in the sun. Plus, the more you dip, the slower you eat. Since it takes your stomach about 20 minutes to tell your brain that it's full, a few extra minutes at the table will add up to fewer calories in your belly.

CONDIMENT CATASTROPHE

Papa John's Dipping Sauces

One of the greatest pitfalls of ordering Papa John's is those little sauce cups they cram in nearly every pizza box. The most common, the Special Garlic Sauce, also happens to be the worst, with 150 calories, 17 grams of fat, and 310 milligrams of sodium in one tiny tub. Isn't pizza fatty and saucy enough? If you must dip, choose the 20-calorie pizza sauce, which is actually made from real produce rather than an amalgam of oils and additives.

P.F. Chang's

D+

A plague of quadruple-digit entrées turns Chang's menu into a nutritional minefield. Noodle dishes and foods from the grill all come with dangerously high fat and calorie counts, while traditional stir-fries are sinking in a sea of excess sodium. Chang's does have a great variety of low-cal appetizers and an ordering flexibility that allows for easy substitutions and tweaks, like the great low-fat "wok velveted" option.

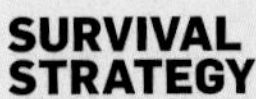

SURVIVAL STRATEGY

Order a lean appetizer like an order of dumplings or the Seared Ahi Tuna for the table, and resolve to split one of the more reasonable entrées between two people. Earn bonus points by tailoring your dish to be light on the oil and sauce.

Eat This

Asian Marinated NY Strip Steak

558 calories
30 g fat (12 g saturated)
864 mg sodium

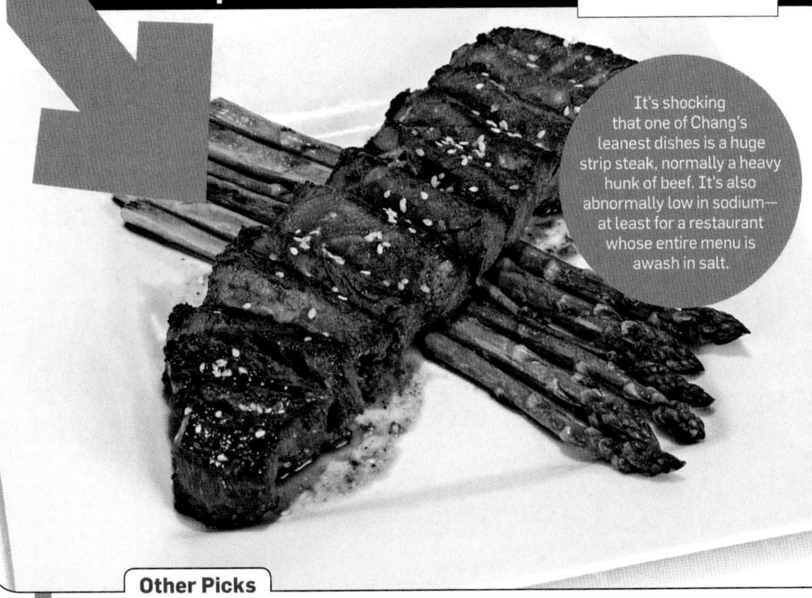

It's shocking that one of Chang's leanest dishes is a huge strip steak, normally a heavy hunk of beef. It's also abnormally low in sodium—at least for a restaurant whose entire menu is awash in salt.

Other Picks

Wild Alaskan Salmon
Steamed with Ginger

250 calories
28 g fat (64g saturated)
1,066 mg sodium

Almond & Cashew Chicken
with Brown Rice Lunch Bowl

294 calories
10 g fat (2 g saturated)
15 g protein, 1,694 mg sodium
34 g carbohydrates

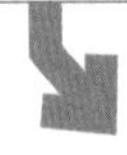

Seared Ahi Tuna

176 calories
4 g fat
1,340 mg sodium

850 calories
30 g fat
(15 g saturated)
10,045 mg sodium

Not That!

Wok Charred Beef

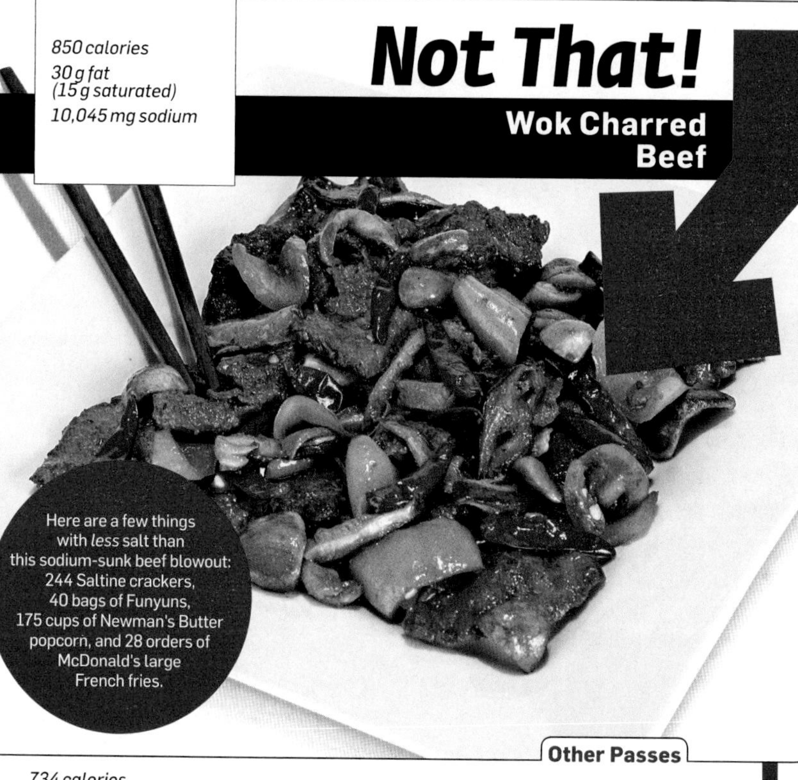

Here are a few things with *less* salt than this sodium-sunk beef blowout: 244 Saltine crackers, 40 bags of Funyuns, 175 cups of Newman's Butter popcorn, and 28 orders of McDonald's large French fries.

Other Passes

734 calories
32 g fat (14 g saturated)
1,306 mg sodium

Wild Alaskan Citrus Soy Salmon

979 calories
27 g fat (4 g saturated)
49 g protein, 2,492 mg sodium
135 g carbohydrates

Sesame Chicken
with Brown Rice Lunch Bowl

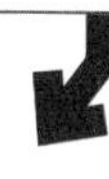

1,448 calories
40 g fat (8 g saturated)
1,778 mg sodium

Salt and Pepper Calamari

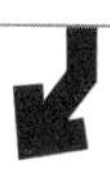

GUILTY PLEASURE

Sweet & Sour Pork

759 calories
27 g fat (15 g saturated)
1,728 mg sodium

Believe it or not, this is one of the leanest entrées on the menu. We'd still recommend splitting it (or at least saving some for later), but it's worth noting that eating the entire portion you're served won't cause a *complete* dietary malfunction.

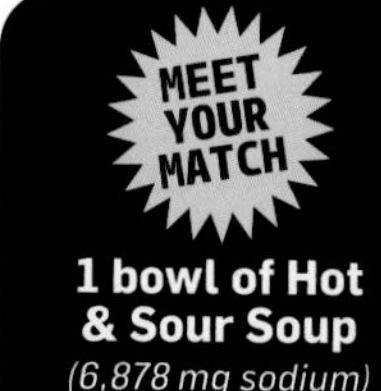

1 bowl of Hot & Sour Soup
(6,878 mg sodium)

=

168 Saltine crackers

FOOD COURT

THE CRIME
Dan Dan Noodles
(full order = 1,888 calories)

THE PUNISHMENT
3 hours and 32 minutes of cross-country skiing

Pizza Hut

In an attempt to push the menu beyond the ill-reputed pizza, Pizza Hut expanded into pastas, salads, and something called a P'Zone. Sound like an improvement? Think again. Calzone-like P'Zones all pack more than 1,200 calories a piece. The salads aren't much better, and the pastas are actually worse. The thin crust pizzas and the Fit 'N Delicious offer redemption with sub-200-calorie slices. Eat a couple of those, and you'll do just fine.

Eat This

Thin 'N Crispy Quartered Ham and Pineapple

14" (2 slices)

480 calories
18 g fat (8 g saturated)
1,500 mg sodium

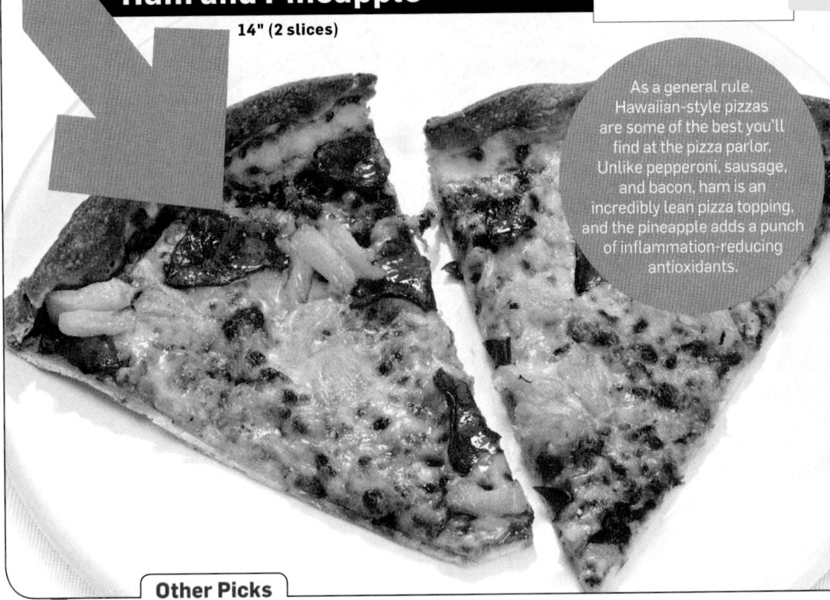

As a general rule, Hawaiian-style pizzas are some of the best you'll find at the pizza parlor. Unlike pepperoni, sausage, and bacon, ham is an incredibly lean pizza topping, and the pineapple adds a punch of inflammation-reducing antioxidants.

Other Picks

Thin 'N Crispy All Natural Pepperoni & Mushroom
12" (2 slices)
380 calories
14 g fat (6 g saturated)
1,060 mg sodium

Fit 'N Delicious Chicken, Red Onion & Green Pepper
(2 slices)
360 calories
9 g fat (3 g saturated)
1,000 mg sodium

Baked Hot Wings
(2)
120 calories
7 g fat (2 g saturated)
500 mg sodium

SURVIVAL STRATEGY

Start with a bowl of Tomato Basil Soup and then turn to a ham or vegetable Thin 'N Crispy pie or anything on the Fit 'N Delicious menu for slices with as little as 150 calories.

Not That!

Thin 'N Crispy Cheese

14" (2 slices)

520 calories
22 g fat (12 g saturated)
1,480 mg sodium

Our research found that relatively low-calorie ham and pineapple actually displace some of the cheese, which means that 2 naked cheese slices actually have 50% more saturated fat than the Hawaiian combo. Ultimately, the Thin 'N Crispy cheese slice still holds one of the top slots on Pizza Hut's menu, but if you can add ham and pineapple *and* save calories, why wouldn't you?

Other Passes

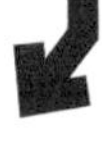

All Natural Sausage and Red Onion
12" pan (2 slices)

520 calories
22 g fat (9 g saturated)
1,100 mg sodium

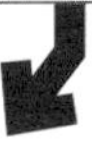

Veggie Lover's Personal Pan Pizza

550 calories
20 g fat (8 g saturated)
1,190 mg sodium

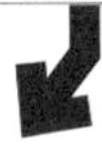

Stuffed Pizza Rolls
(1)

230 calories
11 g fat (5 g saturated)
590 mg sodium

WEAPON OF MASS DESTRUCTION
Meaty P'Zone

1,480 calories
66 g fat (30 g saturated, 2 g trans)
3,680 mg sodium

On July 10, 2007, master competitive eater Joey Chestnut broke the world record by consuming 4.82 pounds of Pizza Hut P'Zones in 6 minutes. By our calculations, Chestnut ate his way through 6,027 calories' worth of P'Zones in those 360 seconds. We doubt you have the intestinal fortitude to tussle with Chestnut, but put down just one of these massive meat pockets and you'll be taking in more calories than you'd find in 7 Krispy Kreme original glazed doughnuts.

FOOD COURT

THE CRIME
2 slices
(14") Meat Lover's Stuffed Crust Pizza (960 calories)

THE PUNISHMENT
1,590 sit-ups at a rate of one sit-up every 4 seconds

Quiznos

C-

Submarine sandwiches can only be so bad, right? We thought so, too, until we saw some of the outrageous offerings on the Quiznos menu. The bigger subs can easily supply a full day's worth of saturated fat and close to 2 days' worth of sodium, and the oversize salads aren't much better. Good thing Quiznos also provides an alternative. The sub shop's Sammies are served on flatbreads and all fall between 200 and 300 calories apiece.

SURVIVAL STRATEGY
Avoid the salads, large subs, and soups that come in bread bowls. Stick with a small sub (at 310 calories, the Honey Bourbon Chicken is easily the best), or pair a Sammie with a cup of soup.

Eat This

Roadhouse Steak Sammies
(2)

390 calories
8 g fat
(2 g saturated)
1,150 mg sodium

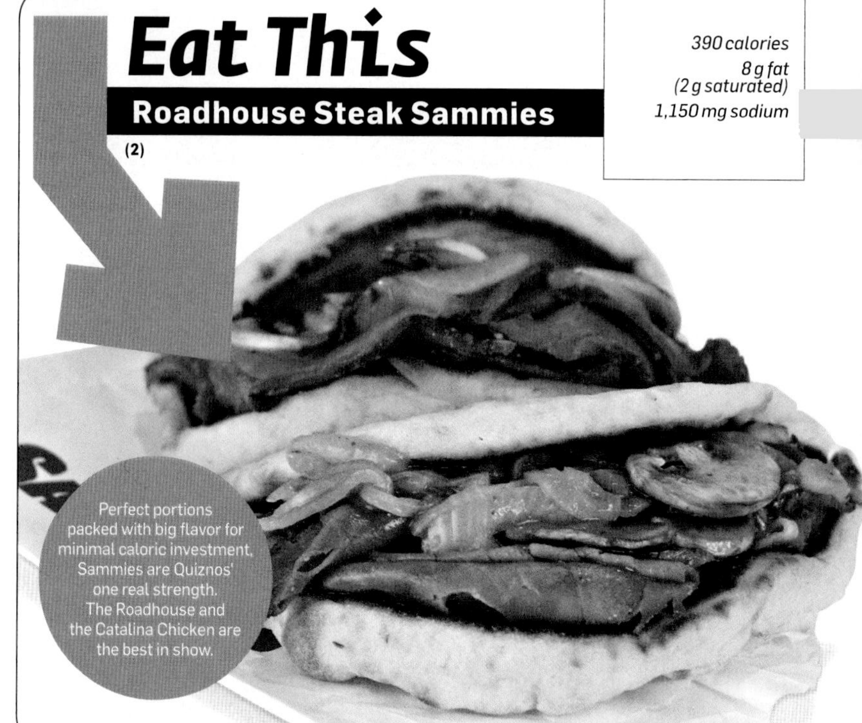

Perfect portions packed with big flavor for minimal caloric investment, Sammies are Quiznos' one real strength. The Roadhouse and the Catalina Chicken are the best in show.

Other Picks

Steakhouse Beef Dip
(small)

440 calories
18 g fat (3.5 g saturated)
1,900 mg sodium

Honey Bourbon Chicken Sandwich
(small)

320 calories
4.5 g fat (0.5 g saturated)
920 mg sodium

Black Angus Steak and Cheddar Breakfast Sandwich

390 calories
17.5 g fat (9 g saturated)
1,040 mg sodium]

750 calories
55.5 g fat
(10.5 g saturated)
930 mg sodium

Not That!

Small Tuna Melt Sub

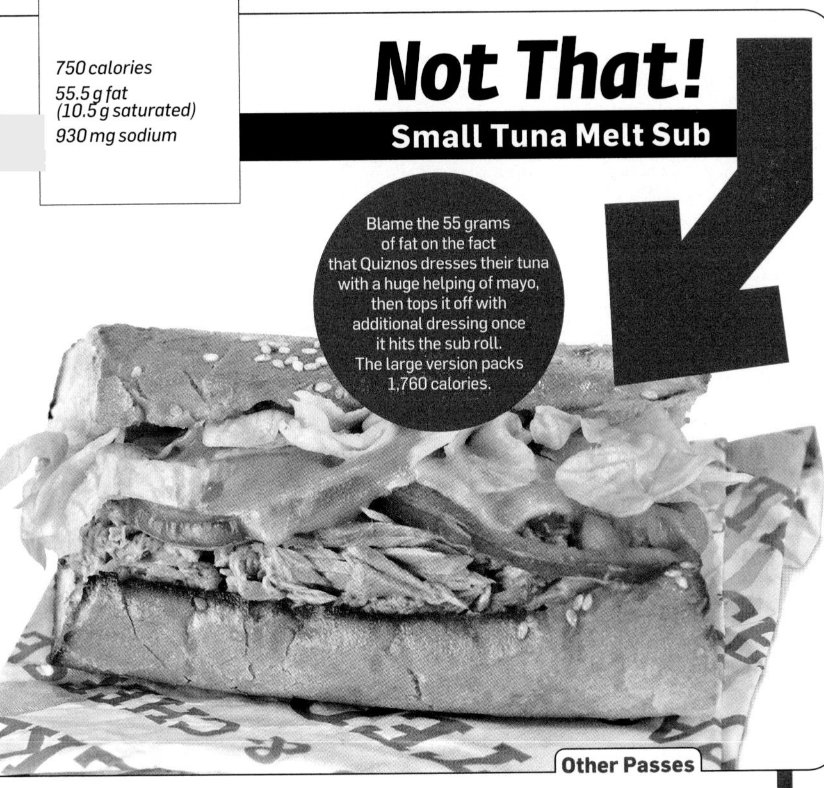

Blame the 55 grams of fat on the fact that Quiznos dresses their tuna with a huge helping of mayo, then tops it off with additional dressing once it hits the sub roll. The large version packs 1,760 calories.

Other Passes

670 calories
41 g fat (10 g saturated, 1 g trans)
1,085 mg sodium

Prime Rib Cheesesteak **(small)**

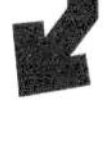

530 calories
26 g fat (5.5 g saturated)
1,085 mg sodium

Honey Mustard Chicken Sandwich **(small)**

440 calories
25.5 g fat (12 g saturated)
1,120 mg sodium

Bacon, Egg, and Cheddar Breakfast Sandwich

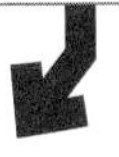

HIDDEN DANGER

Roasted Chicken with Honey Mustard Flatbread Salad

Just another example of how salads aren't always the best choice: This one has a huge load of calories and a ton of saturated fat. You're much better off with the Black & Bleu salad, or better yet, a sandwich.

1,070 calories
71 g fat
(13.5 g saturated)
1,770 mg sodium

STEALTH HEALTH FOOD

Cup of Chili

185 calories
8 g fat (2 g saturated)
760 mg sodium

Look beyond the sandwich menu. The hearty combo of meat and beans fills your belly, and the roasted peppers, onions, and tomatoes provide immune-boosting doses of vitamins A and C. Pair with a Sammie for a filling lunch with an all-star nutritional profile.

Red Lobster

A- Like a lot of chain restaurants, Red Lobster was slow to offer up its nutritional secrets, refusing to tell consumers what, exactly, they were eating. This past year, however, the chain relented—and they deserve credit for doing so. Turns out that with a strong roster of low-calorie, high-protein fish and seafood entrées, plus a number of healthy sides, Red Lobster has earned the distinction of being America's healthiest chain restaurant.

SURVIVAL STRATEGY
Avoid calorie-heavy Cajun sauces, combo dishes, and anything labeled "crispy." And tell the waiter to keep those biscuits for himself. You'll never go wrong with simple broiled or grilled fish and a vegetable side.

Eat This

Blackened Mahi Mahi

with mashed potatoes and asparagus

685 calories
14.5 g fat (5.5 g saturated)
1,570 mg sodium

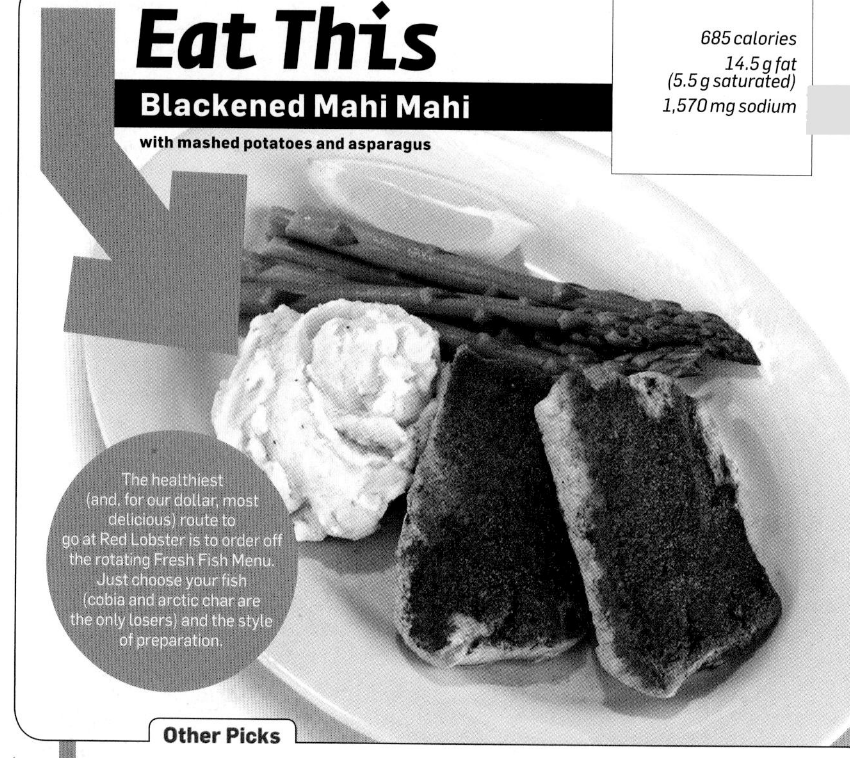

The healthiest (and, for our dollar, most delicious) route to go at Red Lobster is to order off the rotating Fresh Fish Menu. Just choose your fish (cobia and arctic char are the only losers) and the style of preparation.

Other Picks

Center-Cut NY Strip Steak
480 calories
26 g fat (11 g saturated)
820 mg sodium

Live Maine Lobster
(1¼ lb, steamed)
45 calories
0.5 g fat
350 mg sodium

Chilled Jumbo Shrimp Cocktail
120 calories
1 g fat
590 mg sodium

Not That!

Maui Lau Shrimp and Salmon

with rice pilaf and broccoli

1,015 calories
19.5 g fat (4 g saturated)
3,000 mg sodium

The shrimp and salmon by themselves have 790 calories and more than 2,000 milligrams of sodium—hardly the type of healthy eating you expect from 2 of the finest sources of protein out there.

Other Passes

Steak Lobster-and-Shrimp Oscar

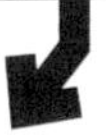

990 calories
60 g fat (26 g saturated)
2,410 mg sodium

North Pacific King Crab Legs **(steamed)**

390 calories
3 g fat
3,570 mg sodium

Crispy Calamari and Vegetables

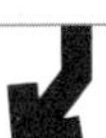

1,520 calories
98 g fat (12 g saturated)
3,060 mg sodium

WEAPON OF MASS DESTRUCTION
Traditional Lobsterita

890 calories
183 g carbohydrates

Think a little predinner libation won't hurt? Think again. By the time you take your first bite of cheddar biscuit, you'll have consumed nearly half a day's worth of calories—almost entirely from added sugar.

HIDDEN DANGER
Cheddar Bay Biscuits

Just because Red Lobster gives them away doesn't mean they're free; these biscuits have a caloric price that can bankrupt an otherwise decent meal. Do your table a favor and ask your server to cut you off after one round.

150 calories
8 g fat
(2.5 g saturated)
250 mg sodium

Romano's Macaroni Gr

D+

This Italian spot serves some of the worst appetizers in the country, offers just a handful of dinner entrées with fewer than 800 calories, and hosts no fewer than 40 menu items that contain more than a full day's sodium intake. But we will give credit to Macaroni Grill for the recent additions of healthier fare like the spiedinis and the 525-calorie Seafood Linguine.

SURVIVAL STRATEGY

Take advantage of the build-your-own-pasta option. Ask for the marinara over a bed of the restaurant's whole wheat penne, and then top it with grilled chicken and steamed vegetables. If you stick to the regular menu, choose the Pollo Magro, the Capellini Pomodoro, or the Shrimp Portofino.

Eat This

Chicken Cannelloni

(lunch portion)

590 calories
29 g fat (17 g saturated)
1,710 mg sodium

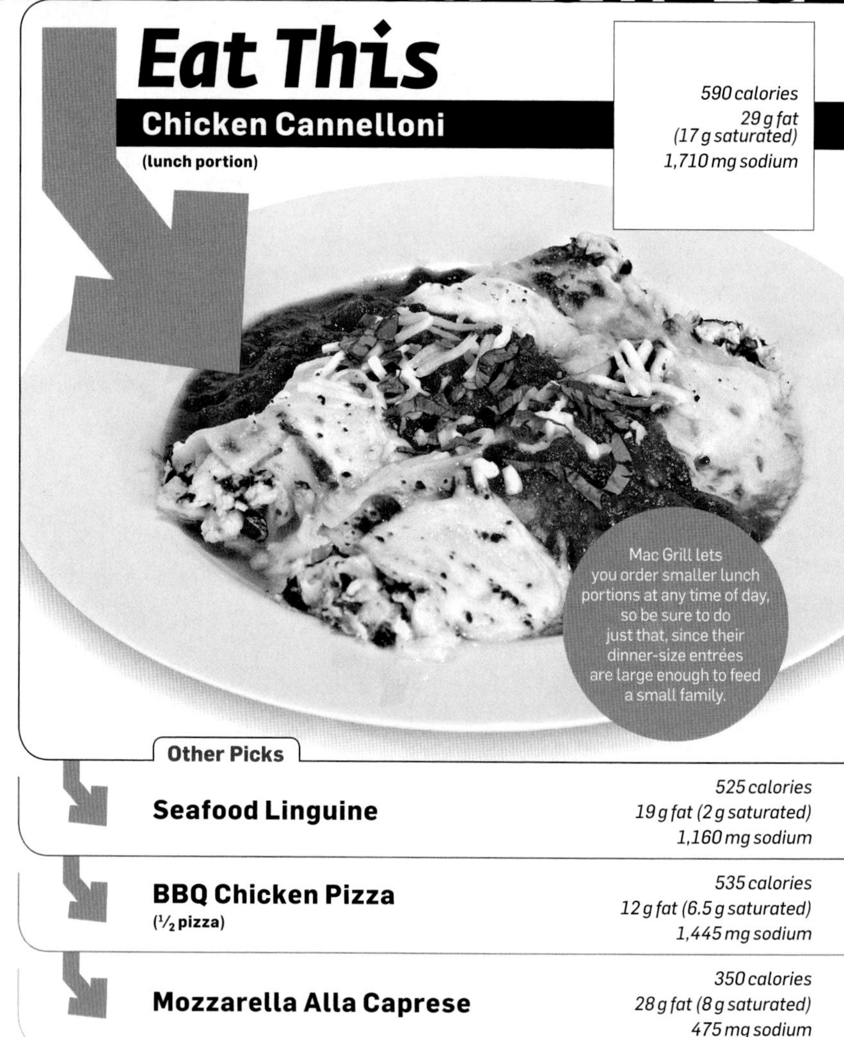

Mac Grill lets you order smaller lunch portions at any time of day, so be sure to do just that, since their dinner-size entrées are large enough to feed a small family.

Other Picks

Seafood Linguine

525 calories
19 g fat (2 g saturated)
1,160 mg sodium

BBQ Chicken Pizza
(½ pizza)

535 calories
12 g fat (6.5 g saturated)
1,445 mg sodium

Mozzarella Alla Caprese

350 calories
28 g fat (8 g saturated)
475 mg sodium

Not That!

Pasta Milano

1,530 calories
98 g fat (44 g saturated)
4,350 mg sodium

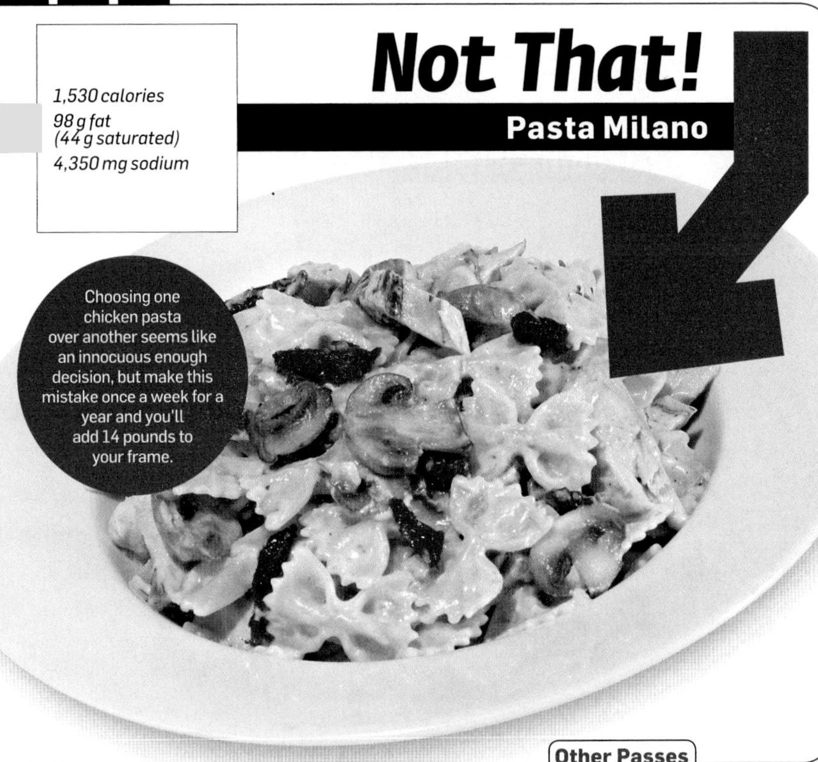

Choosing one chicken pasta over another seems like an innocuous enough decision, but make this mistake once a week for a year and you'll add 14 pounds to your frame.

Other Passes

Lobster Ravioli

1,350 calories
84 g fat (40 g saturated)
2,320 mg sodium

Pesto Chicken Pizza (½ pizza)

900 calories
49.5 g fat (15.5 g saturated)
1,395 mg sodium

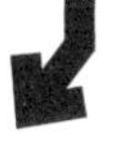

Mozzarella Fritta

900 calories
71 g fat (18 g saturated)
1,620 mg sodium

WEAPON OF MASS DESTRUCTION Parmesan-Crusted Sole (dinner portion)

2,190 calories
141 g fat (58 g saturated)
2,980 mg sodium

This meal posts some grim numbers: more than a day's worth of sodium, more than a day's worth of calories, and as much saturated fat as you should eat in 3 full days. Goes to show that even fish can be a rotten meal when exposed to the combined forces of oil-soaked breading and viscous buttery topping.

MENU DECODER

SPIEDINI: Literally "skewer" in Italian, this new addition to the Macaroni Grill menu is a welcome change from the seemingly endless parade of bloated bowls of pasta and misleading salads. The Jumbo Shrimp version has just 294 calories, making it the best item on the menu.

Ruby Tuesday

D+

The chain earned its infamy off a hearty selection of hamburgers. The problem is, they average 76 grams of fat apiece—more than enough to exceed your recommended daily limit. Even the veggie and turkey burgers have more than 900 calories! The menu is rounded out with appetizers that hover around 1,000 calories, a cadre of high-impact entrées (like potpie and ribs), and a selection of salads that are just as bad.

SURVIVAL STRATEGY
Solace lies in the 3 S's: steak, seafood, and sides. Sirloin, salmon, and shrimp all make for relatively innocuous eating, especially when paired with one of Ruby Tuesday's half-dozen healthy sides, such as mashed cauliflower and baby green beans.

Eat This

Peppercorn Mushroom Sirloin

414 calories
18 g fat
10 g carbohydrates

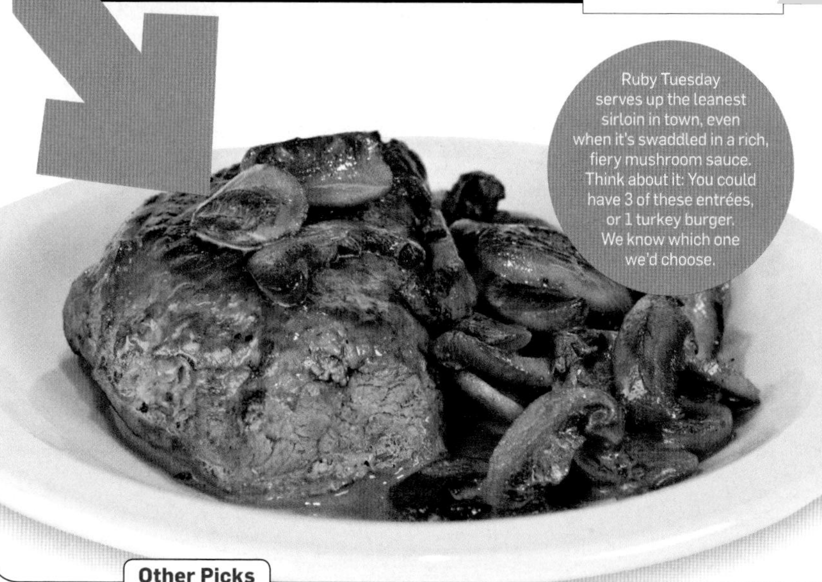

Ruby Tuesday serves up the leanest sirloin in town, even when it's swaddled in a rich, fiery mushroom sauce. Think about it: You could have 3 of these entrées, or 1 turkey burger. We know which one we'd choose.

Other Picks

Chicken Bella
387 calories
17 g fat
6 g carbohydrates

White Bean Chicken Chili
318 calories
11 g fat
29 g carbohydrates

Jumbo Lump Crab Cakes
272 calories
16 g fat
12 g carbohydrates

1,130 calories
68 g fat
62 g carbohydrates

Not That!

Avocado Turkey Burger

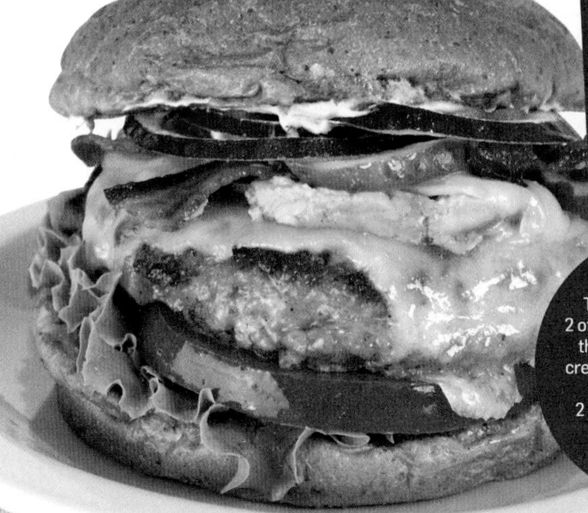

Read it and weep. Turkey and avacado—2 of the healthiest foods on the planet—conspire to create a single burger with more calories than 2 Big Macs and more fat than 8 scoops of Breyers ice cream.

Other Passes

1,167 calories
55 g fat
90 g carbohydrates

Chicken & Broccoli Pasta

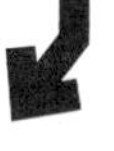

403 calories
29 g fat
21 g carbohydrates

Broccoli Cheese Soup

1,416 calories
80 g fat
80 g carbohydrates

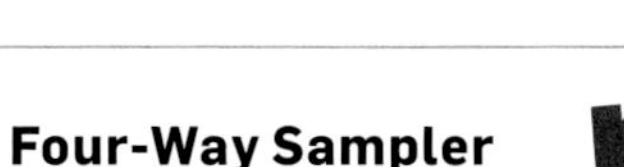

Four-Way Sampler

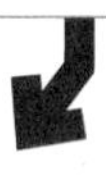

SMART SIDES

Creamy Mashed Cauliflower

136 calories
8 g fat
9 g carbohydrates

Like broccoli and brussels sprouts, cauliflower contains an organic compound called sinigrin, which has been shown to help kill off tumor cells. Plus, when you order the Creamy Mashed Cauliflower, you don't have to worry about accidentally getting one of Ruby's less-forgiving sides—like the 668-calorie Side Loaded Baked Potato.

LITTLE TRICK

The wrap is redeemed at Ruby's! Order your next burger with a wrap instead of a bun and save up to 339 calorie and 29 grams of fat.

BAD BREEDS

Minis

Don't let the name fool you—there's nothing mini about Ruby Tuesday's sliders. The best you can do on this part of the menu is 856 calories and 47 grams of fat (for the Mini Trio).

Sbarro

F Please welcome Sbarro to the list of restaurants that refuse to disclose their food facts. As of this writing, the nutritional information on Sbarro's Web site is frozen in a permanent state of "under construction." Sounds like a pizza pie to the face of anyone who cares about healthy eating. We'll be happy to revise that grade once Sbarro cleans up the scaffolding and jackhammers and reveals a site notable for its nutritional transparency. For now, proceed with caution.

SURVIVAL STRATEGY
Sbarro serves up massive New York–style slices, so keep it to one and be sure to make it of the thin-crust variety. Round out the meal with a side of fruit or a tomato-and-cucumber salad.

Eat This

Cheese New York Style Thin Pizza

*460 calories**

*Sbarro refuses to offer full nutritional information for their menu items.

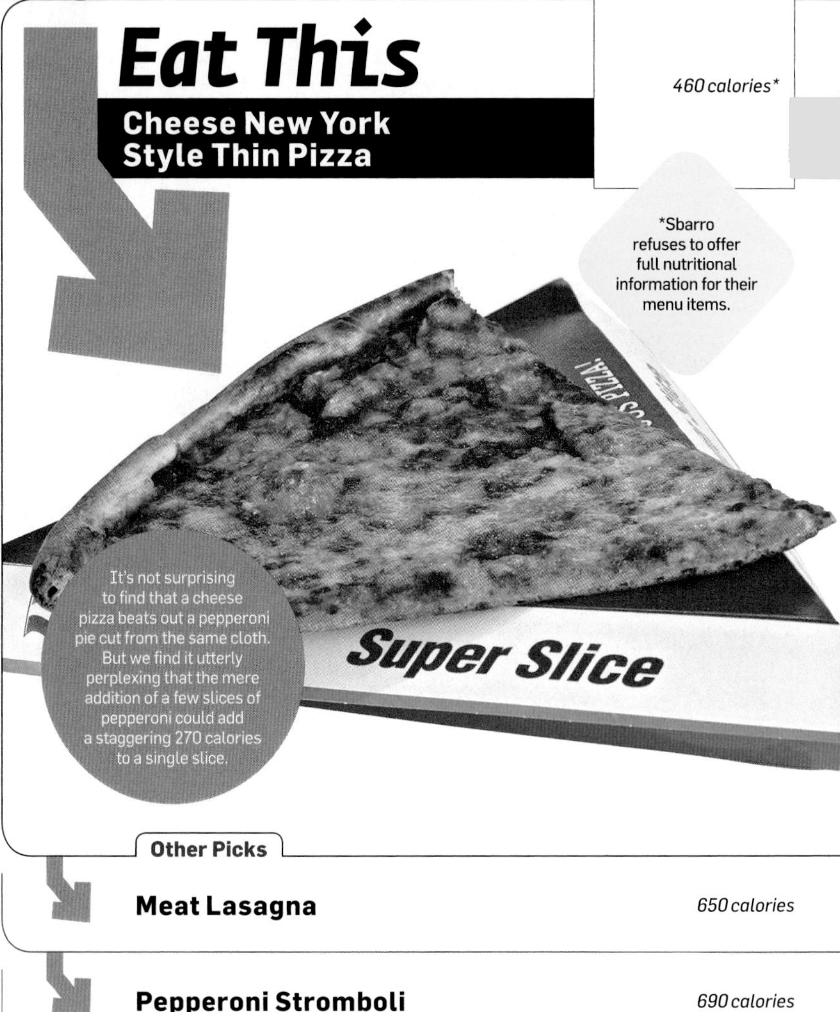

It's not surprising to find that a cheese pizza beats out a pepperoni pie cut from the same cloth. But we find it utterly perplexing that the mere addition of a few slices of pepperoni could add a staggering 270 calories to a single slice.

Other Picks

Meat Lasagna *650 calories*

Pepperoni Stromboli *690 calories*

730 calories*

Not That!

Pepperoni New York Style Thin Pizza

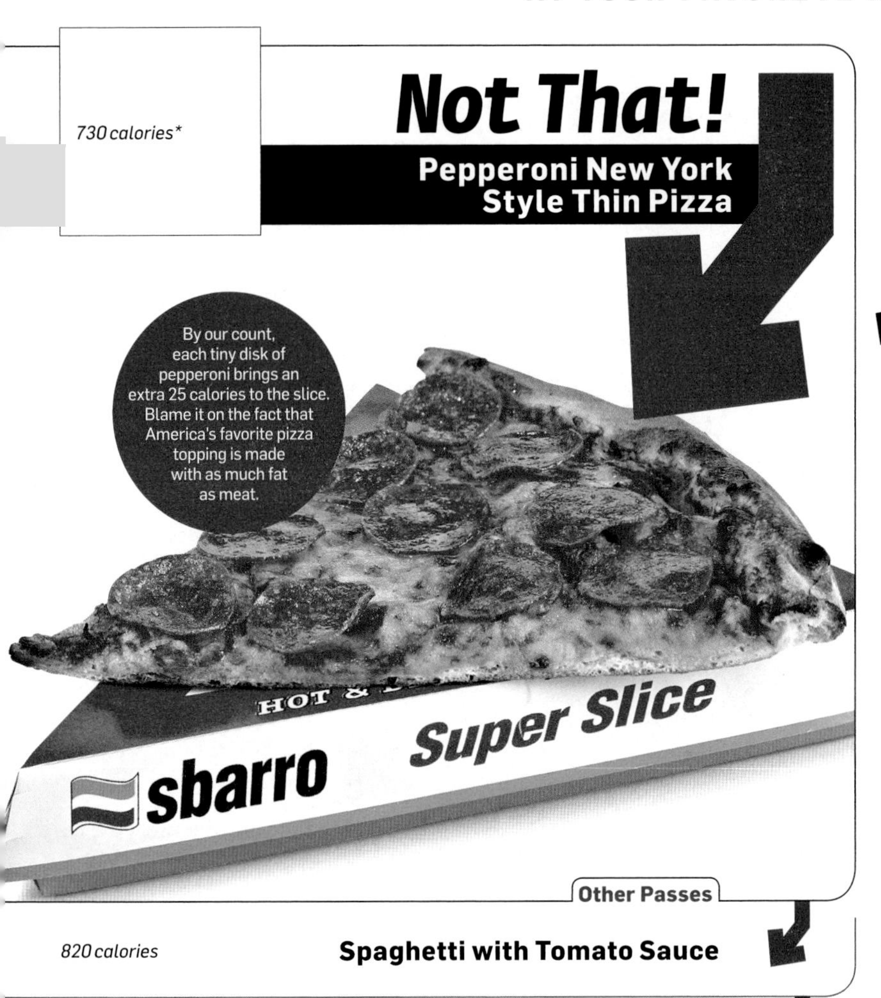

By our count, each tiny disk of pepperoni brings an extra 25 calories to the slice. Blame it on the fact that America's favorite pizza topping is made with as much fat as meat.

Other Passes

820 calories **Spaghetti with Tomato Sauce**

890 calories **Pepperoni Stuffed Pizza**

GUILTY PLEASURE

Meatballs

140 calories

At place like Sbarro's, it's the little victories that matter. In this case, belly-filling meatballs pack 40 fewer calories than boring bread sticks.

FOOD MYTH

Blotting the grease off pizza is the best way to make it healthy.

Obsessive blotting might cut 2 or 3 grams of fat, but the decision to blot (or not) pales next to the decisions you make regarding crust type and toppings. Want to make a healthier pizza? Choose the thinnest crust possible and top it with lean meats like ham and chicken, instead of fatty ones like sausage and pepperoni.

SMART SIDES

Stringbean & Tomato Salad

100 calories

This salad ditches the bowl of lifeless lettuce for brightly colored tomatoes and green beans. Taken together, they provide a big dose of vitamin A and manganese, which promotes good cell communication.

Smoothie King

B- Smoothie King, the older and smaller of the two smoothie titans, suffers from portion problems. The smallest adult option is 20 ounces, which makes it that much harder to keep the calories from sugar remotely reasonable. Added sugars and honey don't make things any better. (Isn't fruit sweet enough?) That being said, the menu boasts a number of great all-fruit smoothies, light options, and an excellent portfolio of smoothie enhancers.

SURVIVAL STRATEGY
Favor the Stay Healthy and Trim Down portions of the menu, and be sure to stick to 20-ounce smoothies made from nothing but real fruit. No matter what you do, avoid anything listed under the "Indulge" section.

Eat This

Mocha Coffee Smoothie

260 calories
2 g fat (0 g saturated)
36 g sugars

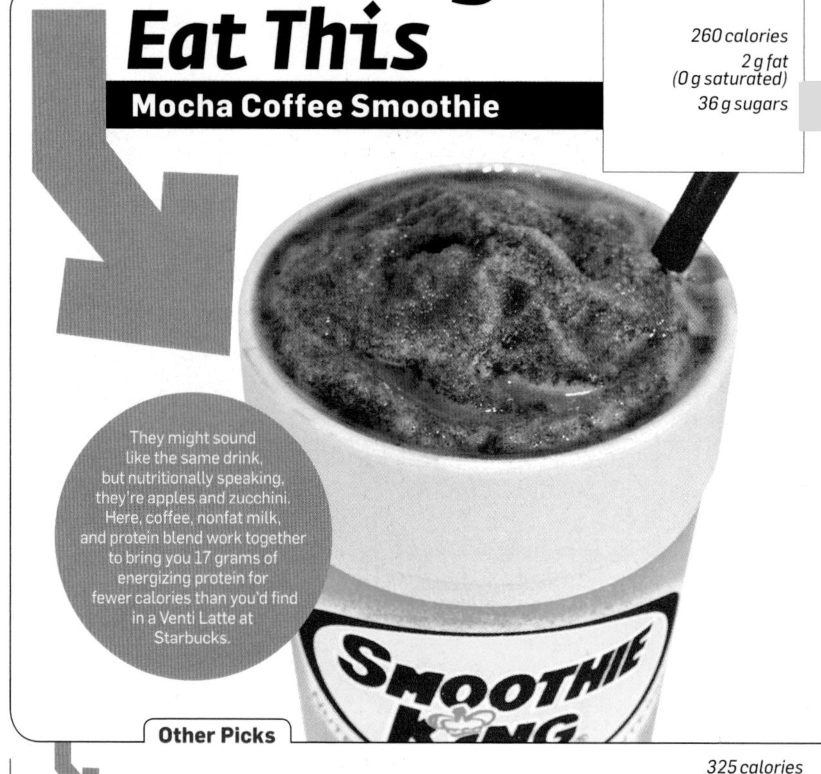

They might sound like the same drink, but nutritionally speaking, they're apples and zucchini. Here, coffee, nonfat milk, and protein blend work together to bring you 17 grams of energizing protein for fewer calories than you'd find in a Venti Latte at Starbucks.

Other Picks

Blueberry Heaven	*325 calories* *1 g fat* *64 g sugars*
High Protein Smoothie—Pineapple	*320 calories* *9 g fat (1 g saturated)* *23 g sugars*
Pineapple Pleasure	*280 calories* *0 g fat* *61 g sugars*

Not That!

Vanilla Mo'Cuccino

551 calories
14 g fat (8 g saturated)
85 g sugars

Wonder where all that sugar comes from? The Mo'Cuccino line replaces milk with ice cream, making this drink more akin to a milk shake than a smoothie or a coffee drink. Ask to "Make It Skinny," and the sugar is sliced to 39 grams while the drink shrinks by 200 calories.

Other Passes

Cranberry Supreme

554 calories
1 g fat
96 g sugars

The Hulk—Strawberry

1,044 calories
35 g fat (16 g saturated)
120 g sugars

Pina Colada Island

600 calories
10 g fat (8 g saturated)
98 g sugars

WEAPON OF MASS DESTRUCTION
Grape Expectations II
(40 oz)

1,096 calories
250 g sugars

The most appalling part of this drink is that you'll find it under the "Snack Right" section of the menu. If you consider a beverage with as much sugar as 53 Oreo cookies to be smart snacking, then you need to have your waistline examined.

MENU DECODER

TURBINADO: One of the 2 sweeteners Smoothie King uses (the other being honey), this raw sugar is made from evaporated cane juice. Don't be fooled by the fancy name, though: It's just as bad for you as normal sugar. Order your smoothie "skinny" and they'll leave it out, eliminating 100 calories from a 20-ounce smoothie.

Starbucks

B+

Starbucks' signature line of drinks typically involves injecting massive loads of sugary syrup and milk into espresso, making 500-calorie concoctions too common for comfort. Plus, their selection of muffins and pastries leaves much to be desired. That said, Starbucks has started offering more nutritious items (like oatmeal and Vivannos), specialty drinks made with skim milk, and in-store nutrition pamphlets.

SURVIVAL STRATEGY
There's no beating a regular cup of joe or unsweetened tea, but if you need a specialty fix, stick with skim milk, sugar-free syrup, and no whipped cream. As for food, go with the Perfect Oatmeal or a Spinach, Roasted Tomato, Feta & Egg White Wrap.

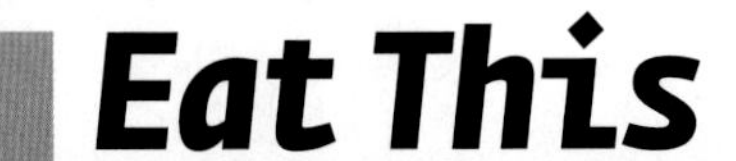

Eat This

Bacon, Gouda, and Egg Frittata

on artisan roll

380 calories
20 g fat
(8 g saturated)
1,050 mg sodium

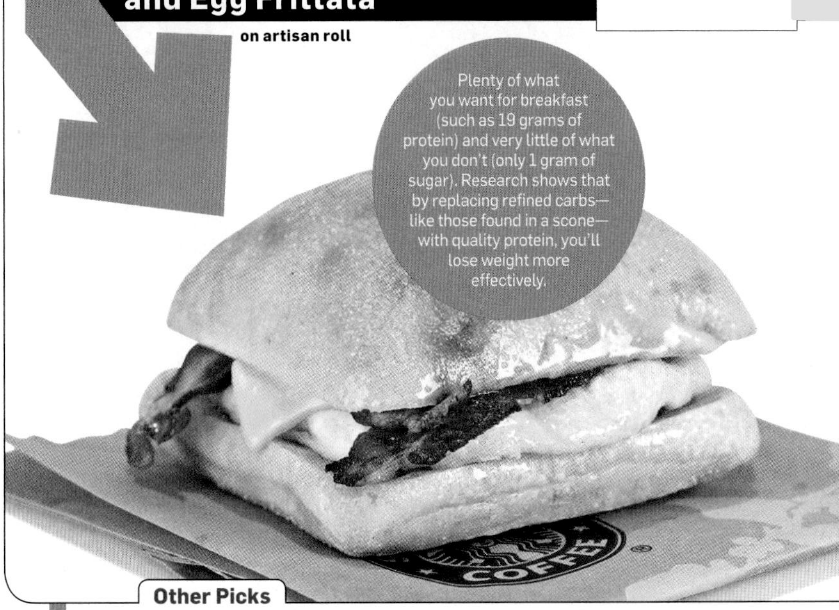

Plenty of what you want for breakfast (such as 19 grams of protein) and very little of what you don't (only 1 gram of sugar). Research shows that by replacing refined carbs—like those found in a scone—with quality protein, you'll lose weight more effectively.

Other Picks

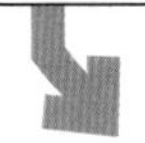

Strawberry Banana Vivanno
(2%)

280 calories
1.5 g fat (1 g saturated)
41 g sugars

Grande Caffe Americano

15 calories
0 g fat
0 g sugars

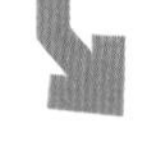

Grande Iced Coffee
with mocha syrup

115 calories
0.5 g fat
24 g sugars

Not That!

Blueberry Scone

460 calories
22 g fat (12 g saturated, 0.5 g trans)
420 mg sodium

With 17 grams of sugar, this harmless-looking scone has twice as much sugar as you'll find in a chocolate doughnut. And it only has 2 grams of fiber to offset that sugar, so you'll be looking at a massive blood sugar spike.

Other Passes

Venti Strawberries and Crème Frappuccino with whipped cream

580 calories
15 g fat (8 g saturated)
78 g sugars

Grande 2% Caffe Latte

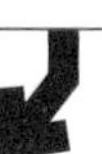

190 calories
7 g fat (4.5 g saturated)
17 g sugars

Grande Java Chip Frappuccino

340 calories
8 g fat (5 g saturated)
52 g sugars

LITTLE TRICK

Personalize your own master brew. Start with black coffee, a few espresso shots, or brewed tea. Add one of a dozen sugar-free syrups, steamed milk, and protein fiber boost and you'll have a first-rate drink for under 150 calories.

STEALTH HEALTH FOOD

Spinach, Roasted Tomato, Feta & Egg White Wrap

270 calories
9 g fat (3.5 g saturated)
1140 mg sodium

You might not think of Starbucks as a great lunch destination, but here's why you should start: This wrap has fewer calories than most of their coffee drinks, contains a massive dose of vitamin A from the tomatoes and spinach, carries a load of protein from the eggs, and is laced with an impressive 8 grams of fiber. Lunch doesn't get much better than that.

Subway

A-

If Jared was able to shed 245 pounds on his own Subway diet, then surely you can find a decent meal here to keep your gut in check. But beware of what researchers call the "health halo": Patrons who believe they're eating in a healthy place tend to reward themselves with extra cheese, mayonnaise, and soda, none of which would have helped Jared lose a single pound. Avoid the halo shine, and you'll be fine at Subway.

SURVIVAL STRATEGY
Trouble lurks in 3 areas at Subway: 1) hot subs, 2) footlongs, 3) chips and soda. Stick to 6-inch cold subs made with ham, turkey, roast beef, or chicken. Load up on veggies, and be extra careful about your condiment choices.

Eat This

Turkey Breast & Black Forest Ham Sandwich

305 calories
4.5 g fat
(1 g saturated)
1,395 mg sodium

(6", on 9-grain wheat bread with lettuce, tomatoes, onions, green peppers, pickles, olives, and mustard)

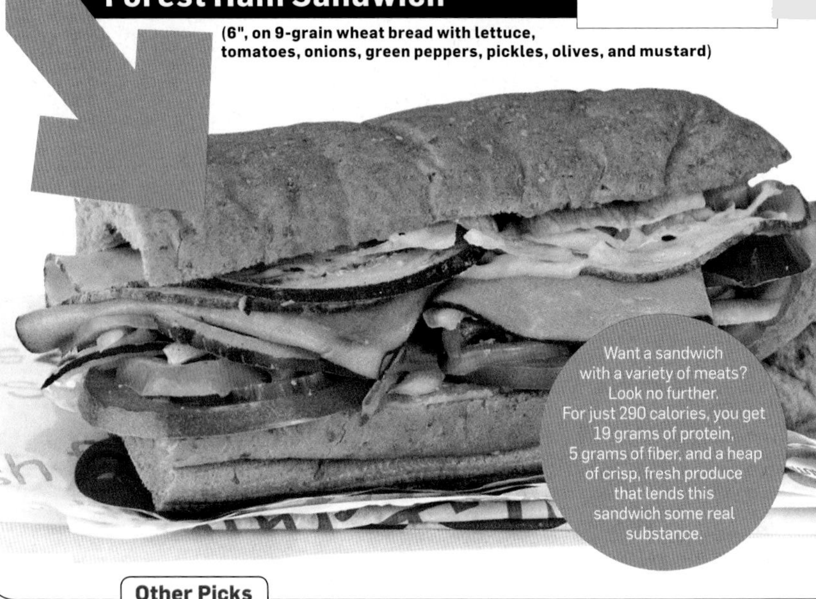

Want a sandwich with a variety of meats? Look no further. For just 290 calories, you get 19 grams of protein, 5 grams of fiber, and a heap of crisp, fresh produce that lends this sandwich some real substance.

Other Picks

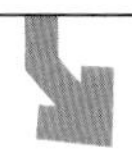

BLT
(6")

360 calories
13 g fat (6 g saturated)
990 mg sodium

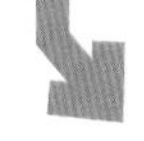

Steak & Cheese
(6")

390 calories
10 g fat (4.5 g saturated)
1,370 mg sodium

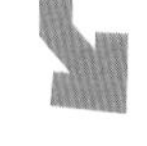

Rosemary Chicken and Dumpling Soup

90 calories
1.5 g fat (0.5 g saturated)
810 mg sodium

530 calories
29 g fat (8 g saturated, 0.5 g trans)
1,670 mg sodium

Not That!

Cold Cut Combo

(6", on 9-grain wheat bread with lettuce, tomatoes, onions, green peppers, pickles, olives, and mayo)

Just because the bologna, ham, and salami used to make this sandwich are all made with turkey doesn't mean they're lean. They pack more calories and sodium than pork ham.

Other Passes

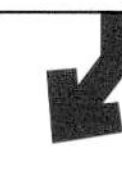

Tuna Sandwich (6")

540 calories
30 g fat (6 g saturated, 0.5 g trans)
1,070 mg sodium

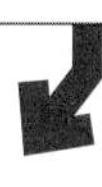

Meatball Marinara with provolone (6")

630 calories
27 g fat (11 g saturated, 1 g trans)
1,785 mg sodium

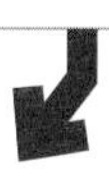

Wild Rice with Chicken Soup

230 calories
11 g fat (3.5 g saturated)
900 mg sodium

CONDIMENT CATASTROPHE

Don't be fooled by the flashy signs touting the subs with "6 grams of fat or less." Subway is nutritionally shrewd, so when they post calorie, fat, and sodium info at their stores, it's in the most flattering light possible: on wheat bread, with nothing but vegetables on the sandwich. Add mayo, cheese, oil or build your sandwich on a different loaf, and you'll need to tack on somewhere between 100 and 300 additional calories.

GUILTY PLEASURE

Footlong Roast Beef Sandwich

580 calories
10 g fat (4.5 g saturated)
1,800 mg sodium

As footlong sandwiches go, this can't be beat. It's relatively low in calories and fat, and it has the least amount of sodium of any footlong meat sandwich at Subway.

LITTLE TRICK

The best cheese at Subway? Swiss. Two triangles have just 30 milligrams of sodium, versus 200 milligrams in the American.

T.G.I. Friday's

F We salute Friday's for one thing and one thing only, and that's their smaller-portions menu. The option to order smaller servings ought to be the new model, dethroning the dogmatic bigger-is-better principle that dominates chain restaurants. But no matter how small they shrink the entrées, we're still forced to fail this chain due to their strict policy of nutritional secrecy.

SURVIVAL STRATEGY

Danger is waiting in every crack and corner of Friday's menu. In fact, there are only 4 entrées with fewer than 800 calories on the menu. Your best bets? The 400-calorie Shrimp Key West, the 480-calorie Dragonfire Chicken, or finding another restaurant entirely.

Eat This

Dragonfire Chicken

*480 calories**

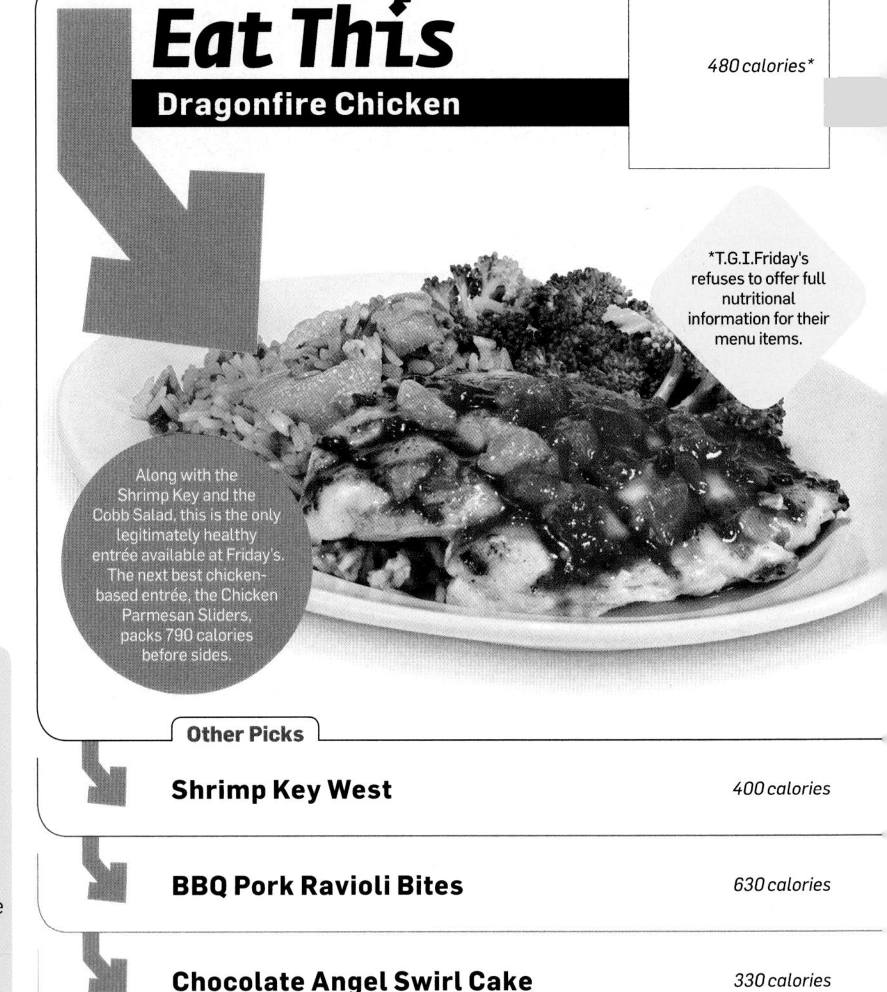

*T.G.I.Friday's refuses to offer full nutritional information for their menu items.

Along with the Shrimp Key and the Cobb Salad, this is the only legitimately healthy entrée available at Friday's. The next best chicken-based entrée, the Chicken Parmesan Sliders, packs 790 calories before sides.

Other Picks

Shrimp Key West — *400 calories*

BBQ Pork Ravioli Bites — *630 calories*

Chocolate Angel Swirl Cake — *330 calories*

1,360 calories*

Not That!

Pecan-Crusted Chicken Salad

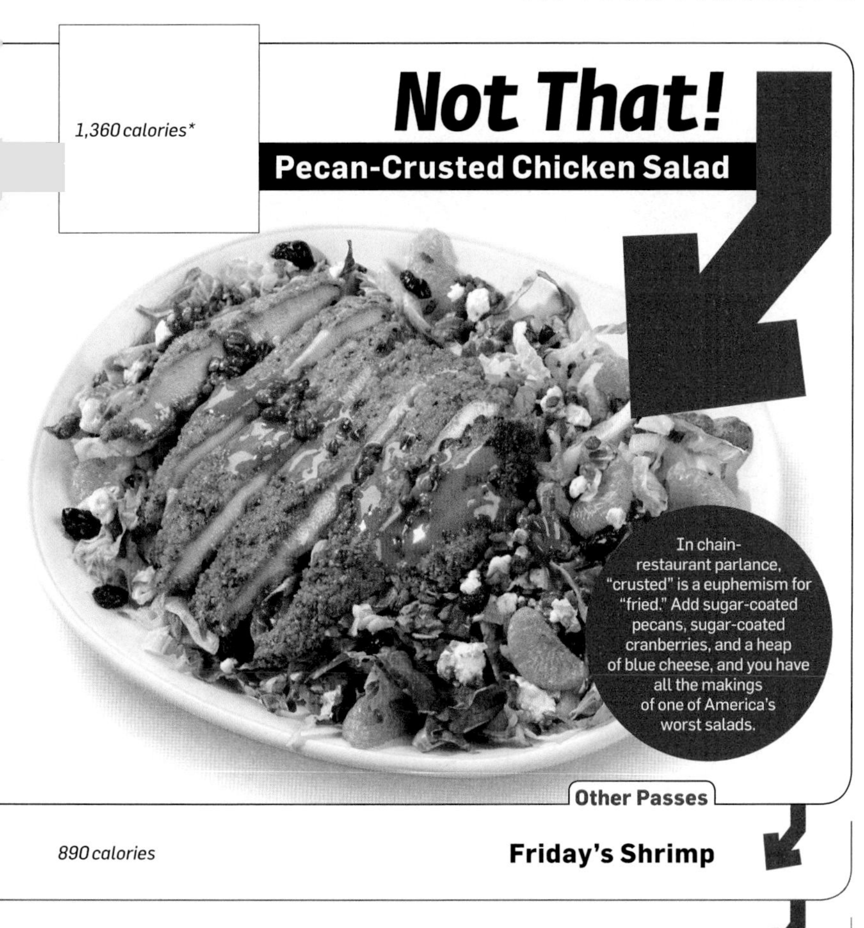

In chain-restaurant parlance, "crusted" is a euphemism for "fried." Add sugar-coated pecans, sugar-coated cranberries, and a heap of blue cheese, and you have all the makings of one of America's worst salads.

Other Passes

890 calories — **Friday's Shrimp**

860 calories — **Green Bean Fries**

1,500 calories — **Brownie Obsession**

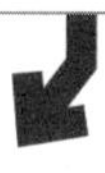

WEAPON OF MASS DESTRUCTION
Loaded Potato Skins

*2,270 calories**

Nothing on the menu indicates that these are anything but your average potato skins, but the calorie count puts them among the worst foods in America. Eating a whole order is like starting your meal with 4 Big Macs. Even if you split these with 3 friends, you're still taking in a meal's worth of calories—*before* you move on to your meal.

GUILTY PLEASURE

Cobb Salad

590 calories

A salad may seem a strange fit for a Guilty Pleasure, but considering that every other entrée-size bowl of greens save one at Friday's has more than 900 calories, this is truly a rare find. Bacon, blue cheese, avocado, and grilled chicken pack plenty of substance—and decadence—into the bowl, but for fewer than a third of the calories found in the Santa Fe.

Taco Bell

B Here's the good news: The next time you run for the border, you don't have to run all the way home to burn off the calories. Taco Bell combines two things with bad nutritional reputations—Mexican food and fast food—but provides plenty of ways for you to keep your meal under 500 calories. The best way to do it is to stick with the Fresco Menu, where no single item exceeds 350 calories.

SURVIVAL STRATEGY
Stay away from Grilled Stuft Burritos, food served in a bowl, and anything prepared with multiple "layers"—they're all trouble. Instead, order any 2 of the following: crunchy tacos, bean burritos, or anything on the Fresco menu.

Eat This

Fresco Ranchero Chicken Soft Tacos (2)

340 calories
8 g fat
(3 g saturated)
1,460 mg sodium

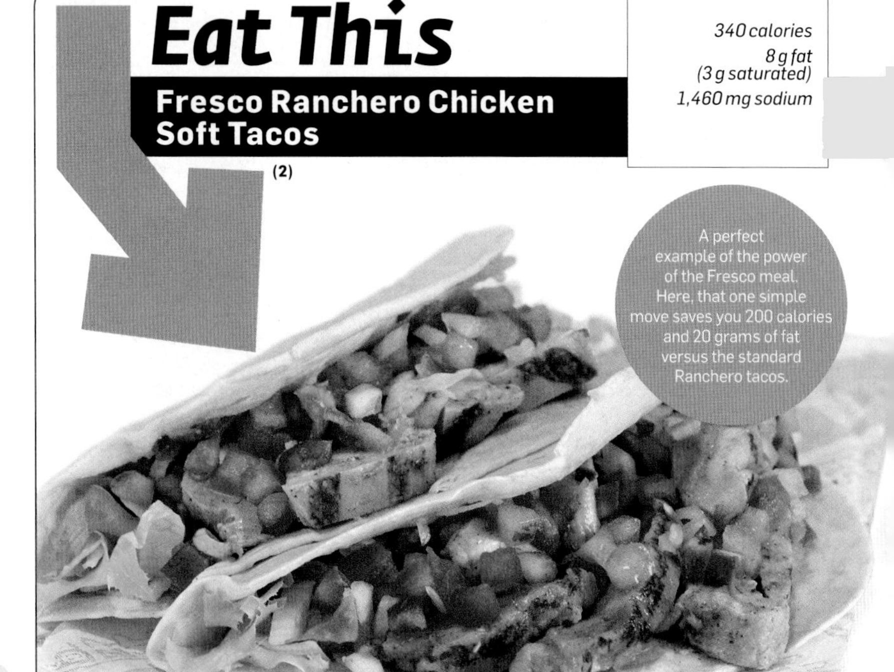

A perfect example of the power of the Fresco meal. Here, that one simple move saves you 200 calories and 20 grams of fat versus the standard Ranchero tacos.

Other Picks

Fresco Fiesta Chicken Burrito
340 calories
8 g fat (2.5 g saturated)
1,240 mg sodium

Steak Taquitos
310 calories
11 g fat (5 g saturated)
930 mg sodium

Pintos 'n Cheese
160 calories
6 g fat (3 g saturated, 0.5 g trans)
670 mg sodium

640 calories
23 g fat (7 g saturated)
2,160 mg sodium

Not That!

Grilled Stuft Burrito

(chicken)

Taco Bell's popular Stuft burritos are among the worst items on its extensive menu. This one suffers from a serious salt issue, with close to a full day's sodium allotment stuffed into the toasty tortilla.

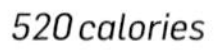

Other Passes

820 calories
43 g fat (10 g saturated, 1.5 g trans)
1,740 mg sodium

Fiesta Taco Salad

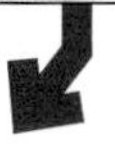

520 calories
28 g fat (12 g saturated, 1 g trans)
1,300 mg sodium

Steak Quesadilla

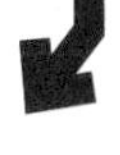

270 calories
16 g fat (2.5 g saturated)
840 mg sodium

Cheesy Fiesta Potatoes

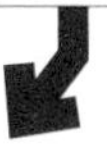

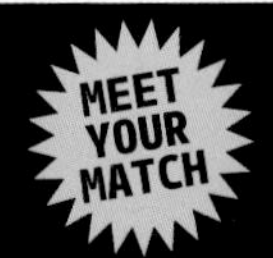

Chipotle Steak Fully Loaded Taco Salad
(960 calories)
=
6 Fresco Crunchy Tacos

GUILTY PLEASURE

Cinnamon Twists

170 calories
7 g fat
10 g sugars

Rare is the restaurant dessert with fewer than 200 calories. These twists, with less sugar than your average bowl of breakfast cereal and a good dose of insulin-stabilizing cinnamon, make a fitting end to a light meal.

1,474

Amount of sodium, in milligrams, in the average burrito at Taco Bell. (That's 61% of your recommended daily intake.)

Tim Horton's

B+ While Tim brings few nutritional superstars to the table, he also manages to avoid the massive calorie land mines that dot nearly every other restaurant menu. In fact, the worst item on the menu is the 470-calorie Frosted Cinnamon Roll. Even though the calorie counts are low, the menu is still littered with refined carbohydrates, from doughnuts to muffins to sugary coffee drinks. Choose wisely.

SURVIVAL STRATEGY

More than ever, it's about the quality of your calories than the quantity. Your best bet at breakfast is the fruit-topped yogurt or brown sugar oatmeal. For lunch, choose either 2 wraps or 1 sandwich and a zero-calorie beverage, and you'll be on solid ground.

Eat This

Apple Fritter Timbits

(4)

200 calories
6 g fat (4 g saturated)
220 g sugars

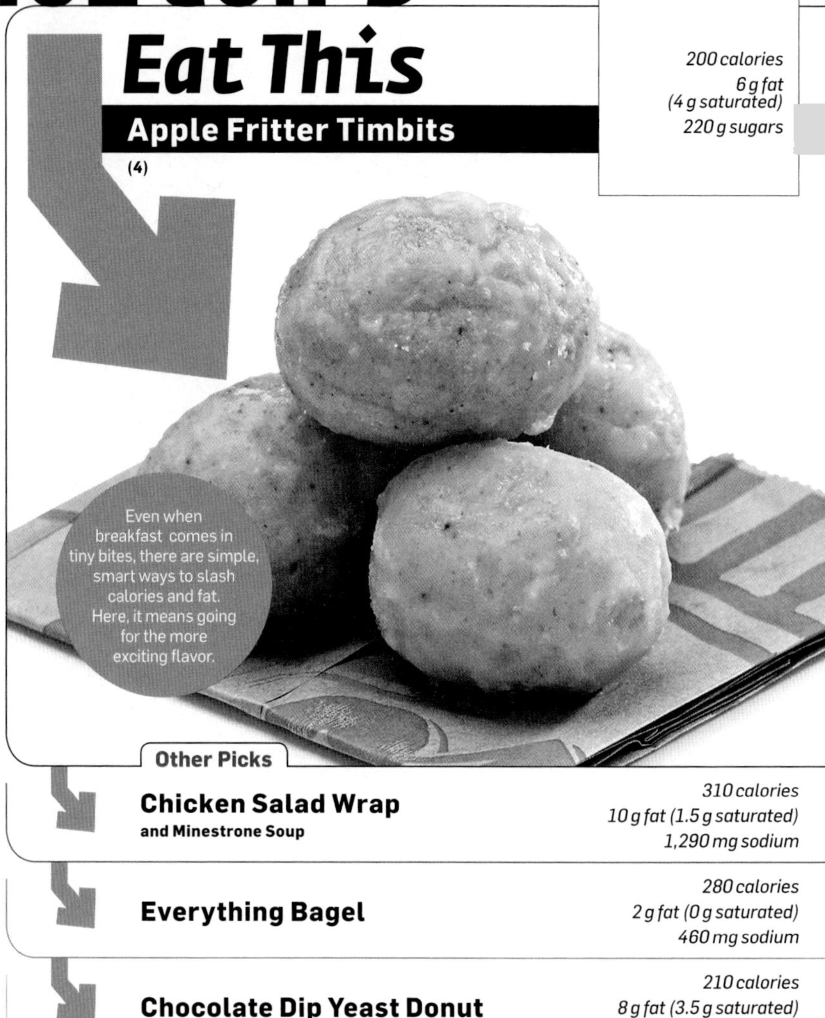

Even when breakfast comes in tiny bites, there are simple, smart ways to slash calories and fat. Here, it means going for the more exciting flavor.

Other Picks

Chicken Salad Wrap
and Minestrone Soup

310 calories
10 g fat (1.5 g saturated)
1,290 mg sodium

Everything Bagel

280 calories
2 g fat (0 g saturated)
460 mg sodium

Chocolate Dip Yeast Donut

210 calories
8 g fat (3.5 g saturated)
8 g sugars

280 calories
20 g fat
(10 g saturated)
240 mg sodium

Not That!

Old Fashioned Plain Timbits

(4)

If you're going to opt for cake-style Timbits, might as well go for the Chocolate Glazed bites, which contain the same amount of calories but with just half the fat. Plus, wouldn't you enjoy chocolate more anyway?

Other Passes

Toasted Chicken Club
440 calories
7 g fat (2.5 g saturated)
1,070 mg sodium

12 Grain Bagel
330 calories
9 g fat (1 g saturated)
580 mg sodium

Walnut Crunch Donut
360 calories
23 g fat (10 g saturated)
9 g sugars

HIDDEN DANGER

Whole Grain Raspberry Muffin

Don't be fooled by the whole grains; this muffin, with as much sugar as 7 Apple Fritter Timbits, is only marginally better for you than a cinnamon roll.

400 calories
17 g fat
(4 g saturated)
26 g sugars

GUILTY PLEASURE

Plain Croissant

200 calories
11 g fat (5 g saturated)

Take joy in the fact that a butter-rich croissant is actually a smarter order than a multigrain bagel or muffin.

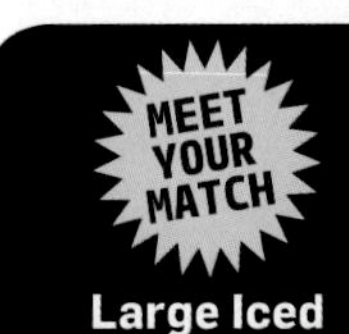

Large Iced Capp Original
(62 g sugars)

14 Chips Ahoy! Chocolate Chip Cookies

Uno Chicago Grill

D+

Uno stikes a curious (if not altogether healthy) balance between oversize sandwiches and burgers, lean grilled steaks and fish entrées, and one of the world's most calorie-dense foods, deep dish pizza, which Uno's invented. They may pride themselves on their nutritional transparency, but the only thing that's truly transparent is that there are far too many dishes here that pack 1,000 calories or more.

SURVIVAL STRATEGY

Stick with flatbread instead of deep-dish pizzas—this one move could save you more than 1,000 calories at a sitting. Beyond that, turn to the Smoke, Sizzle & Splash section of the menu for nutritional salvation.

Eat This

Barbecue Chicken Flatbread

(1/3 pizza)

320 calories
11 g fat (4.5 g saturated)
700 mg sodium

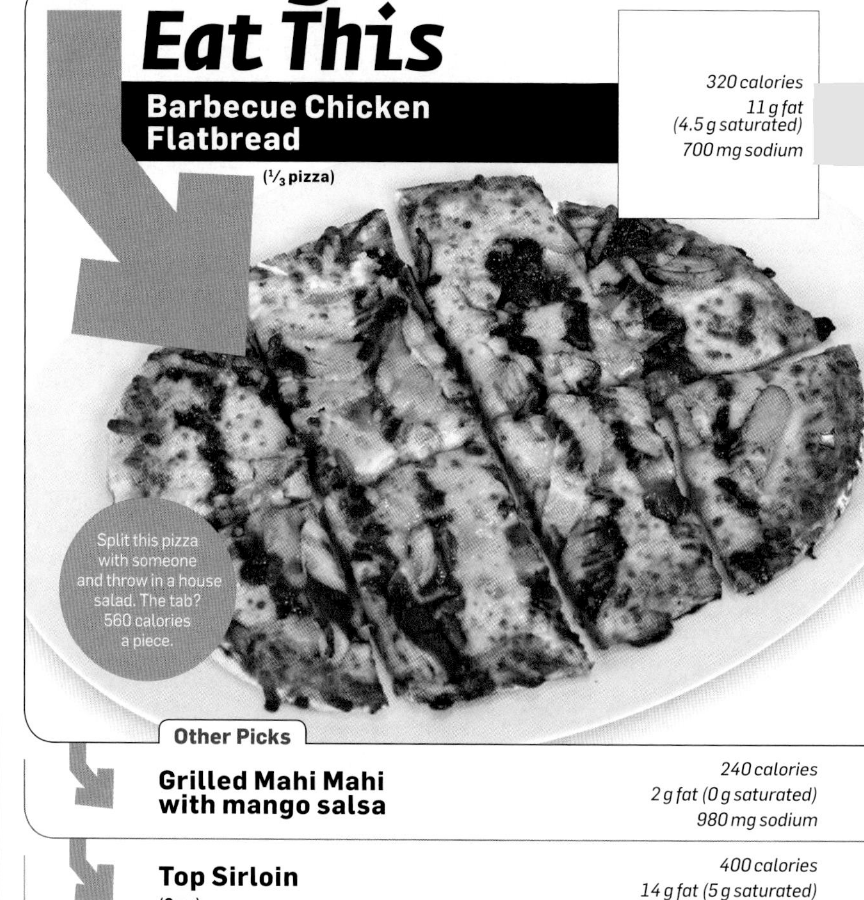

Split this pizza with someone and throw in a house salad. The tab? 560 calories a piece.

Other Picks

Grilled Mahi Mahi with mango salsa

240 calories
2 g fat (0 g saturated)
980 mg sodium

Top Sirloin
(8 oz)

400 calories
14 g fat (5 g saturated)
620 mg sodium

Penne Bolognese

760 calories
18 g fat (7 g saturated)
1,880 mg sodium

Not That!

Roasted Red Pepper and Chicken Deep Dish

(1/3 pizza)

680 calories
43 g fat (12 g saturated)
970 mg sodium

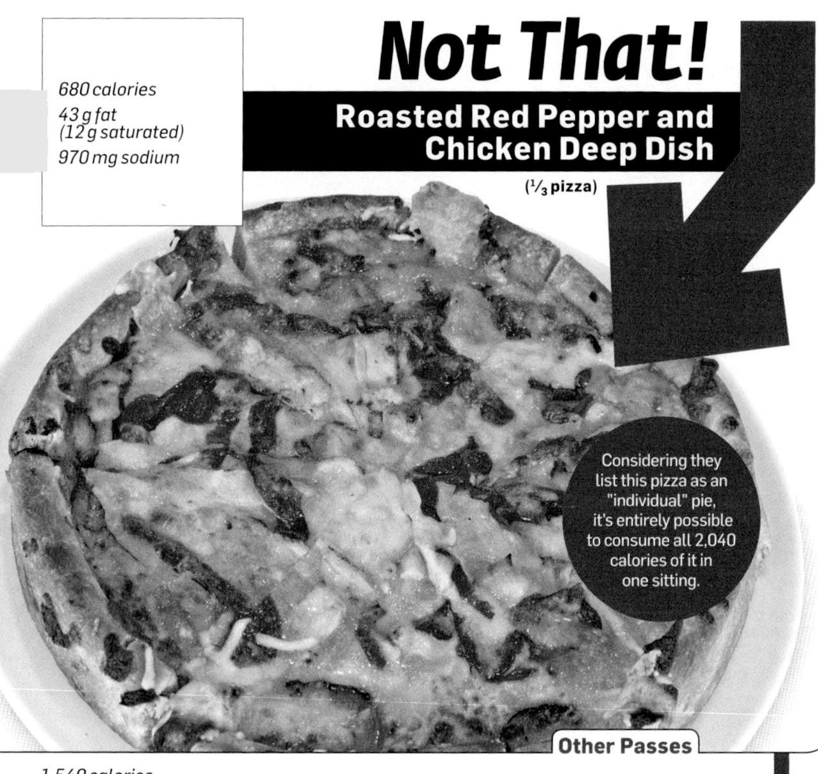

Considering they list this pizza as an "individual" pie, it's entirely possible to consume all 2,040 calories of it in one sitting.

Other Passes

Fisherman's Platter

1,540 calories
110 g fat (14 g saturated)
2,900 mg sodium

Cheddar Burger

1,180 calories
78 g fat (32 g saturated, 3 g trans)
1,840 mg sodium

Chicken Spinoccoli

1,340 calories
66 g fat (30 g saturated)
3,020 mg sodium

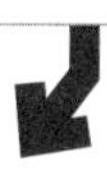

WEAPON OF MASS DESTRUCTION
Mega-Size Deep Dish Sundae

2,800 calories
136 g fat (72 g saturated)
272 g sugars

First rule of portion control: Never eat anything that can be described with a word like "mega." Even if you get 3 people to help you wolf this thing down, you'll still be responsible for 700 calories and 68 grams of sugar.

BAD BREED

Appetizers

Along with Chili's, this is the worst starters menu in America. Not 1 app has fewer than 800 calories, and 2 have more than 2,000. Skip straight to the main event.

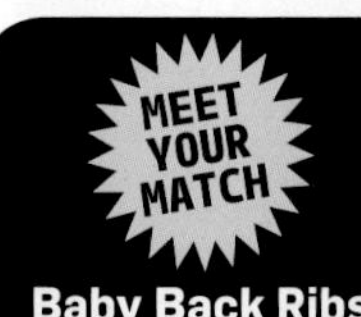

Baby Back Ribs
(110 g sugars)
=
9 bowls of Froot Loops

Wendy's

B+ Scoring a decent meal at Wendy's is just about as easy as scoring a bad one, and that's a big compliment to pay a burger joint. Options such as chili and mandarin oranges offer the side-order variety that's missing from less-evolved fast-food chains like Dairy Queen and Carl's Jr. Plus, Wendy's offers a handful of Jr. Burgers that don't stray far above 300 calories. Where Wendy's errs is in the expanded line of desserts and the roster of double- and triple-patty burgers.

SURVIVAL STRATEGY
Choose a grilled chicken sandwich or a wrap—they don't exceed 320 calories. Or opt for a small burger and pair it with chili or a side salad.

Eat This

Double Stack

with Small Chili

550 calories
24 g fat (10.5 g saturated, 1 g trans)
1,640 mg sodium

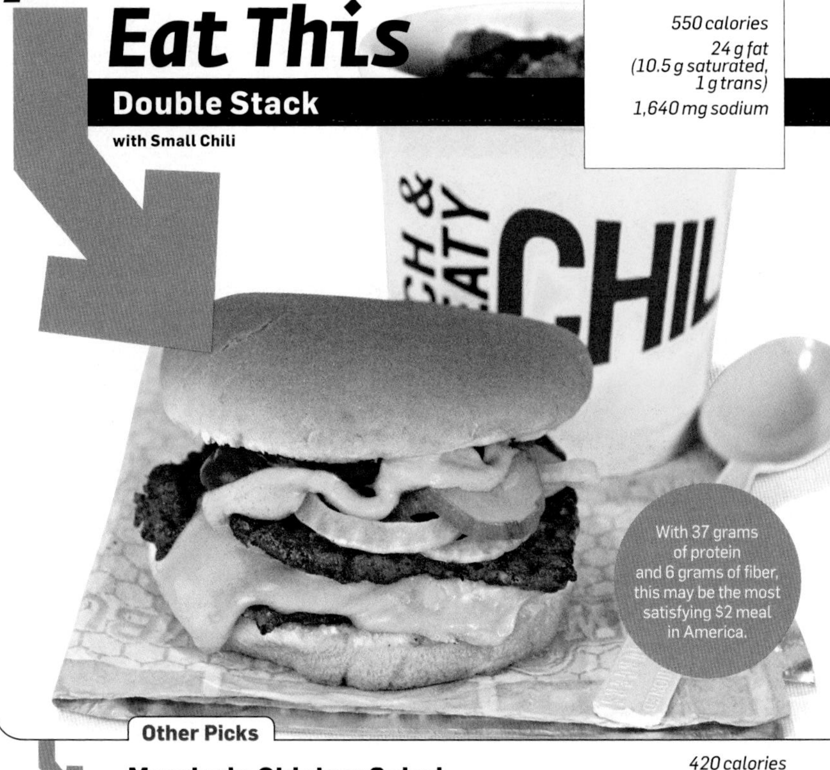

With 37 grams of protein and 6 grams of fiber, this may be the most satisfying $2 meal in America.

Other Picks

Mandarin Chicken Salad
with crispy noodles and oriental sesame dressing

420 calories
14.5 g fat (2 g saturated)
1,180 mg sodium

Ultimate Chicken Grill Sandwich

320 calories
7 g fat (1.5 g saturated)
950 mg sodium

Chocolate Frosty
(small)

320 calories
8 g fat (5 g saturated)
41 g sugars

700 calories
40 g fat (17 g saturated, 2 g trans)
1,440 mg sodium

Not That!

Double with Everything

and cheese

In the pantheon of fast-food burgers, this cannot compete with the atrocities wrought by the Double Whoppers and Six Dollar Burgers of the world. But there are too many burgers at Wendy's to end up with this mistake.

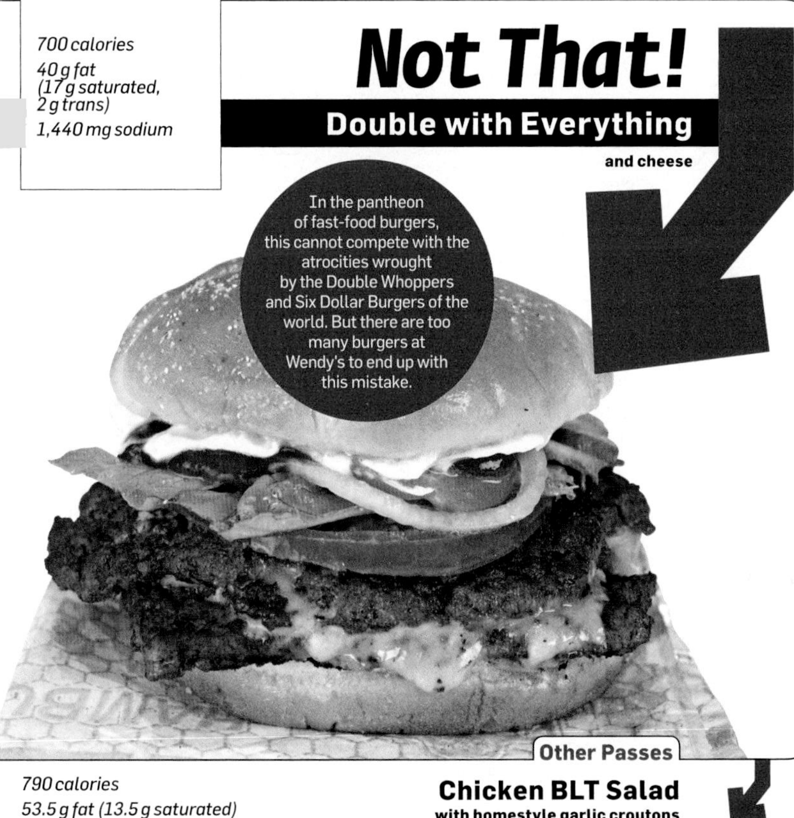

Other Passes

790 calories
53.5 g fat (13.5 g saturated)
1,735 mg sodium

Chicken BLT Salad
with homestyle garlic croutons and honey Dijon dressing

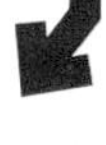

550 calories
26 g fat (8 g saturated)
1,290 mg sodium

Chicken Club Sandwich

550 calories
21 g fat (15 g saturated, 0.5 g trans)
68 g sugars

Coffee Twisted Frosty
(chocolate)

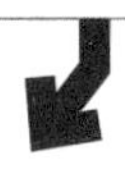

GUILTY PLEASURE

Spicy Chicken Fillet Sandwich

440 calories
16 g fat (3 g saturated)

Despite being fried and topped with mayonnaise, this superpopular Wendy's sandwich brings the heat without a whole lot of calories. In fact, the Spicy Chicken comes in around 200 calories lighter than similar sandwiches offered at other fast-food joints.

BAD BREED

French Fries

Wendy's fries are more caloric, fattier, and saltier than McDonald's. Stick with one of their healthier sides, such as chili, mandarin oranges, or a baked potato.

LITTLE TRICK

Order a baked potato and a small chili for lunch, and then pour the chili on top of the spud. This combination has nearly as much protein as a hamburger, but with about six times as much fiber. All for just 460 calories.

4

Eat This, Not That!

AT THE SUPERMARKET

Quantum physics.

Middle East politics. Jack Bauer's daily planner.

What do these three things have in common? Each of them is easier to grasp than the average American supermarket.

No matter how meticulously edited our shopping lists are, it's hard not to be overwhelmed the minute we set foot into the electric blue fluorescent glow of the grocery store. More than 50,000 packaged goods line the shelves of the average supermarket, and that's before you take into account the meat, fish, deli, and cheese counters; the produce section, with its exotic greens and 30 different kinds of apples; the precooked quickie dinner area; and the little server with the latex gloves offering a taste of chorizo and bourbon mustard or whatever else they're pushing that day. Go in with a plan to buy 35 items, and you'll come out with 50 of them—and wonder the next day how they ever crept into your kitchen.

And the power of supermarkets (and, um, supermarketers) to have their way with us has never been greater. A February 2009 poll by MINTEL found that

79 percent of Americans say they're trying to eat at home more, to save money. But are we saving? An April 2009 survey by *Better Homes and Gardens* found that women were spending $34 more every single week at the supermarket. Why? In part because food manufacturers are so sneaky about the ways they trick us into buying their products. That's why it's important for your wallet—and the part of your body that sits on it—to be smart about supermarket strategies.

Nobody wants to have to exercise discipline every time they go on a shopping trip, especially when it comes to the visceral happiness that food can bring us. Yet giving in to temptation or bad judgment at the supermarket can have consequences that last a lifetime. Because we're creatures of habit, we tend to simply grab the same brands every time we hit the store. That's fine, as long as we've chosen wisely. But the wrong choices can cost us thousands, maybe tens of thousands, of calories every year.

Consider this: Let's say that every night you have a modest dessert of two cookies, and your favorite is Oreo Cakesters Chocolate Crème. That means every night you're taking in 250 calories for dessert. Not a terrible nutritional crime by any means—more like a misdemeanor. But if your regular choice was Oreo Fudgees instead of the Cakesters, and you ate the same two cookies every night, by the end of a year you would have saved yourself more than 40,000 calories—the equivalent of a whopping 11½ pounds.

Amazing, right? But every single choice you make in the supermarket comes with the same potential long-term consequences. Think of all the things you and your family consume on a daily or weekly basis—staples like peanut butter, bread, nacho chips, canned fruit, salad dressings, and ice cream. Each choice can add an unnecessary 10, 50, 100 calories or more to your day—and that can very quickly add up. (Imagine those calories were dollars. You'd want to know if you were spending 100 extra dollars every day on something you didn't have to, right?)

So in this chapter, we've surveyed the supermarket shelves and found caloric savings here, there, and everywhere. Some are little savings; some are dramatic, however, and you will be shocked by how quickly and easily they will change your life. Regardless, start rewriting your shopping list—and try these strategies to better stick to it.

STRATEGY #1

STAY AWAY FROM THE SOFT, CREAMY CENTER. That would be the soft, creamy center of the supermarket—aisles 3 through 11, in most grocery stores. While the healthy stuff like dairy, produce, meat, and seafood is usually located around the edges, the interior of the supermarket is almost always packed with highly processed foods made with corn and soy and the 3,000 or more additives manufacturers use to make things that are edible but aren't actually food.

STRATEGY #2

AVERT YOUR EYES! On any grocery shelf, the most highly processed, most caloric, and often most highly priced products are about 5 feet off the ground. Why? Because that's about where your eyes are. That's very valuable real estate, and since supermarkets charge manufacturers for that placement, you can bet that the food marketers are figuring out a way to pass that cost on to you—either by trimming nutrition or amping up cost, or both. Reach up and kneel down, and you'll find both price points and nutrition labels that make a lot more sense.

STRATEGY #3

GET BACK TO THE EARTH. On one hand, we have an apple, a chicken, and a potato. On the other hand, a jar of applesauce, a bag of chicken nuggets, and some chips. Which hand is healthier?

Pretty simple, right? The apple has more nutrients than the sauce, the chicken has fewer carbohydrates than the nuggets, and the potato has less fat than the chips. And the apple/chicken/potato hand is a lot cheaper, too. It's a simple rule: The closer food is to its natural form, the healthier it is for you. So until they start growing apples inside little plastic containers, stick with what Mother Nature gave you.

STRATEGY #4

EAT MORE FOOD, EAT FEWER INGREDIENTS. Another important thing to keep in mind: the fewer ingredients, the better something typically is for you. (Foods with five or fewer deserve a special place in your pantry.) When apples turn into applesauce, they can often double their caloric load because of the addition of high-fructose corn syrup (HFCS). Which would you rather eat: an apple, or a combination of apples, water, and HFCS for twice the calories?

STRATEGY #5

WATCH WHO'S ON FIRST. Reading an ingredients label is like reading a baseball box score: It has plenty of information, but you need to understand what the stats mean. If you know what OBP and ERA mean, you have a good understanding of what's happening in the game. If not, a box score just reads like a bunch of gibberish.

Nutrition labels are the same. There are two things to keep an eye on: The first is the order of ingredients—labels by law must list them in order of volume. So if the number one ingredient is, say, "spinach," that's good. If it's "sugar" or "high-fructose corn syrup" or "canary droppings," that's probably bad. The second thing to look at is the servings per container. You'd be amazed by how a 200-calorie dish really becomes a 400-calorie dish when the little tiny dish supposedly contains two servings—even though you know you're going to eat the whole thing.

Join today! For more fat-melting, money-saving tips, become a member of the EAT THIS, NOT THAT! Premium Web site. Join at **EATTHIS.COM** *and you can personalize grocery lists, print out recipes, and have access to an exclusive database containing thousands of restaurant and supermarket items.*

STRATEGY #6

ELIMINATE THE DRIVE-BY. A recent study found that shoppers who made "quick trips" to the store purchased an average of 54 percent more merchandise than they planned. Instead, be smart about your trips. Bring a list—and a pen to cross off what you've already dropped into your cart. And try doing your shopping on Wednesday evening—that's when supermarkets are the most abandoned, which means a shorter trip and less time in the checkout aisle, eyeing the latest Jen/Brad/Angie brouhaha and those enticing little chocolate-covered crispy crackers that you don't mean to buy, but the kids are complaining and you're hungry and...

Cereal

Eat This

Kashi GoLean
(1 cup)
140 calories
1 g fat (0 g saturated)
10 g fiber
6 g sugars

An astounding 13 grams of protein in every bowl.

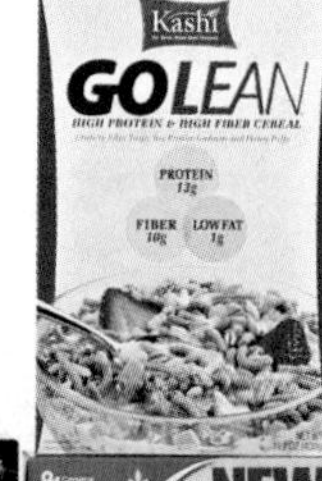

Quaker Instant Oatmeal Lower Sugar Maple & Brown Sugar
(1 packet, 34 g)
120 calories
2 g fat
3 g fiber
4 g sugars

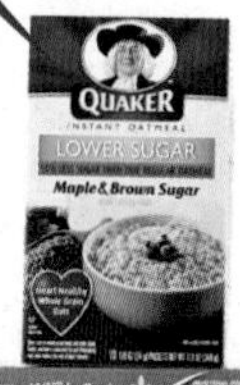

Kashi GoLean Creamy Instant Hot Cereal Truly Vanilla
(1 packet, 40 g)
150 calories
2 g fat
7 g fiber
6 g sugars

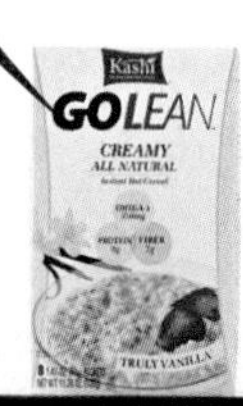

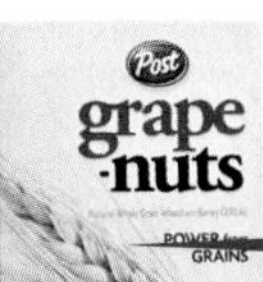

Grape-Nuts
(½ cup)
200 calories
1 g fat
(0 g saturated)
7 g fiber
4 g sugars
Calorie-dense, but packed with plenty of fiber and protein. Try adding to a cup of Greek yogurt and some fruit.

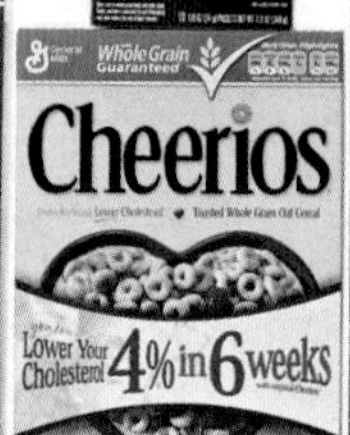

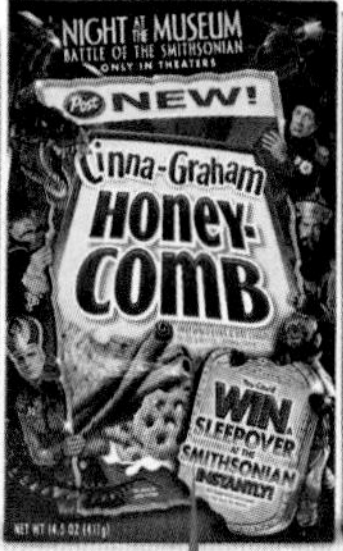

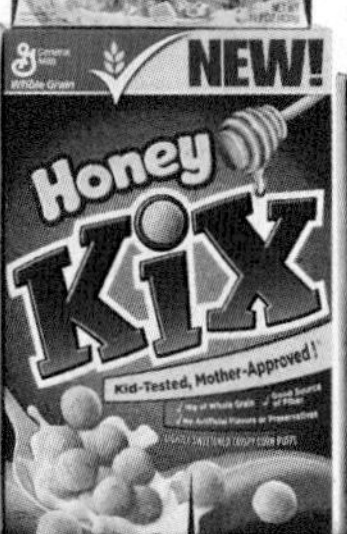

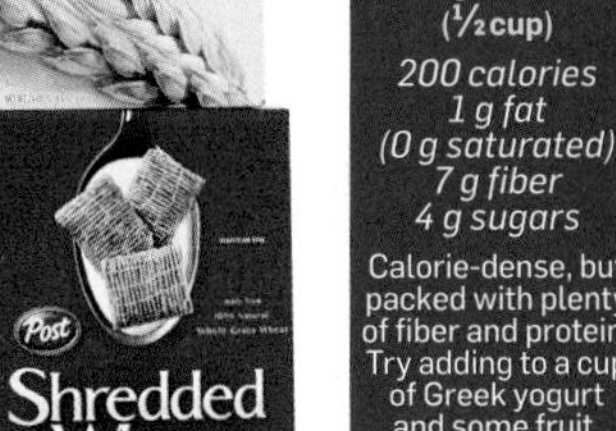

Kellogg's Froot Loops
(1 cup, 29 g)
110 calories
1 g fat
(0.5 g saturated)
<1 g fiber
12 g sugars
If you're going to keep a dessertlike cereal in the house, this is your best bet.

Cheerios
(1 cup)
100 calories
2 g fat
3 g fiber
1 g sugars
A solid staple for any pantry. Blend with ground flaxseed and raisins for a nutritionally powerful breakfast.

Cinna-Graham Honey-Comb
(1 cup)
87 calories
1 g fat
(0.5 g saturated)
1.5 g fiber
7 g sugars
As far as sweet cereals go, this ranks at the top.

Honey Kix
(1 cup)
96 calories
1 g fat
(0 g saturated)
2.5 g fiber
5 g sugars
The air inside puffed cereals gives them a huge caloric advantage over flakes and Oh's.

Post Shredded Wheat Spoon Size Original
(1 cup, 49 g)
170 calories
1 g fat
(0 g saturated)
6 g fiber
0 g sugars
An all-time favorite.

Not That!

Kellogg's Smart Start Original Antioxidants
(1 cup)
190 calories
0.5 g fat (0 g saturated)
3 g fiber
14 g sugars

The smattering of vitamins in this cereal doesn't make it worth the heavy calorie and sugar loads.

Quaker Simple Harvest Multigrain Instant Hot Cereal Vanilla, Almond, and Honey (1 packet)
160 calories
3 g fat
4 g fiber
9 g sugars

Cream of Wheat Instant Hot Cereal Maple Brown Sugar
(1 packet, 35 g)
130 calories
0 g fat
1 g fiber
13 g sugars
Almost pure carbs.

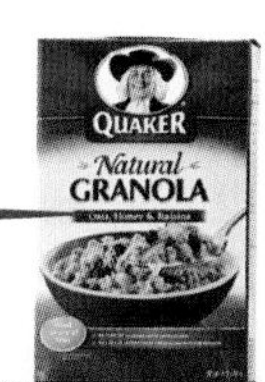

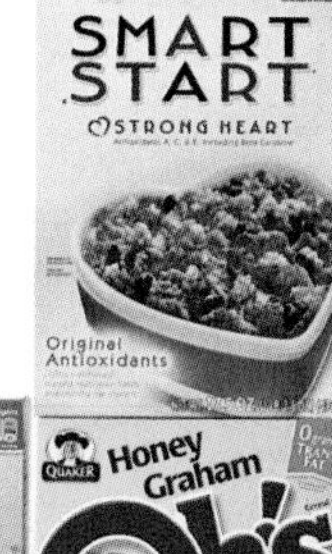

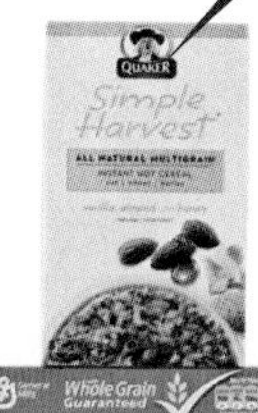

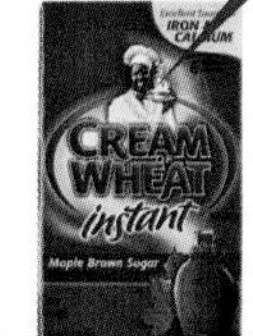

Quaker Natural Granola Oats, Honey & Raisins
($^1/_2$ cup)
210 calories
6 g fat
(3.5 g saturated)
3 g fiber
15 g sugars

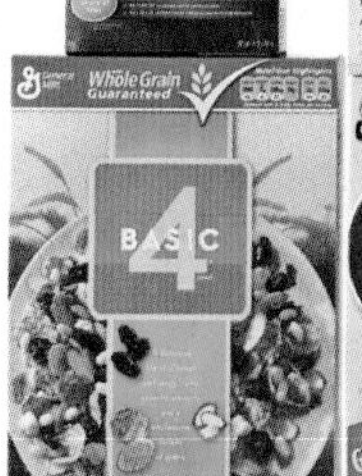

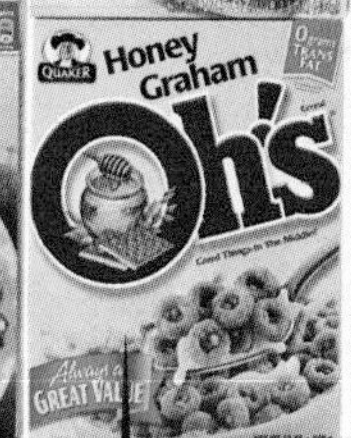

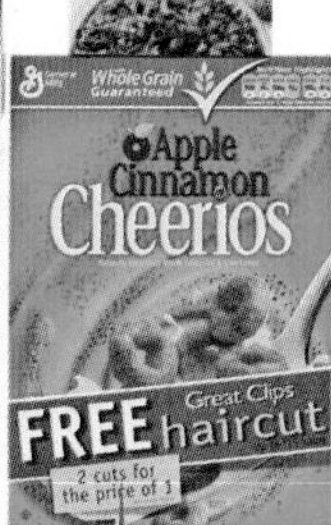

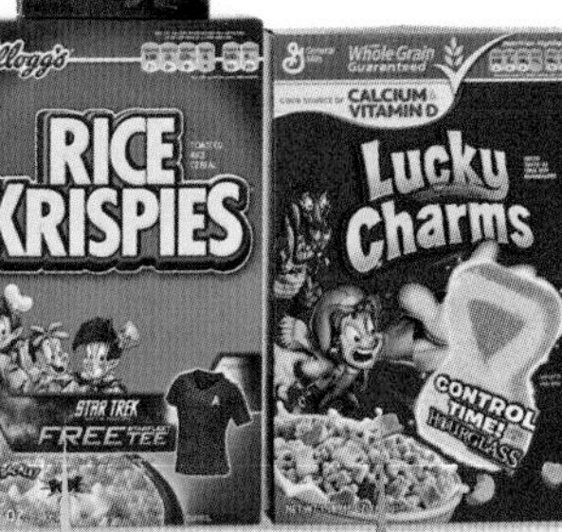

General Mills Basic 4
(1 cup, 55 g)
200 calories
2 g fat
(1 g saturated)
3 g fiber
14 g sugars
Looks healthy, right? Not with more sugar than a bowl of ice cream.

Honey Graham Oh's
(1 cup)
147 calories
3 g fat
(2 g saturated)
1.5 g fiber
16 g sugars
Oh's are more sugar-loaded than Froot Loops, Lucky Charms, or Trix.

Apple Cinnamon Cheerios
($^3/_4$ cup, 30 g)
120 calories
1.5 g fat
1 g fiber
12 g sugars
Cheerios are great, but the sugary spin-offs aren't.

Rice Krispies
(1 cup)
120 calories
0 g fat
0 g fiber
3 g sugars
Even Cookie Crisp and Lucky Charms contain a bit of fiber, but this iconic breakfast bowl? Not a shred of it.

General Mills Lucky Charms
(1 cup, 36 g)
147 calories
1.5 g fat
1.5 g fiber
15 g sugars
One of the most caloric cereals in the supermarket.

Breakfast Breads

Eat This

Sure, the low calorie load is impressive, but the true boon is the 8 grams of fiber added to each muffin. This is the best breakfast bread in the supermarket.

Thomas' Multi-Grain Light English Muffins
(1 muffin, 57 g)
100 calories
1 g fat (0 g saturated)
8 g fiber
<1 g sugars

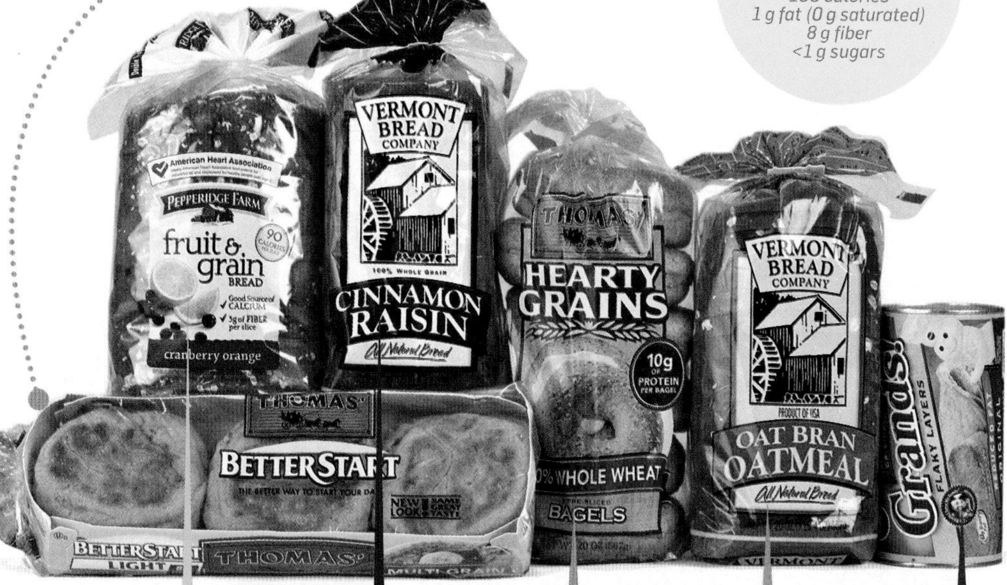

Pepperidge Farm Fruit & Grain Cranberry Orange
(1 slice, 40 g)
90 calories
1.5 g fat
(0 g saturated)
3 g fiber
5 g sugars
Packed with real fruit.

Vermont Bread Company Cinnamon Raisin
(1 slice, 31 g)
70 calories
0 g fat
2 g fiber
6 g sugars
Boost the fiber and protein with a tablespoon of peanut butter.

Thomas Hearty Grains 100% Whole Wheat
(1 bagel, 95 g)
240 calories
2 g fat
(0.5 g saturated)
7 g fiber
7 g sugars
With bagels, nothing but 100% whole wheat will do.

Vermont Bread Company Oat Bran Oatmeal
(1 slice, 31.5 g)
70 calories
1 g fat
(0 g saturated)
2 g fiber
2 g sugars
The first ingredient is whole wheat flour, the mark of a great bread.

Pillsbury Grands! Biscuits Flaky Layers Reduced Fat Original
(1 biscuit, 58 g)
160 calories
6 g fat
(2 g saturated)
4 g sugars
One of the few Pillsbury cans without trans fat.

Not That!

Too many nutritional advancements have been made to the English muffin to continue to fall back on this subpar version.

Thomas' Original English Muffins
(1 muffin, 57 g)

120 calories
1 g fat (0 g saturated)
1 g fiber
1 g sugars

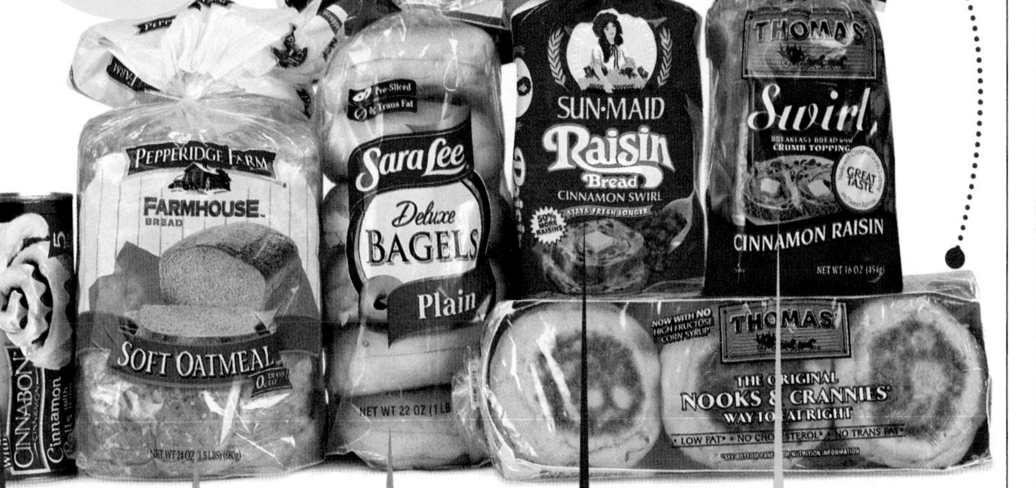

Pillsbury Grands! Cinnamon Rolls with Icing
(1 biscuit, 99 g)

310 calories
9 g fat
(2 g saturated, 2.5 g trans)
23 g sugars

A flood of sugar and dangerous fats.

Pepperidge Farm Farmhouse Soft Oatmeal
(1 slice, 43 g)

120 calories
1.5 g fat
(0.5 g saturated)
1 g fiber
3 g sugars

If it's made with oats, then where's the fiber?

Sara Lee Deluxe Bagels Plain
(1 bagel, 104 g)

270 calories
1.5 g fat
(0.5 g saturated)
2 g fiber
3 g sugars

Too many calories and carbs and too little fiber is a recipe for elevated blood sugar.

Sun-Maid Raisin Cinnamon Swirl
(1 slice, 32 g)

100 calories
1.5 g fat
(0.5 g saturated)
1 g fiber
7g sugars

Drop an easy 30 calories from each slice by choosing Vermont instead.

Thomas Cinnamon Raisin Swirl with Crumb Topping
(1 slice, 38 g)

120 calories
2 g fat
(1 g saturated)
1 g fiber
9 g sugars

Yogurt

Eat This

Stonyfield Farm Oikos Greek Vanilla
(1 cup, 150 g)
110 calories
0 g fat
11 g sugars

This cup has 16 grams of protein, about the same amount as two glasses of 2% milk. The difference is, it has about 125 fewer calories than the milk.

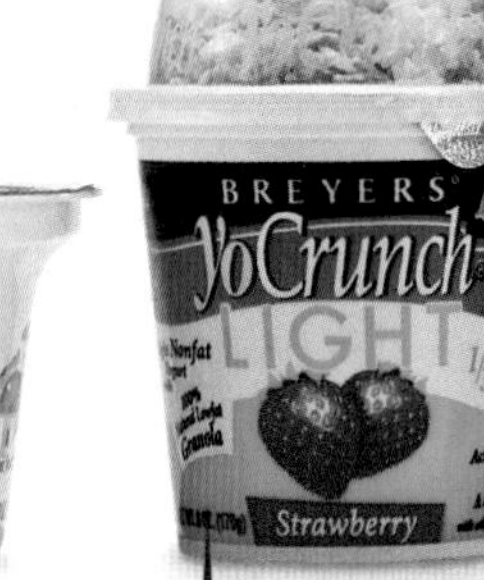

Breyers YoCrunch Light Strawberry with Granola
(1 cup, 170 g)
120 calories
1 g fat
(0 g saturated)
11 g sugars
This is the perfect dessert yogurt.

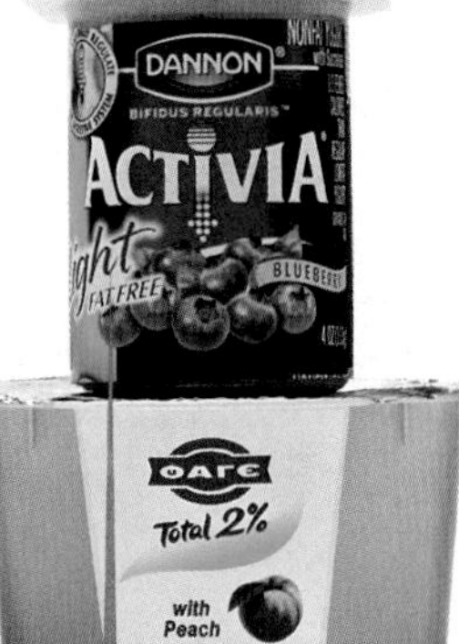

Dannon Activia Light Fat Free Blueberry
(1 cup, 113 g)
70 calories
0 g fat
9 g sugars
Dannon is fortified with 3 grams of inulin fiber, which teams up with the protein to beat back hunger.

Fage Total 2% with Peach
(1 container, 150 g)
130 calories
2.5 g fat
(1.5 g saturated)
17 g sugars
An impressive 15 grams of protein per cup. Plus the fruit here is real (which is rarer than you'd think).

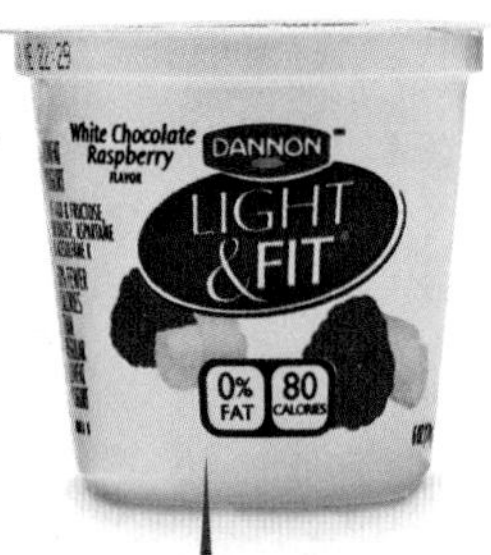

Dannon Light & Fit White Chocolate Raspberry
(1 cup, 170 g)
80 calories
0 g fat
11 g sugars
Yogurt doesn't get any lighter than this.

Not That!

Dannon All Natural Lowfat Vanilla
(1 cup, 170 g)
150 calories
2.5 g fat (1.5 g saturated)
25 g sugars

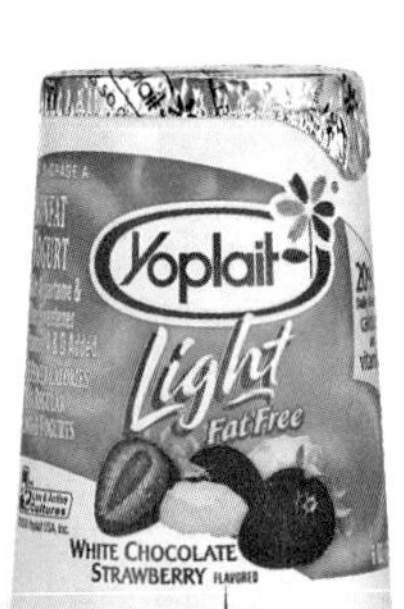

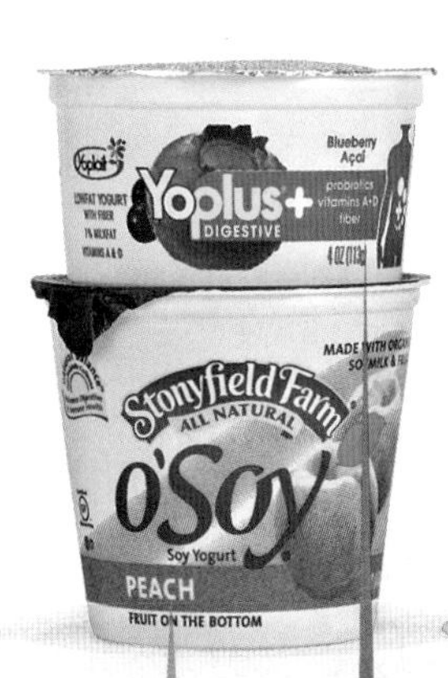

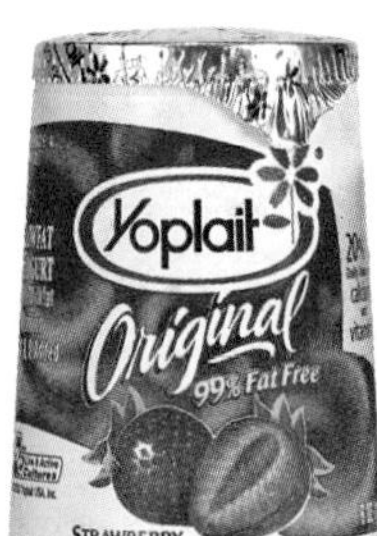

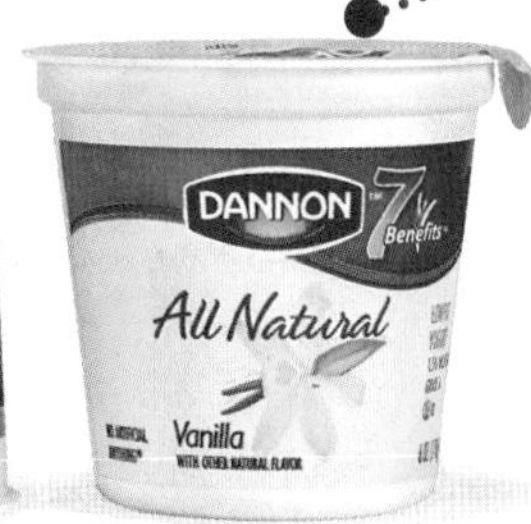

Yoplait Light Fat Free White Chocolate Strawberry
(1 cup, 170 g)
100 calories
0 g fat
14 g sugars
Yoplait will rarely be your best bet for calorie savings.

Stonyfield Farm All Natural O'Soy Peach
(1 container, 170 g)
170 calories
2.5 g fat
(0 g saturated)
28 g sugars
There are dramatically better peach yogurts and soy yogurts. Don't settle for this.

Yoplait Blueberry Acai Yoplus Digestive
(1 cup, 113 g)
110 calories
1.5 g fat
(1 g saturated)
16 g sugars
Nearly 60% of the calories are from sugar.

Yoplait Original 99% Fat Free Strawberry
(1 cup, 170 g)
170 calories
1.5 g fat
(1 g saturated)
27 g sugars
Who cares if it's "99% Fat Free" if it has more sugar than a Kit Kat bar?

Less than half the protein and more than twice the sugar as in Stonyfield's Greek yogurt.

Cheese

Eat This

Kraft Singles 2% Milk (1 slice, 19 g)

45 calories
2.5 g fat (1.5 g saturated)
260 mg sodium

With 4 grams of protein and a quarter of your day's calcium, this is one of the best cheese slices in the cooler.

Athenos Natural Feta Cheese Crumbled (¼ cup, 34 g)

90 calories
7 g fat
(4 g saturated)
380 mg sodium

Feta rules in the crumbled category.

Sargento Artisan Blends Parmesan (2 tsp, 5 g)

20 calories
1.5 g fat
(1 g saturated)
55 mg sodium

The best cheese for topping pasta.

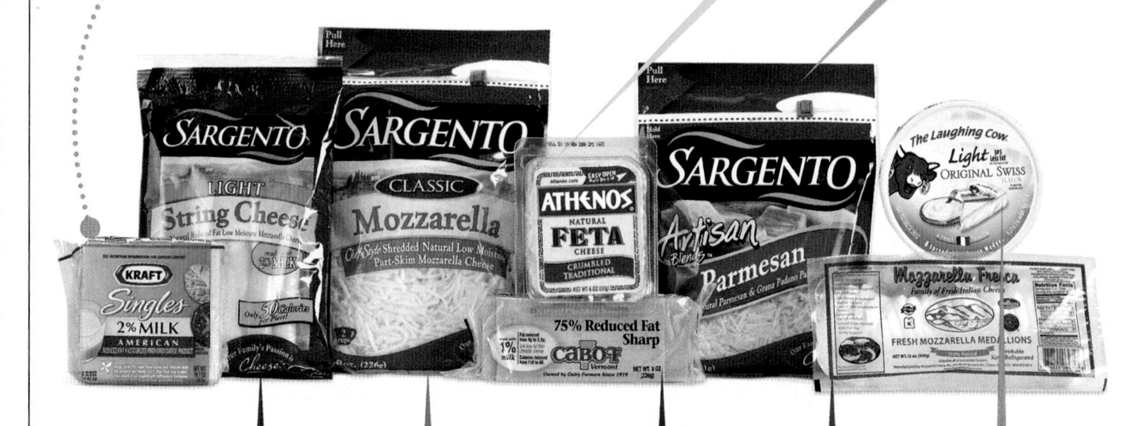

Sargento Light String (1 stick, 21 g)

50 calories
2.5 g fat
(1.5 g saturated)
180 mg sodium

The 6 grams of protein and 15% of your daily calcium make this an ideal light snack.

Sargento Classic Mozzarella (¼ cup, 28 g)

80 calories
5 g fat
(3.5 g saturated)
190 mg sodium

Melts easily and adds 7 grams of protein to your meal.

Cabot 75% Reduced Fat Sharp Cheddar (28 g)

60 calories
2.5 g fat
(1.5 g saturated)
200 mg sodium

Protein accounts for 60% of the calories in this cheese.

Mozzarella Fresca (28 g)

60 calories
4.5 g fat
(2.5 g saturated)
25 mg sodium

Fresh mozzarella has a low butterfat content, making it one of the lightest cheeses in the cooler.

The Laughing Cow Light Original Swiss (1 wedge, 21 g)

35 calories
2 g fat
(1 g saturated)
260 mg sodium

Add Triscuits for a belly-filling snack.

Not That!

Kraft Deli Deluxe American (1 slice, 19 g)
70 calories
6 g fat (3.5 g saturated)
310 mg sodium

More than twice the fat concentration found in Kraft's 2% Singles.

Kraft Macaroni & Cheese Topping (2 tsp, 6 g)
25 calories
1 g fat
(0 g saturated)
270 mg sodium
Half the protein, five times the salt of Sargento.

Kraft Blue Cheese Crumbles (¼ cup, 32 g)
110 calories
9 g fat
(6 g saturated)
430 mg sodium
Fat alone provides nearly two-thirds of the calories in blue cheese.

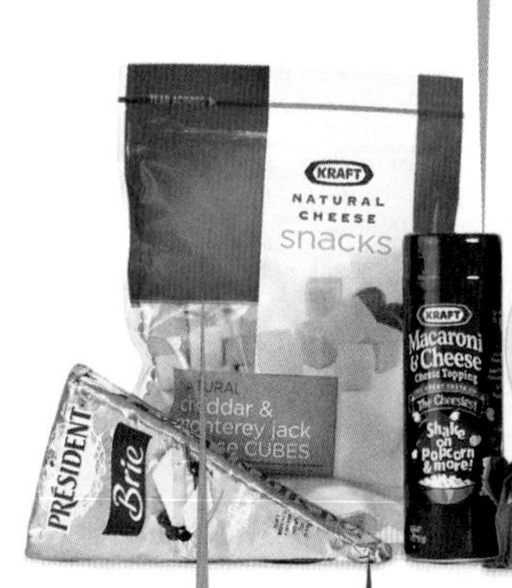

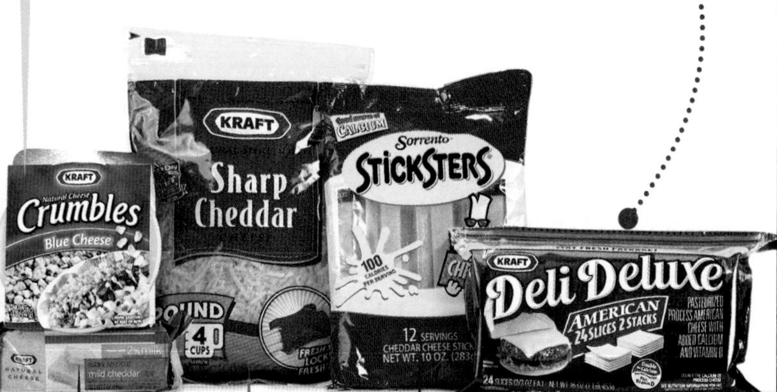

Kraft Snackables Cubes Cheddar & Monterey Jack (7 pieces, 30 g)
120 calories
10 g fat
(6 g saturated)
200 mg sodium

President Soft-Ripened Brie (28 g)
100 calories
9 g fat
(4 g saturated)
120 mg sodium
Tasty brie may be, but light it is not. Save this one for special occasions.

Kraft 2% Milk Mild Cheddar block (28 g)
90 calories
7 g fat
(4.5 g saturated)
220 mg sodium
Even with 2% milk, this cheese earns 70% of its calories from fat.

Kraft Sharp Cheddar Natural Shredded (¼ cup, 28 g)
110 calories
9 g fat
(6 g saturated)
180 mg sodium
Swiss and mozz trounce Cheddar.

Sorrento Sticksters Cheddar (1 stick, 24 g)
100 calories
8 g fat
(4.5 g saturated)
150 mg sodium
You don't want a snack that eats up 20% of your day's saturated fat.

Deli Meats

Eat This

Hormel Natural Choice Oven Roasted Deli Turkey
(56 g)
50 calories
1 g fat (0 g saturated)
490 mg sodium

Hormel's Natural Choice is one of the only nitrite-free lines of deli meats in the cooler.

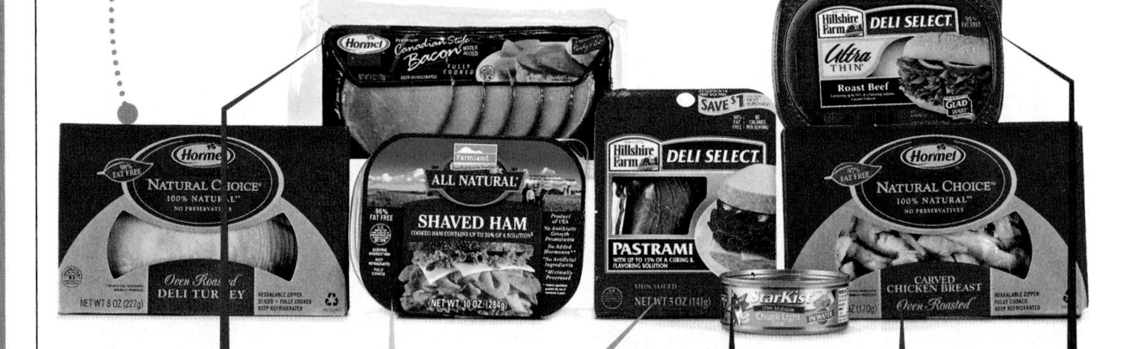

Hormel Natural Choice Canadian Bacon
(1 slice, 28 g)
35 calories
1 g fat
(0.5 g saturated)
340 mg sodium
Save 105 calories!

Farmland All Natural Shaved Ham
(6 slices, 57 g)
60 calories
1 g fat
(0 g saturated)
530 mg sodium
One of the few deli-meat lines to eschew dangerous preservatives.

Hillshire Farm Deli Select Pastrami
(7 slices, 58 g)
60 calories
1 g fat
(0.5 g saturated)
750 mg sodium
The leanest pastrami out there.

StarKist Low Sodium Chunk Light Tuna in Water
($^{1}/_{2}$ can, 112 g)
100 calories
1 g fat
(0 g saturated)
250 mg sodium
Chunk light has lower toxin levels.

Hormel Natural Choice 100% Natural Oven-Roasted Chicken Breast (56 g)
60 calories
1.5 g fat
(0.5 g saturated)
340 mg sodium

Hillshire Farm Deli Select Ultra Thin Roast Beef
(56 g)
70 calories
3 g fat
(1 g saturated)
550 mg sodium
The best in the beef category.

Not That!

Buddig The Original Deli Thin Turkey
(56 g)
90 calories
5 g fat (2 g saturated)
600 mg sodium

Buddig consistently offers the worst deli cuts in the cooler.

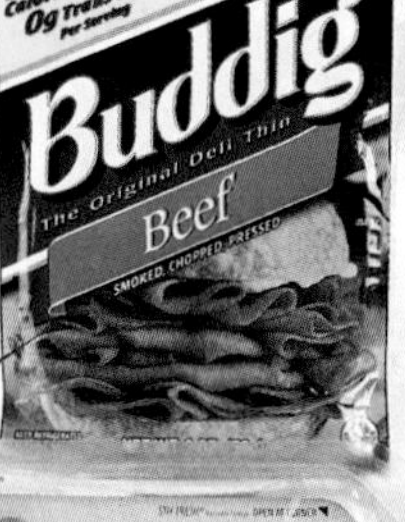

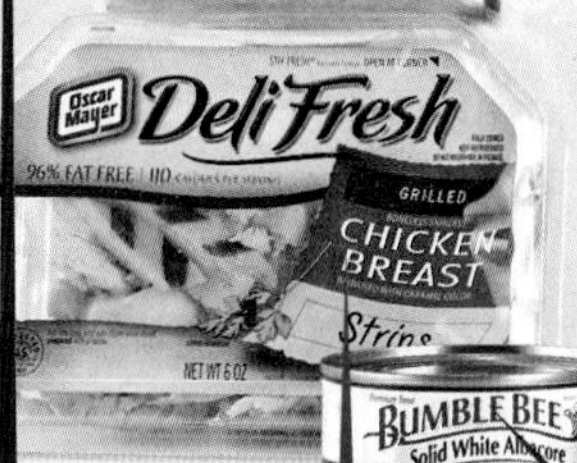

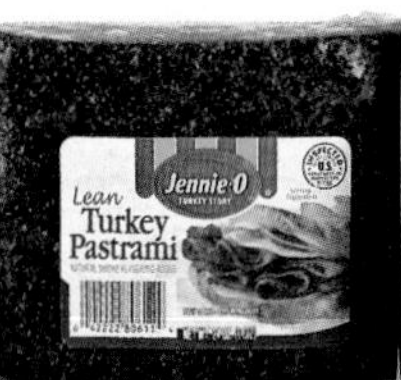

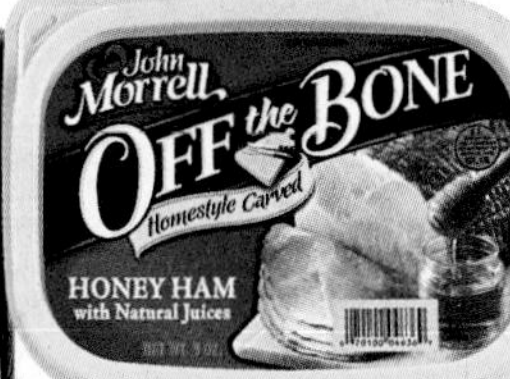

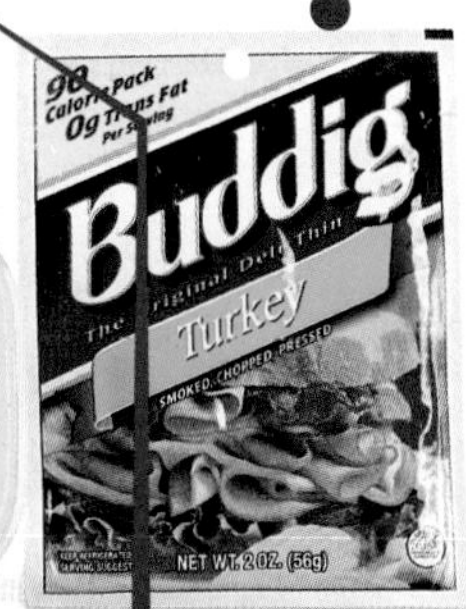

Buddig Beef The Original Deli Thin
(1 pack, 56 g)
90 calories
5 g fat
(2 g saturated)
790 mg sodium
This is one of the fattiest cuts we've come across.

Oscar Meyer Deli Fresh Grilled Chicken Breast Strips
(56 g)
73 calories
1 g fat
(0.5 g saturated)
460 mg sodium
Loaded with fillers.

Bumble Bee Solid White Albacore Tuna in Vegetable Oil
(1/2 can, 112 g)
180 calories
6 g fat
(1 g saturated)
360 mg sodium
Avoid albacore.

Jennie-O Lean Turkey Pastrami (56 g)
80 calories
4 g fat
(1 g saturated)
640 mg sodium
Just remember, there's no guarantee that turkey's going to be the lightest option.

John Morrell Off the Bone Honey Ham
(56 g)
80 calories
3 g fat
(1 g saturated)
610 mg sodium
Each serving provides more than a quarter of your day's sodium.

Armour Pepperoni Italian Style
(17 slices, 29 g)
140 calories
13 g fat
(5 g saturated)
530 mg sodium
Pepperoni is the worst among all pizza and sandwich toppings.

Hot Dogs and Sausages

Eat This

Applegate Farms Andouille Sausage
(1 sausage, 85 g)

120 calories
6 g fat (2 g saturated)
620 mg sodium

Applegate offers up more protein for less than half the calories and a third of the fat found in the ever-popular Johnsonville brats.

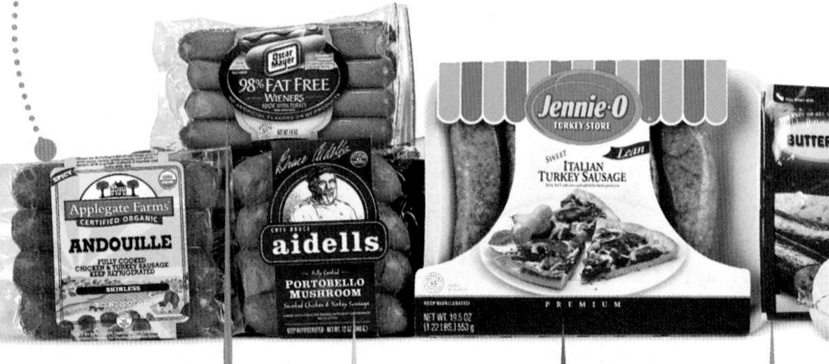

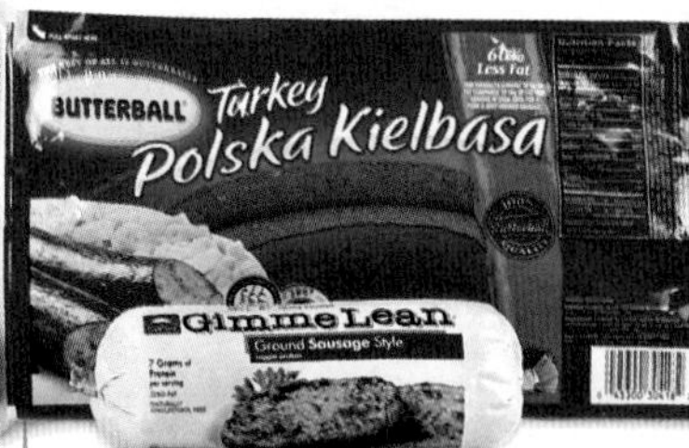

Oscar Mayer 98% Fat Free Wieners
(1 frank, 50 g)

40 calories
0.5 g fat
(0 g saturated)
470 mg sodium

A lighter frank doesn't exist—a full 50% of the calories are from protein.

Aidells Portobello Mushroom Chicken & Turkey Sausage
(1 sausage, 85 g)

140 calories
8 g fat
(2.5 g saturated)
540 mg sodium

First-class food.

Jennie-O Sweet Italian Turkey Sausage
(1 link, 109 g)

160 calories
10 g fat
(2.5 g saturated)
650 mg sodium

This swap of turkey for beef will save you 14 grams of fat per sausage.

Butterball Turkey Polska Kielbasa (56 g)

100 calories
6 g fat
(2 g saturated)
610 mg sodium

You'll gain 33% more protein by choosing turkey over beef-and-pork sausages.

Lightlife Gimme Lean Ground Sausage Style Veggie Protein
(71 g)

75 calories
0 g fat
388 mg sodium

Veggie sausage is made from soy protein and seasoned to taste like the real thing.

Not That!

Johnsonville Brats Original Bratwurst
(1 sausage, 85 g)

270 calories
22 g fat (8 g saturated)
810 mg sodium

This all-meat amalgam earns 198 of its calories from fat.

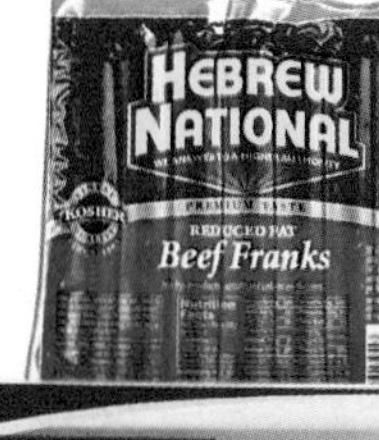

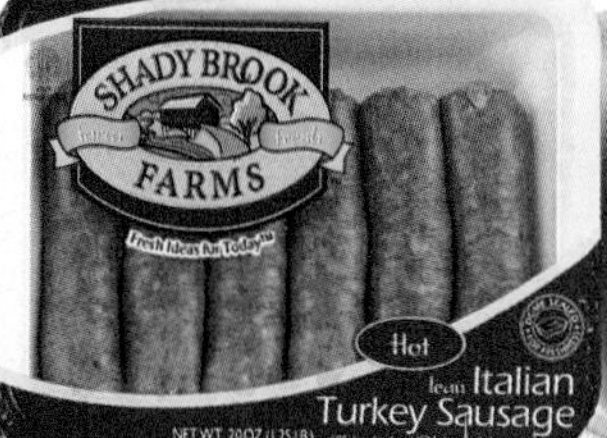

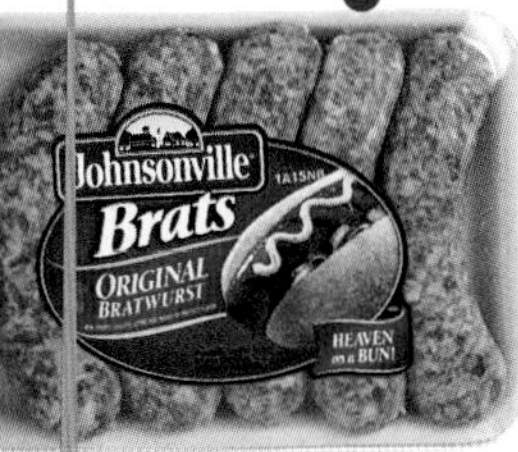

Morningstar Farms Veggie Sausage Links
(3 links, 67.5 g)

120 calories
4.5 g fat
(1 g saturated)
450 mg sodium

Sure it's better than real sausage, but there are lighter faux meats on the market.

Hillshire Farm Beef Smoked Sausage (56 g)

170 calories
15 g fat
(6 g saturated, 1 g trans)
520 mg sodium

Never settle for any packaged meat riddled with trans fat.

Ballpark Grillmaster Smokehouse Franks
(1 link, 82 g)

270 calories
24 g fat
(9 g saturated)
940 mg sodium

Nearly half a day's saturated fat per link.

Shady Brook Farms Lean Italian Turkey Sausage Hot
(1 link, 93 g)

160 calories
9 g fat
(2.5 g saturated)
620 mg sodium

Not the best turkey link in the cooler.

Hebrew National Reduced Fat Beef Franks
(1 frank, 45 g)

110 calories
9 g fat
(3.5 g saturated)
490 mg sodium

"Reduced fat" has very little meaning in the supermarket.

Condiments

Eat This

Kraft Mayo with Olive Oil
(1 Tbsp, 15 g)
45 calories
4 g fat (0 g saturated)
95 mg sodium

Although it says only "olive oil" on the label, this spread is actually made with both olive and canola oils. And that's good news; it means you're getting a variety of heart-healthy fatty acids from monounsaturates and omega-3s.

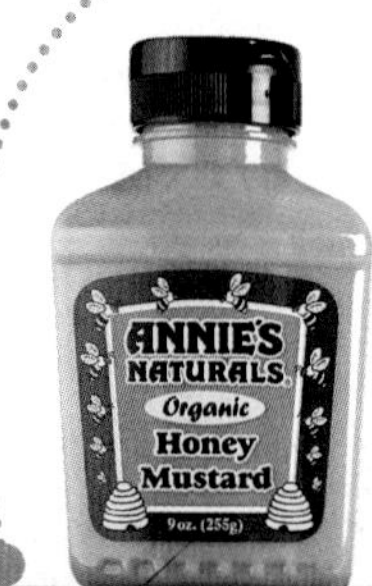

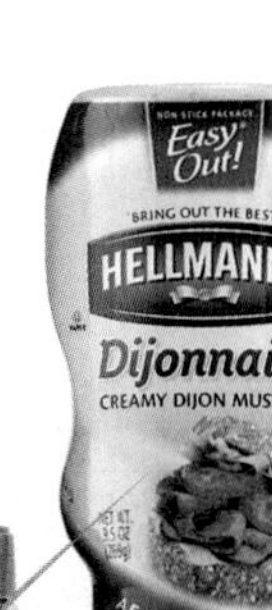

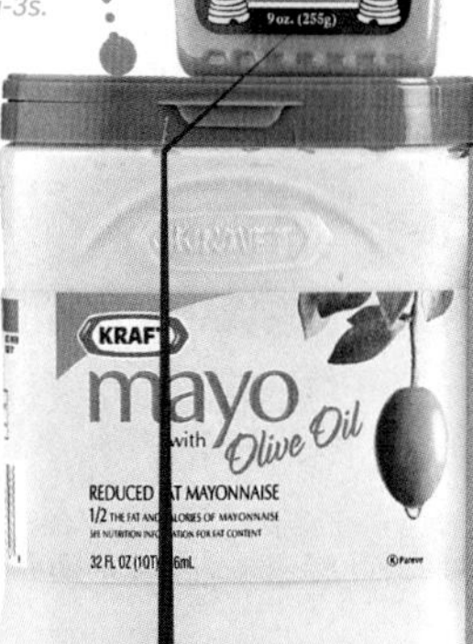

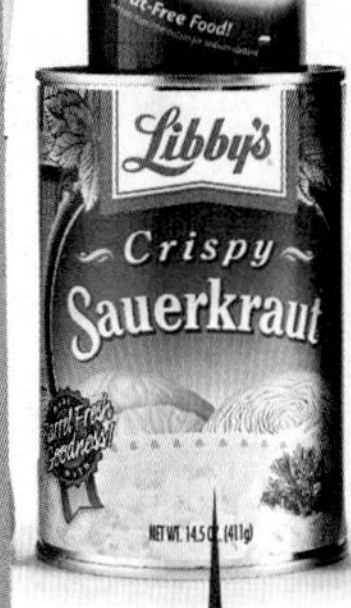

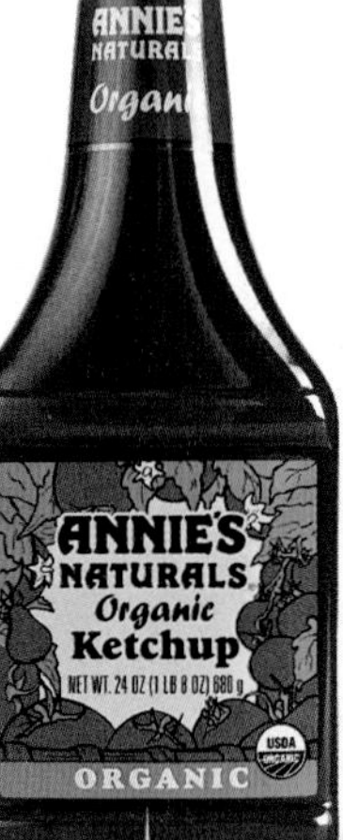

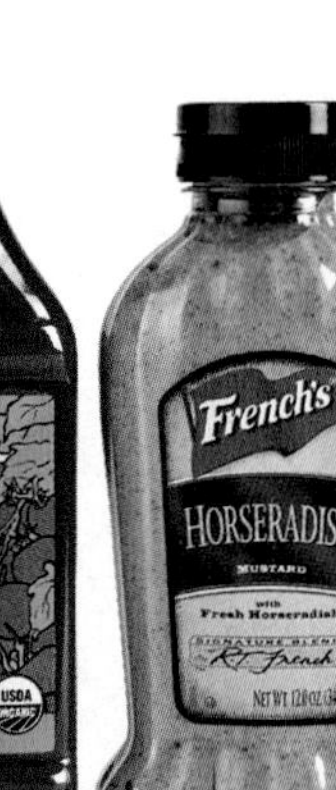

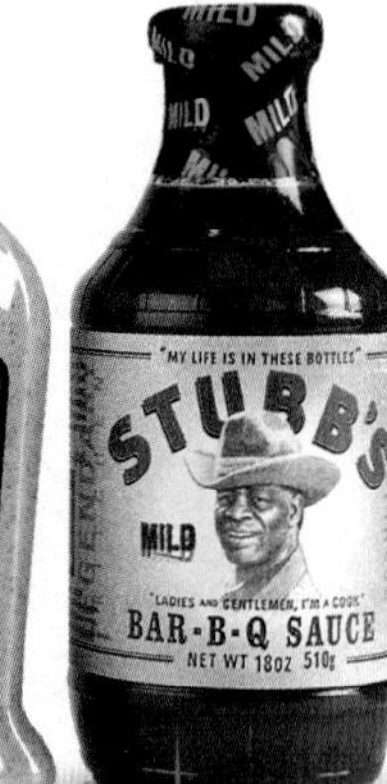

Annie's Naturals Organic Honey Mustard
(1 Tbsp, 18 g)
30 calories
0 g fat
120 mg sodium
Mustard seeds are rich in omega-3s and the antioxidant selenium.

Hellmann's Dijonnaise
(1 Tbsp, 15 g)
15 calories
0 g fat
210 mg sodium
The Dijonnaise is actually more mustard than mayo, making it far safer than the name implies.

Libby's Crispy Sauerkraut
(2 Tbsp, 30 g)
5 calories
0 g fat
200 mg sodium
Cut calories and sodium in one fell swoop.

Annie's Naturals Organic Ketchup
(1 Tbsp, 17 g)
15 calories
0 g fat
150 mg sodium
Research shows that organic ketchup packs more lycopene.

French's Horseradish Mustard
(2 Tsp, 10 g)
10 calories
0 g fat
160 mg sodium
Get the same kick as horseradish sauce, but without the glut of soybean oil.

Stubb's Mild Bar-B-Q Sauce
(2 Tbsp, 32 g)
30 calories
0 g fat
220 mg sodium
You'd be hard pressed to find a better barbecue sauce in the supermarket.

Not That!

Hellman's Light
(1 Tbsp, 13 g)
90 calories
10 g fat (1.5 g saturated)
70 mg sodium

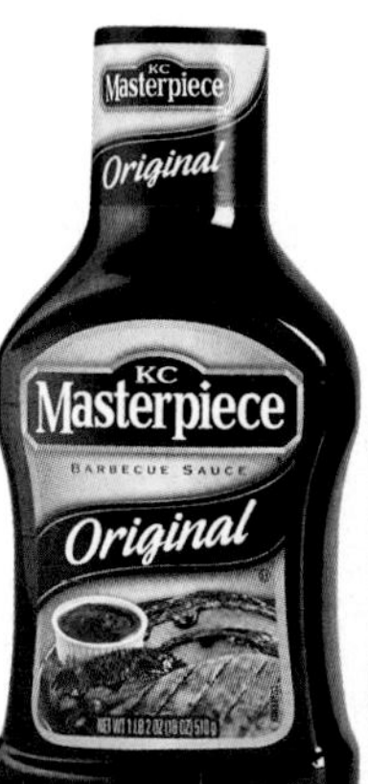

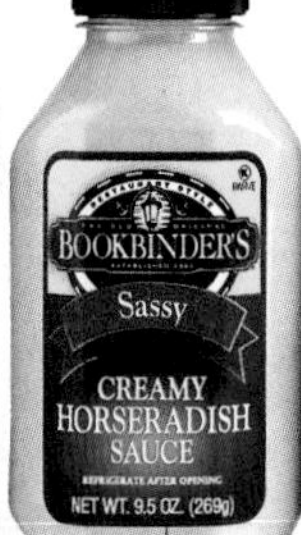

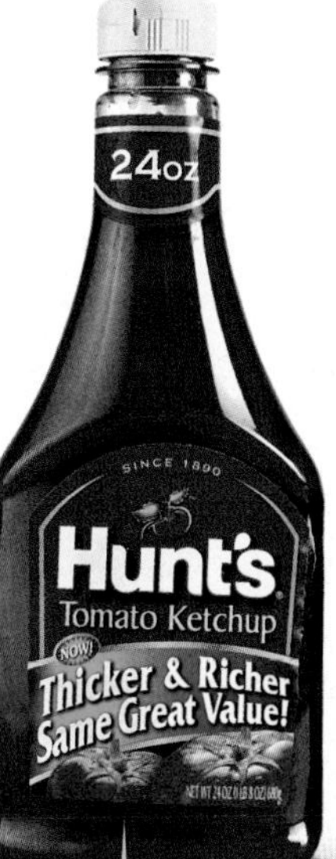

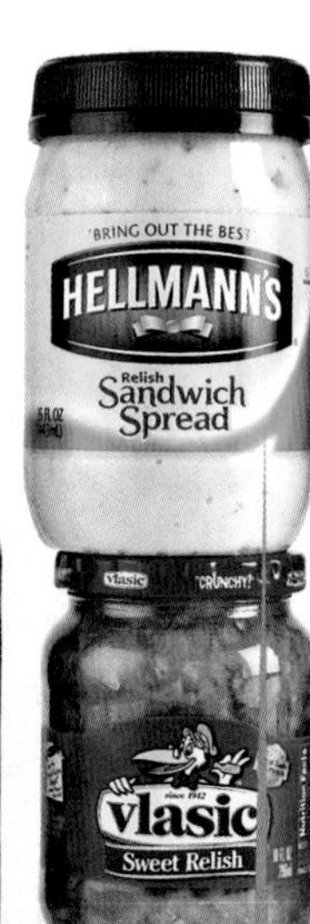

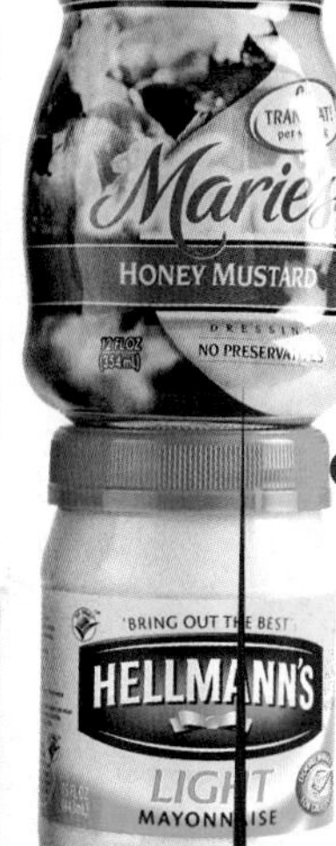

Even "light" mayo (made with cheap soybean oil) loses out to the new olive oil mayos. If you're a Hellmann's devotee, never fear—they also make a great olive-oil based mayonnaise.

KC Masterpiece Barbecue Sauce Original
(2 Tbsp, 36 g)
60 calories
0 g fat
240 mg sodium
Ten grams of sugar per serving, mostly from high-fructose corn syrup.

Bookbinder's Sassy Creamy Horseradish Sauce
(2 tsp, 10 g)
30 calories
2 g fat
80 mg sodium
There's more oil than horseradish in this second-rate sauce.

Hunt's Tomato Ketchup
(1 Tbsp, 17 g)
20 calories
0 g fat
190 mg sodium
Organic isn't always worth the extra cash (at least nutritionally), but with ketchup it definitely is.

Vlasic Sweet Relish
(2 Tbsp, 30 g)
30 calories
0 g fat
280 mg sodium
Each serving of relish tarnishes your dog with 8 grams of corn sugar.

Hellmann's Relish Sandwich Spread
(1 Tbsp, 15 g)
60 calories
5 g fat
(1 g saturated)
200 mg sodium
"Spread" = fatty mayonnaise hybrid.

Marie's Honey Mustard Dressing
(1 Tbsp, 15 g)
70 calories
6.5 g fat
(1 g saturated)
110 mg sodium
Comprised almost entirely of oil.

Breads

Eat This

Martin's Whole Wheat
(2 slices, 45 g)

140 calories
2 g fat (0 g saturated)
8 g fiber

Each slice packs 4 grams of fiber and 6 grams of protein. For our money, this is the best bread in America.

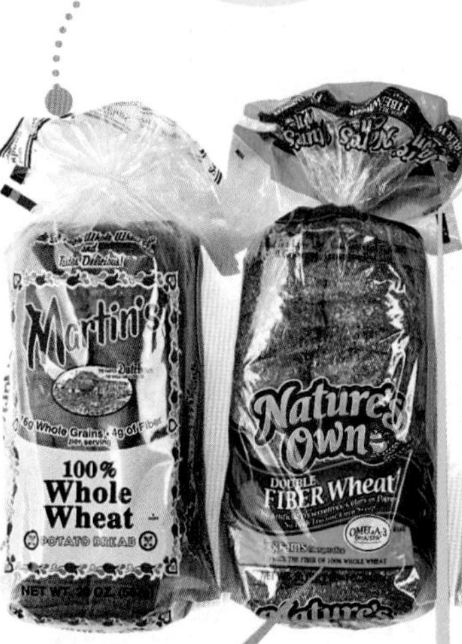

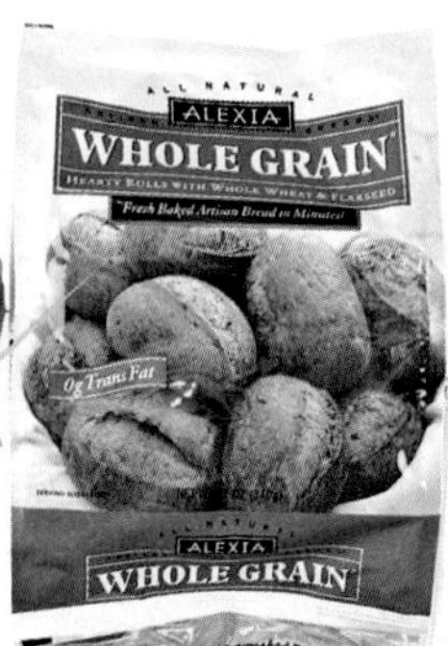

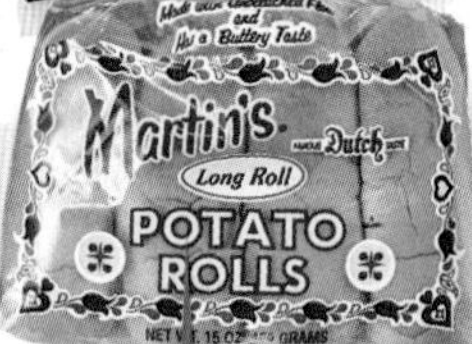

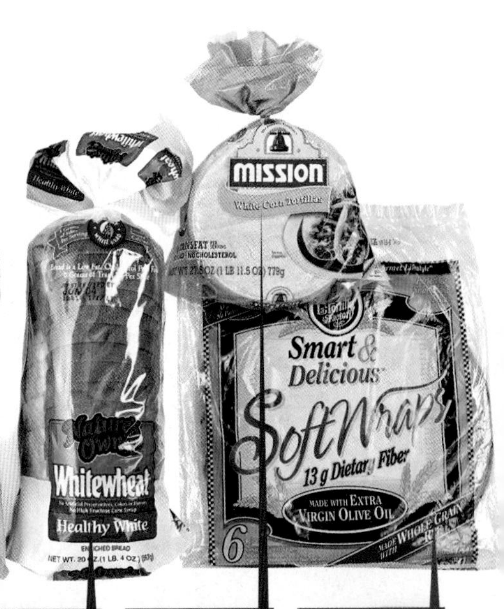

Nature's Own Double Fiber Wheat
(2 slices, 56 g)

100 calories
1 g fat
(0 g saturated)
10 g fiber

Great breads have a favorable fiber-to-calorie ratio. Few can beat this.

Alexia Whole Grain Hearty Rolls
(1 roll, 43 g)

90 calories
1 g fat
(0 g saturated)
2 g fiber

The best roll in the supermarket is actually hiding in the freezer section.

Martin's Long Roll Potato Rolls
(1 bun, 53 g)

130 calories
1.5 g fat
4 g fiber

Martin mines the spud to come up with more fiber than you'll find in whole wheat buns.

Nature's Own Whitewheat
(2 slices, 52 g)

100 calories
2 g fat
(0.5 g saturated)
5 g fiber

There's no longer any excuse to grab a typical, low-fiber white bread.

Mission White Corn
(2 tortillas, 51 g)

110 calories
1.5 g fat
(0 g saturated)
3 g fiber

With more fiber and fewer calories, corn trumps flour every time in the tortilla showdown.

La Tortilla Factory Smart & Delicious Low Carb Whole Wheat
(1 wrap, 62 g)

90 calories
3 g fat
(0 g saturated)
13 g fiber

Not That!

You'd have to be a nut to find this bread healthy. It has one of the worst fiber-to-calorie ratios in the bread aisle.

Arnold Health Nut
(2 slices, 60 g)
160 calories
2 g fat (0 g saturated)
2 g fiber

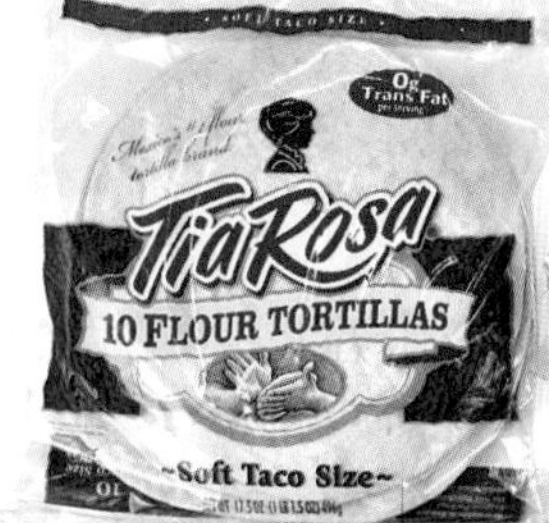

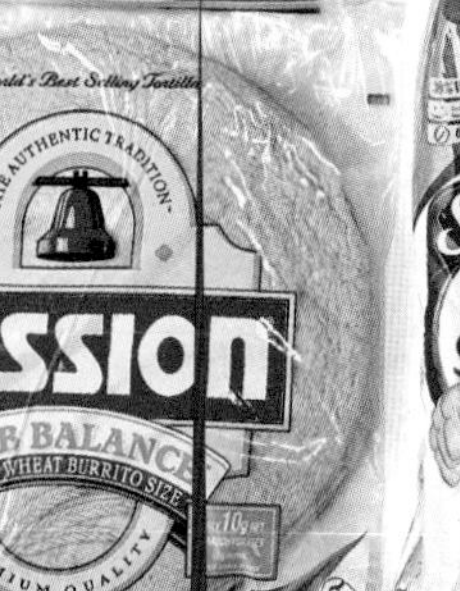

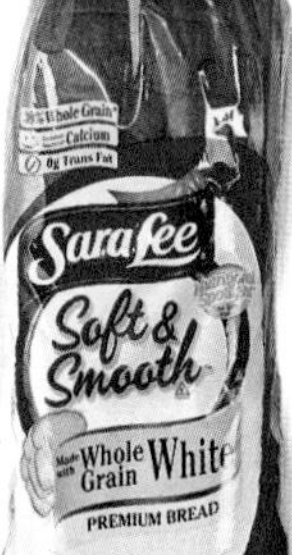

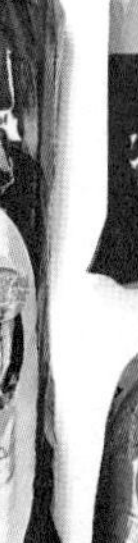

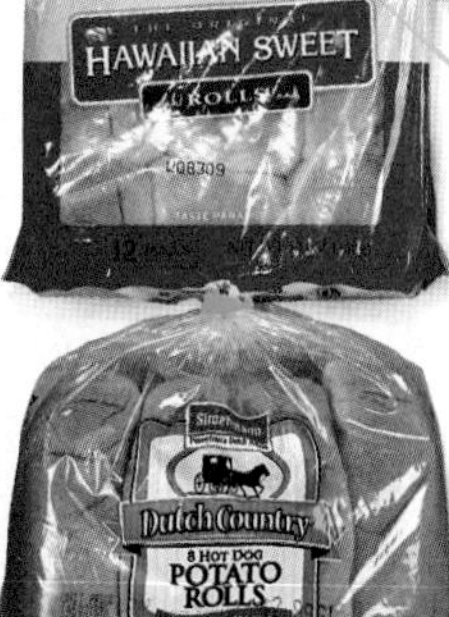

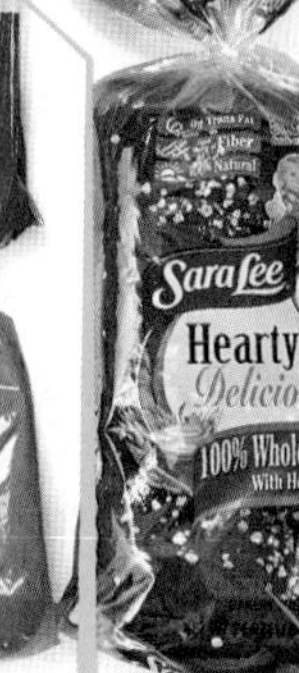

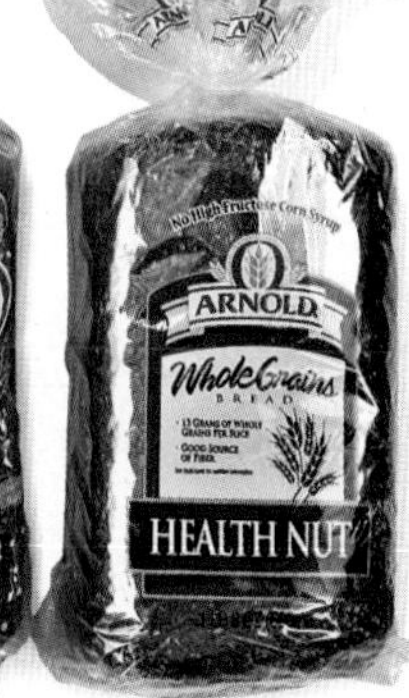

Mission Carb Balance Whole Wheat Burrito Size
(1 tortilla, 70 g)
200 calories
4.5 g fat
(1 g saturated)
21 g fiber
Fiber-rich, but calorie-dense.

Tia Rosa Soft Taco Size Flour
(1 tortilla, 50 g)
150 calories
4.5 g
(2.5 g saturated)
1 g fiber
Made from oil and refined white flour. Any questions?

Sara Lee Soft & Smooth Made with Whole Grain White
(2 slices, 57 g)
150 calories
2 g fat
(0.5 g saturated)
3 g fiber

Stroehmann Dutch Country Hot Dog Potato Rolls
(1 roll, 53 g)
150 calories
2 g fat
1 g fiber
Don't settle for subpar buns.

King's Hawaiian Sweet Rolls
(1 roll, 28 g)
100 calories
2.5 g fat
(1.5 g saturated)
1 g fiber
Less fiber and five times the sugar as Alexia's Whole Grain Roll.

Sara Lee Hearty & Delicious 100% Whole Wheat with Honey
(2 slices, 86 g)
240 calories
3 g fat
(1 g saturated)
6 g fiber

Grains and Noodles

Eat This

Bob's Red Mill Organic Whole Grain Quinoa
(¼ cup, 46 g)
170 calories
2.5 g fat (0 g saturated)
3 g fiber

Kashi 7 Whole Grain Pilaf
(½ cup cooked)
110 calories
2 g fat
(0 g saturated)
3.5 g fiber
A tasty, nutrient-rich grain that deserves to be a staple at home.

Fantastic World Foods Organic Whole Wheat Couscous
(¼ cup dry, 45 g)
170 calories
0.5 g fat
(0 g saturated)
6 g fiber

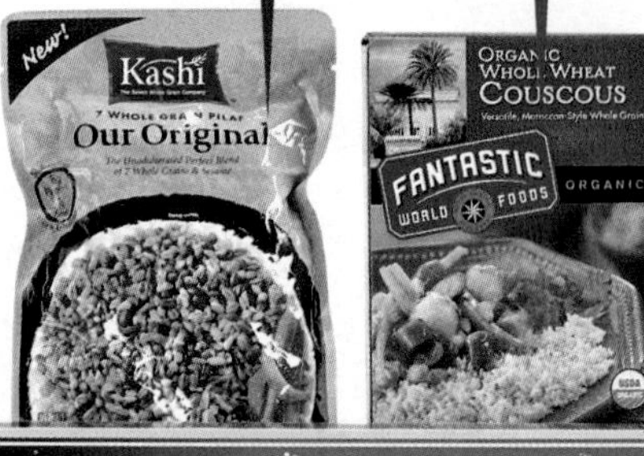

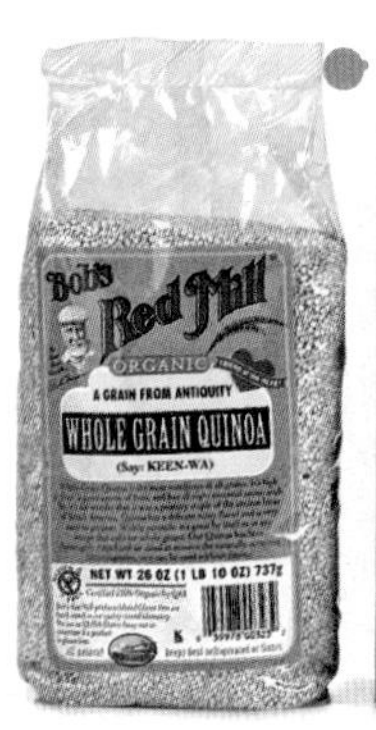

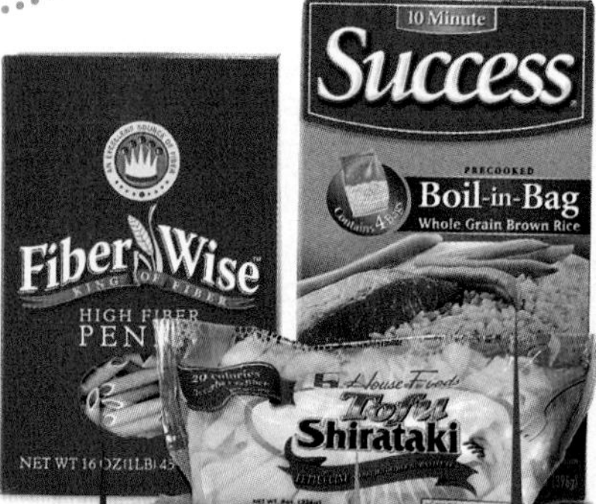

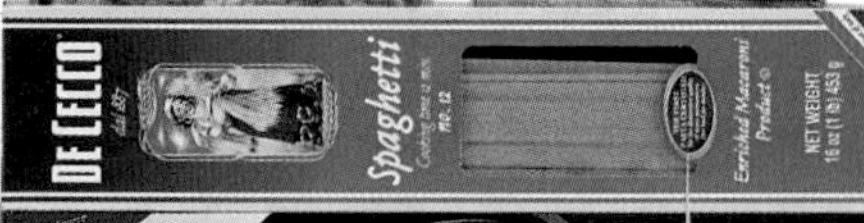

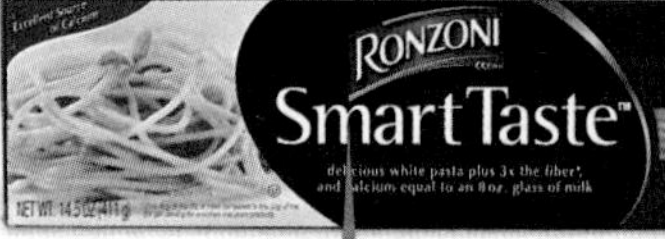

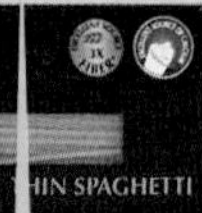

Quinoa is the king of grains in that it's loaded with protein, fiber, and healthy fats—the nutrients that promote long-lasting energy.

Fiber Wise High Fiber Penne (57 g)
170 calories
1 g fat
(0 g saturated)
12 g fiber
This blend earns its abundance of fiber by incorporating pea and flax flour into the recipe.

House Foods Tofu Shirataki Fettuccine
(113 g)
20 calories
0.5 g fat
(0 g saturated)
2 g fiber
Popular in Japanese cuisine, these noodles are nearly carb-free.

Success Boil-in-Bag Whole Grain Brown Rice
(½ cup, about 1 cup cooked)
150 calories
1 g fat
(0 g saturated)
2 g fiber

Ronzini Smart Taste Thin Spaghetti
(56 g)
180 calories
1 g fat
(0 g saturated)
6 g fiber
Our favorite noodle in the market.

De Cecco Spaghetti No. 12 (57 g)
200 calories
1 g fat
(0 g saturated)
2 g fiber
When you eat pasta as much as Americans do, every calorie and fiber gram counts.

RiceSelect Couscous Tri-Color (¼ cup dry, 43 g)

150 calories
0 g fat
2 g fiber

Why tamper with a perfect food? Whole wheat trumps tri-color every time.

RiceSelect Royal Blend Whole Grain (¼ cup dry)

160 calories
1.5 g fat
(0 g saturated)
2 g fiber

Too many calories and too little fiber to be considered a good blend.

Not That!

Uncle Ben's Natural Whole Grain Brown Rice (¼ cup, 47 g)

170 calories
1.5 g fat (0 g saturated)
2 g fiber

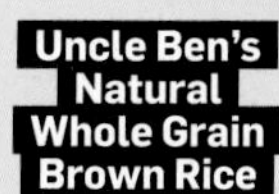

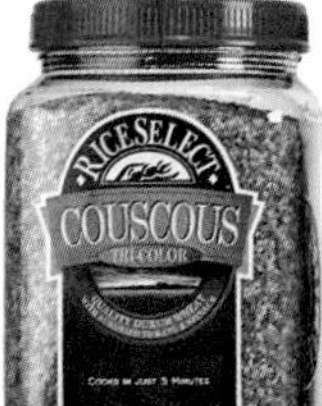

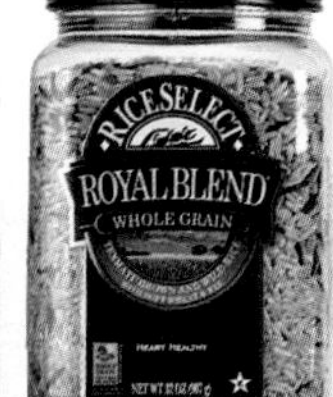

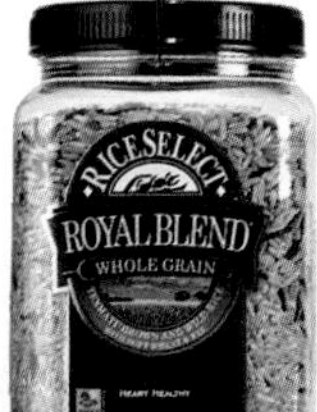

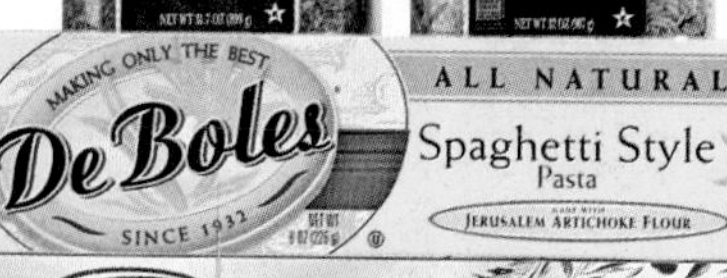

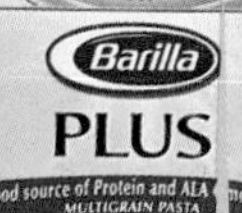

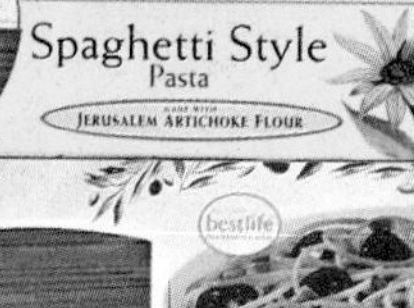

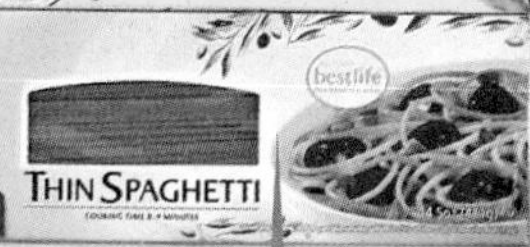

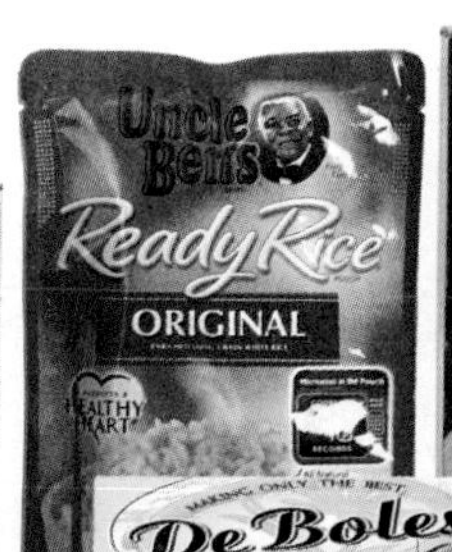

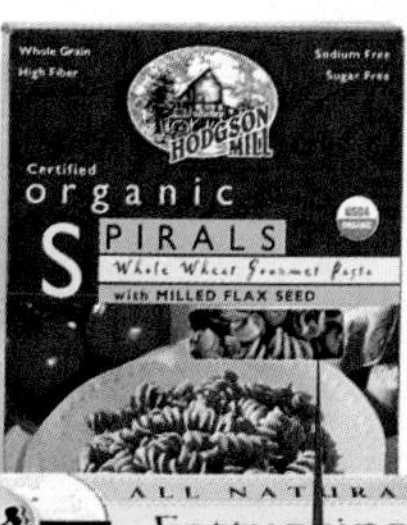

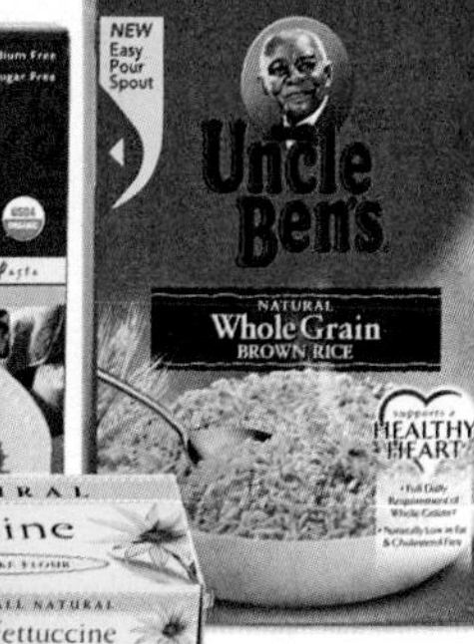

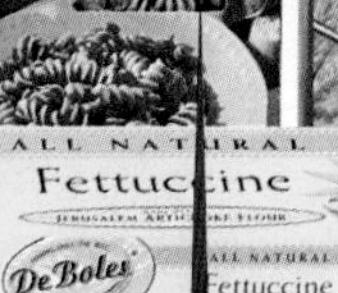

De Boles Spaghetti (57 g)

210 calories
1 g fat
(0 g saturated)
1 g fiber

With so many great, tasty whole wheat pastas on the market, regular spaghetti should be a rare treat.

Barilla Plus Thin Spaghetti (56 g)

210 calories
2 g fat
(0 g saturated)
4 g fiber

While better than normal pasta, it's no match for Ronzini.

Uncle Ben's Ready Rice Original Long Grain Rice (⅓ cup, about 1 cup cooked)

200 calories
2.5 g fat
(0 g saturated)
1 g fiber

Ditch white rice.

DeBoles Fettuccine (57 g)

210 calories
1 g fat
(0 g saturated)
1 g fiber

You should never eat a noodle with fewer than 2 grams of fiber per serving.

Hodgson Mill Organic Spirals Whole Wheat (57 g)

215 calories
2.5 g fat
(0 g saturated)
6 g fiber

Way better than white pasta, but too caloric for whole grain pasta.

Not even "healthy" brown rice can compete with quinoa's fiber load. Need another reason to make the switch? Quinoa also has 50% more protein.

Sauces

Eat This

Classico Tomato & Basil
(½ cup, 125 g)

50 calories
1 g fat (0 g saturated)
380 mg sodium

Classico makes the most reliable line of the store-common widely available pasta sauces.

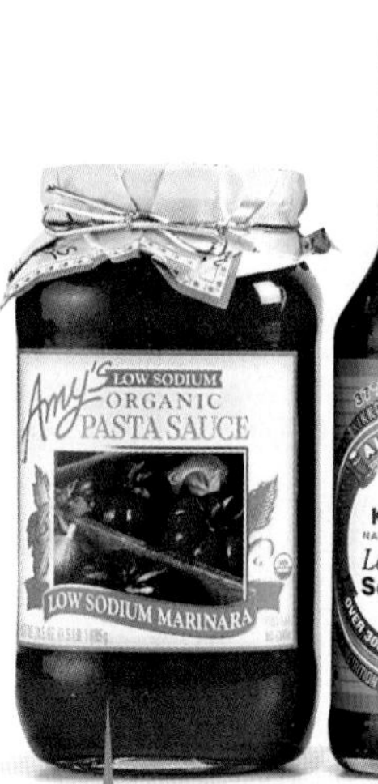

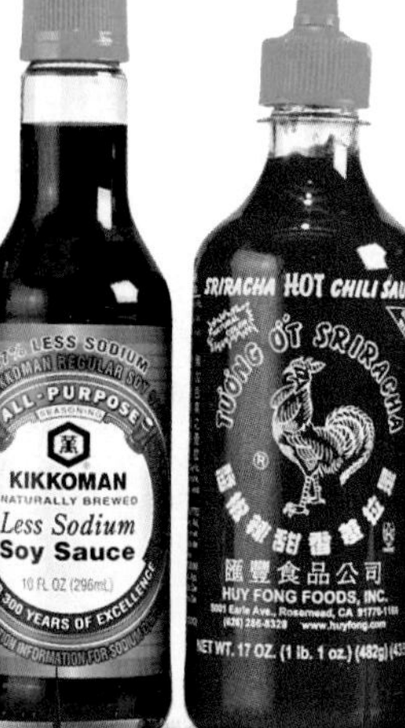

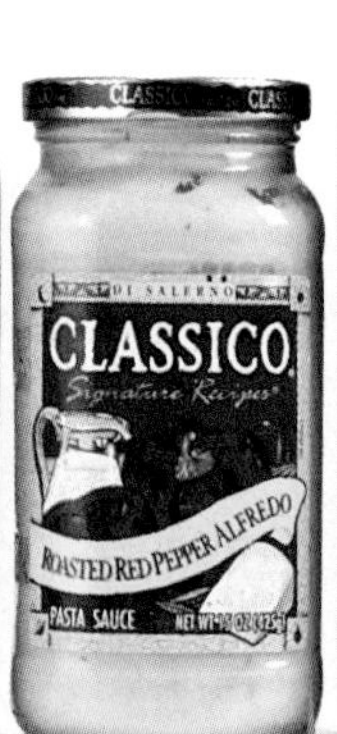

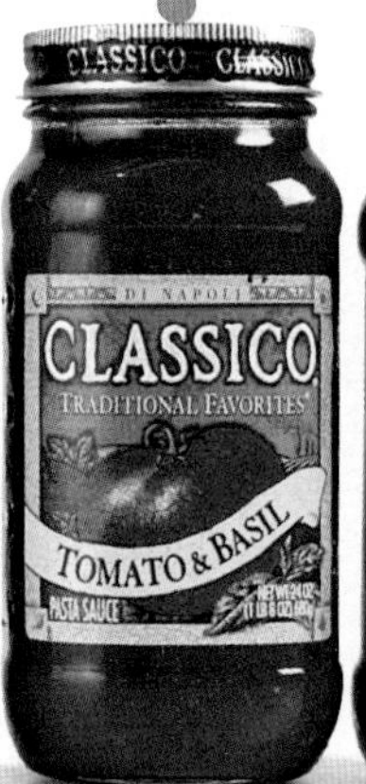

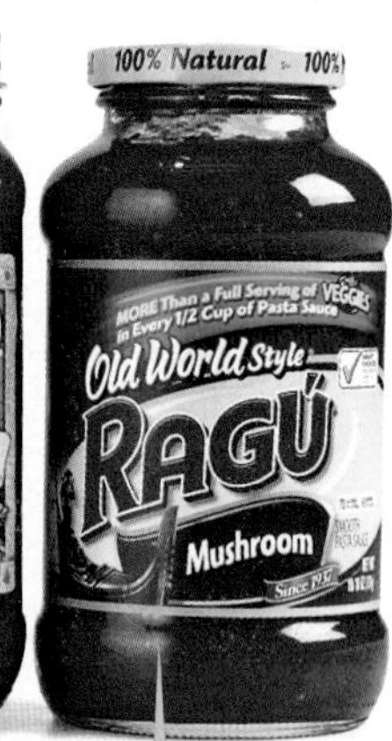

Amy's Low Sodium Organic Marinara
(½ cup, 125 g)

40 calories
1 g fat
(0 g saturated)
100 mg sodium

Not all of Amy's sauces are reliable, but this is one of the healthiest in the store.

Kikkoman Less Sodium Soy Sauce
(1 Tbsp, 15 mL)

10 calories
0 g fat
575 mg sodium

Sodium is the only thing that matters when comparing soy sauces. Stick to this one and you'll be okay.

Huy Fong Sriracha Chili Sauce
(1 Tbsp, 15 g)

15 calories
0 g fat
300 mg sodium
3 g sugars

Loaded with metabolism-boosting, pain-relieving capsaicins.

Classico Roasted Red Pepper Alfredo
(½ cup, 120 g)

120 calories
10 g fat
(6 g saturated)
620 mg sodium

There's no such thing as a "healthy" Alfredo sauce; this one's as close as they come.

Ragu Old World Style Mushroom
(½ cup, 125 g)

70 calories
2.5 g fat
(0 g saturated)
320 mg sodium

The first two ingredients are just what they should be: tomato puree and mushrooms.

Not That!

Newman's Own Tomato & Basil
(½ cup, 125 g)

90 calories
4.5 g fat (0.5 g saturated)
620 mg sodium
12 g sugars

We love many of Newman's products, but this isn't one of them. Sugar is listed as the fourth ingredient, which is why this sauce carries more than twice the sugar load as Classico's.

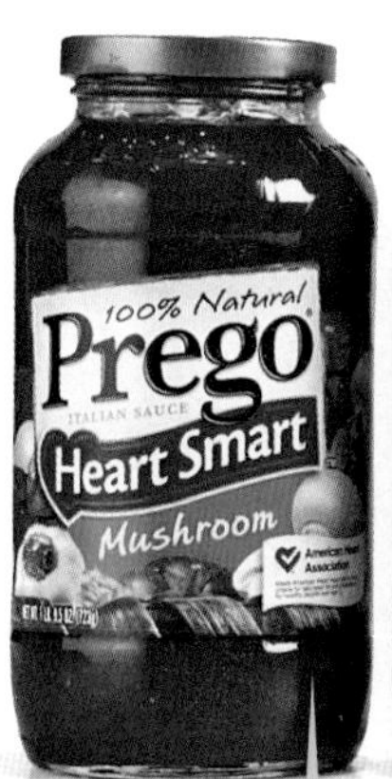

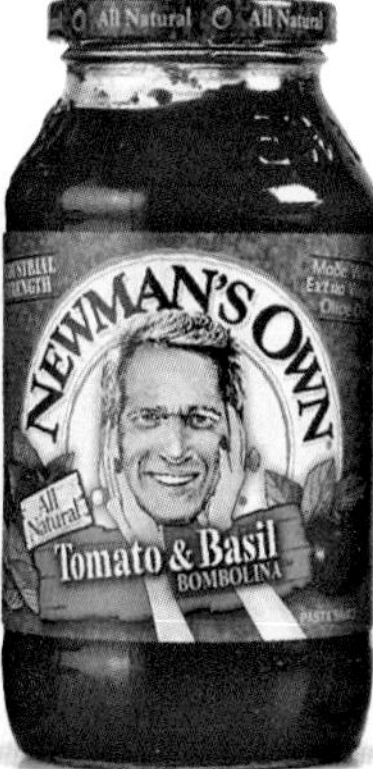

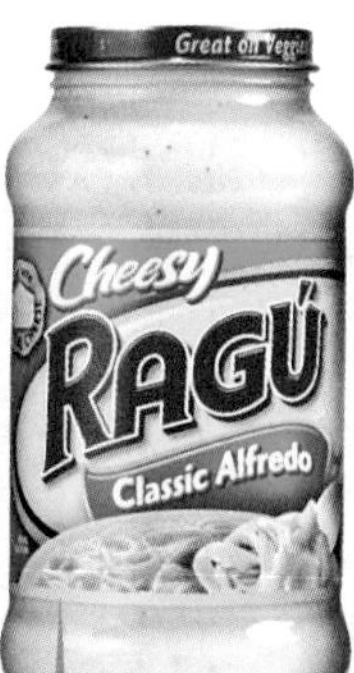

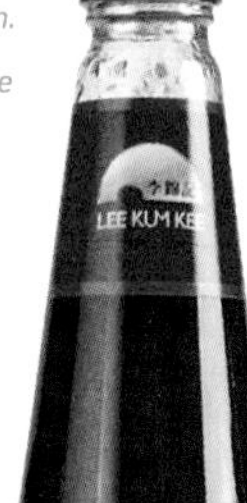

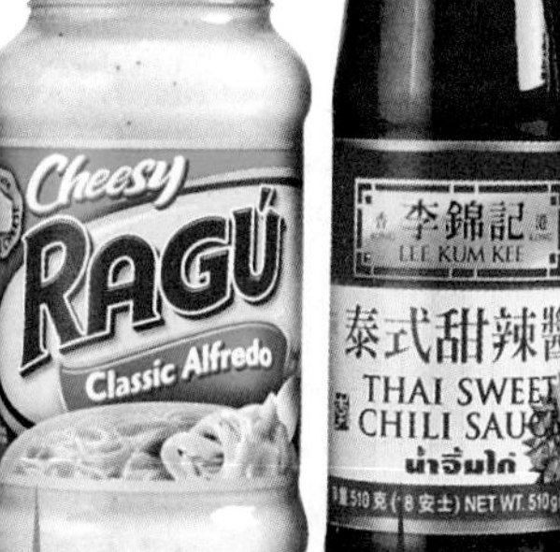

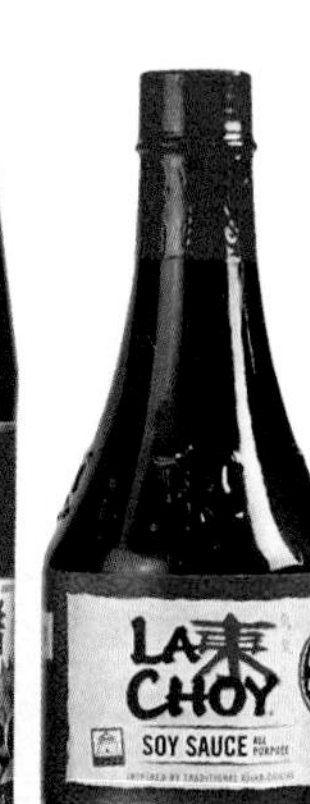

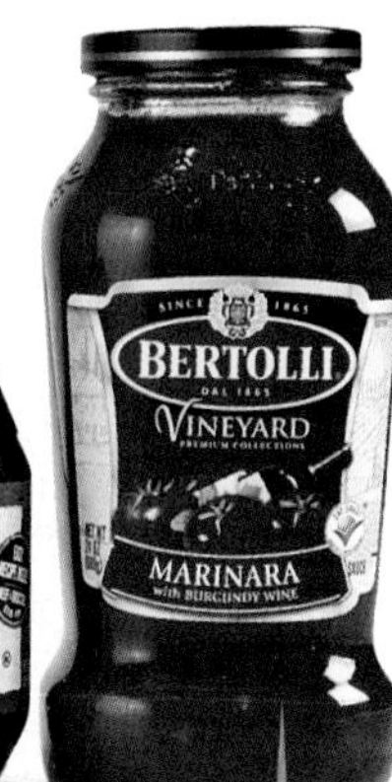

Prego Heart Smart Mushroom
(½ cup, 121 g)

100 calories
3 g fat
(0.5 g saturated)
410 mg sodium

Less sodium than their regular sauces, but still consistently worse than Ragu.

Ragu Cheesy Classic Alfredo
(½ cup, 122 g)

220 calories
20 g fat
(7 g saturated)
700 mg sodium

Typical Alfredo sauces have enough cheese, butter, and cream to put a dairy farmer's kids through college.

Lee Kum Kee Thai Sweet Chili Sauce
(1 Tbsp, 15 g)

40 calories
0 g fat
210 mg sodium
8 g sugars

The first three ingredients in this sauce are sugar, water, and corn syrup.

La Choy Soy Sauce
(1 Tbsp, 15 mL)

10 calories
0 g fat
1,160 mg sodium

This is, hands down, the briniest bottle of soy in the supermarket. Get half your day's sodium in 1 tablespoon.

Bertolli Vineyard Marinara with Burgundy Wine
(½ cup, 136 g)

80 calories
2 g fat
(0 g saturated)
500 mg sodium

Invest the caloric savings in a glass of vino.

Soups

Eat This

Campbell's Healthy Request Condensed Chicken Noodle
(1 cup prepared)
60 calories
2 g fat
(0.5 g saturated)
480 mg sodium
Just like the classic can, only better.

Campbell's Chunky Chili with Beans, Grilled Steak
(1 cup)
200 calories
3 g fat (1 g saturated)
870 mg sodium

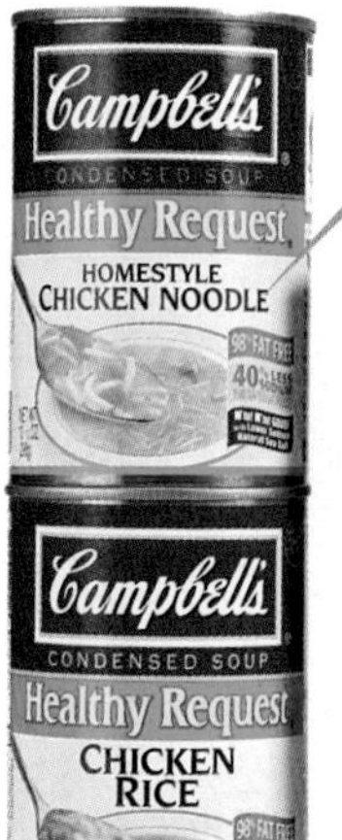

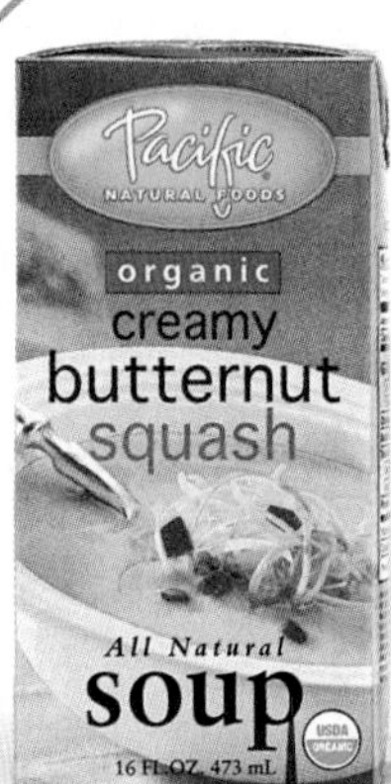

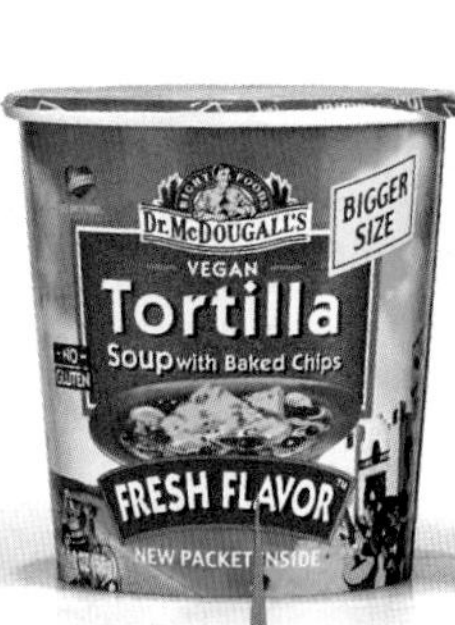

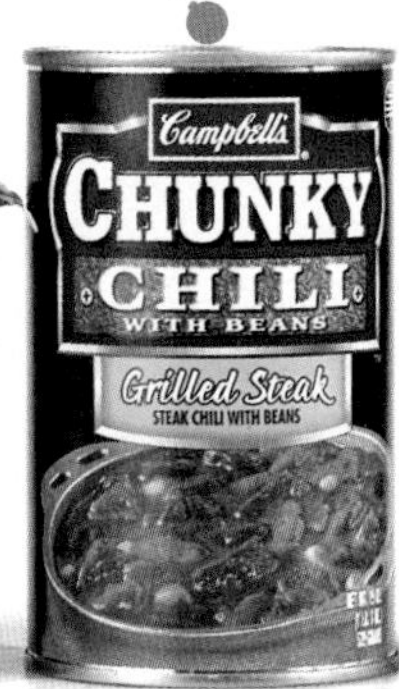

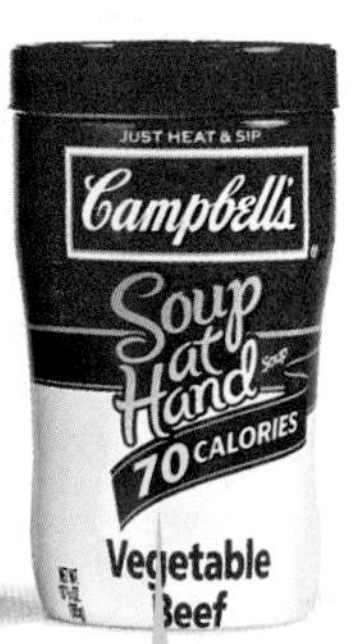

Campbell's Healthy Request Condensed Chicken Rice
(1 cup prepared)
70 calories
1.5 g fat
(0.5 g saturated)
480 mg sodium
Save calories, sodium, and cash.

Pacific Natural Foods Organic Creamy Butternut Squash
(1 cup prepared)
90 calories
2 g fat
(0 g saturated)
550 mg sodium
Loaded with vitamin A.

Dr. McDougall's Vegan Tortilla with Baked Chips
(1 cup prepared)
100 calories
1 g fat
310 mg sodium
Just eat it: A full container packs 10 grams of protein and 6 grams of fiber for 200 calories.

The fiber- and potassium-rich beans help combat the effects of the elevated sodium count.

Campbell's Soup at Hand Vegetable Beef
(1 container)
70 calories
1 g fat
930 mg sodium
Throw in a side salad and a piece of fruit, and you've got a super lean lunch in your hands.

Not That!

Hormel Chili with Beans
(1 cup)
260 calories
7 g fat (3 g saturated)
1,200 mg sodium

Go for seconds and you've just eaten a day's worth of sodium in one meal.

Progresso Traditional Chicken Noodle
(1 cup prepared)
100 calories
2.5 g fat
(0.5 g saturated)
690 mg sodium
Slurp the whole can and you'll be taking in more than half your day's sodium intake.

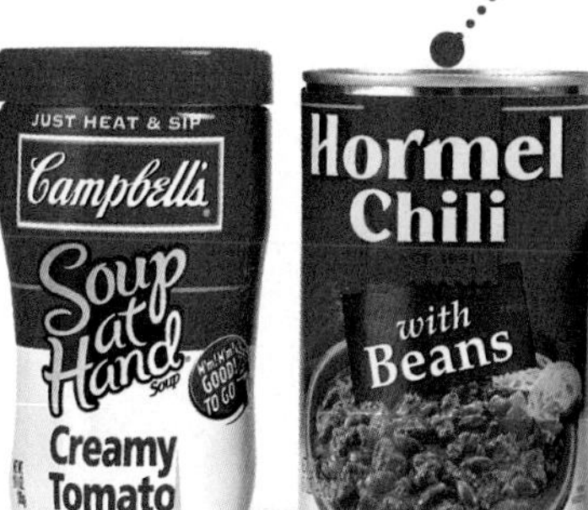

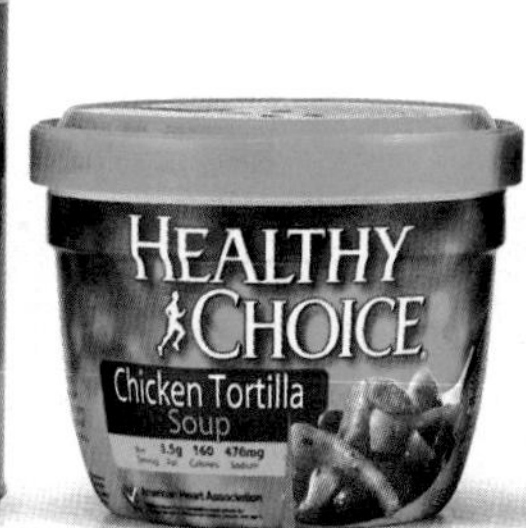

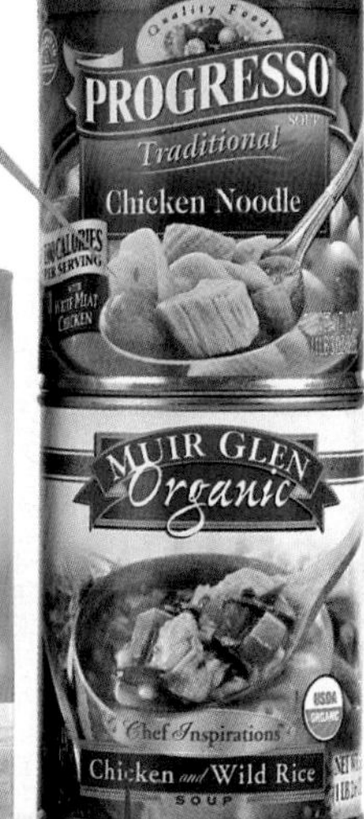

Campbell's Soup at Hand Creamy Tomato
(1 container)
190 calories
4 g fat
940 mg sodium
It's not just the cream driving up the calories here—it's also a glut of added sugar.

Healthy Choice Chicken Tortilla
(1 cup prepared)
160 calories
1.5 g fat
470 mg sodium
Not a disastrous cup of soup, but there are better products on the market.

V8 Golden Butternut Squash
(1 cup prepared)
140 calories
2 g fat
(1 g saturated)
750 mg sodium
35% more sodium and 55% more calories than Pacific Foods Butternut Soup.

Muir Glen Organic Chicken and Wild Rice
(1 cup prepared)
90 calories
2 g fat
(0.5 g saturated)
860 mg sodium
The fact that this soup is organic does nothing to counter the assault of sodium.

Bars

Eat This

Larabar Jŏcalat Chocolate
(1 bar, 48 g)
190 calories
10 g fat (2 g saturated)
5 g protein
5 g fiber
18 g sugars

Larabar proves that even indulgences can be good for you. This bar is made from exactly 6 ingredients: dates, almonds, walnuts, cocoa powder, cocoa mass, and cashews.

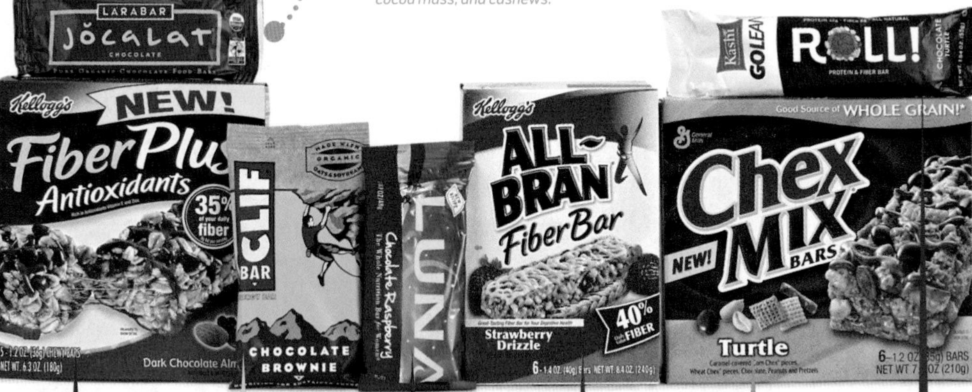

Kellogg's Fiber Plus Antioxidants Dark Chocolate Almond
(1 bar, 36 g)
130 calories
5 g fat
9 g fiber
7 g sugars

Clif Bar Chocolate Brownie
(1 bar, 68 g)
240 calories
5 g fat
(1.5 g saturated)
10 g protein
5 g fiber
22 g sugars

Luna Chocolate Raspberry
(1 bar, 48 g)
170 calories
5 g fat
(2.5 g saturated)
9 g protein
5 g fiber
13 g sugars

All-Bran Fiber Bar Strawberry Drizzle
(1 bar, 40 g)
120 calories
2.5 g fat
(1 g saturated)
2 g protein
10 g fiber
9 g sugars

Chex Mix Bars Turtle
(1 bar, 35 g)
130 calories
3.5 g fat
(1 g saturated)
4 g fiber
11 g sugars
Twice the fiber and fewer calories than the Quaker bar.

Kashi GoLean Roll! Chocolate Turtle
(1 bar, 55 g)
190 calories
5 g fat
(1.5 g saturated)
12 g protein
6 g fiber
14 g sugars

Not That!

PowerBar Performance Milk Chocolate Brownie
(1 bar, 65 g)

240 calories
3.5 g fat (0.5 g saturated)
8 g protein
1 g fiber
26 g sugars

The main ingredient in this bar is what PowerBar calls the C2 MAX carbohydrate blend. Translation: 4 different sugars swirled together.

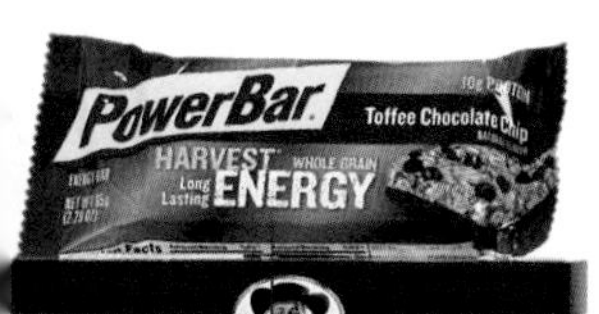

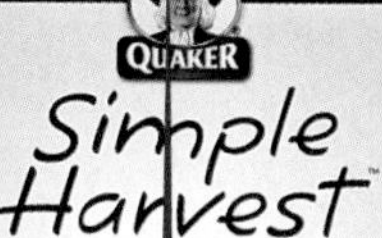

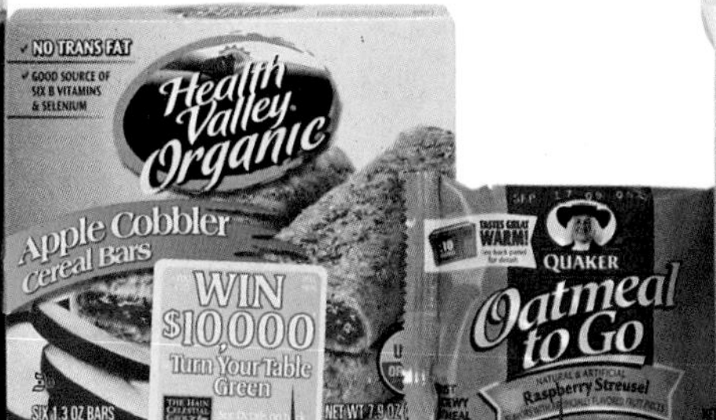

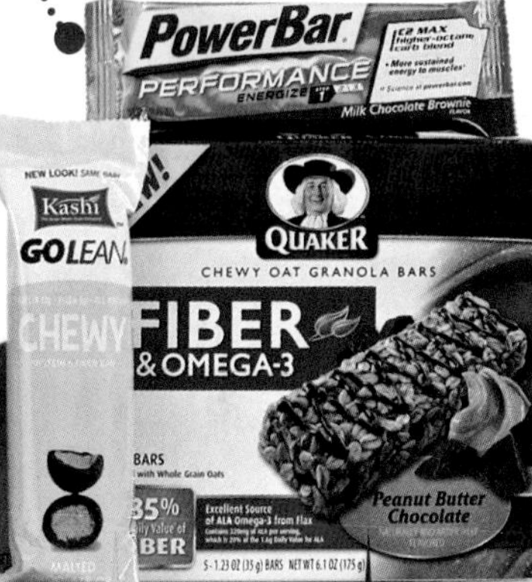

PowerBar Harvest Whole Grain Energy Toffee Chocolate Chip (1 bar, 65 g)
250 calories
5 g fat
(2.5 g saturated)
10 g protein
5 g fiber
20 g sugars

Quaker Simple Harvest Dark Chocolate Chunk
(1 bar, 35 g)
150 calories
4.5 g fat
(1.5 g saturated)
2 g fiber
10 g sugars

Health Valley Apple Cobbler Cereal Bars
(1 bar, 37 g)
140 calories
2.5 g fat
(0 g saturated)
2 g protein
1 g fiber
15 g sugars

Quaker Oatmeal to Go Raspberry Streusel
(1 bar, 60 g)
220 calories
4 g fat
(1 g saturated)
4 g protein
5 g fiber
19 g sugars

Kashi GoLean Malted Chocolate Crisp
(1 bar, 78 g)
290 calories
6 g fat
(4 g saturated)
13 g protein
6 g fiber
35 g sugars

Quaker Fiber & Omega-3 Peanut Butter Chocolate
(1 bar, 35 g)
150 calories
5 g fat
9 g fiber
7 g sugars
Made with hydrogenated oil.

Crackers

Eat This

Unlike most crackers, Triscuits aren't filled with empty carbs, preservatives, or emulsifiers. Instead they rely on a simple nutritious recipe: whole wheat, oil, and salt. And if it's a thinner cracker you're after, look for Triscuits Thin Crisps. They use the Triscuit recipe to create Wheat Thin–size crackers.

Nabisco Triscuit Original
(6 crackers, 28 g)
120 calories
4.5 g fat (1 g saturated)
3 g fiber
180 mg sodium

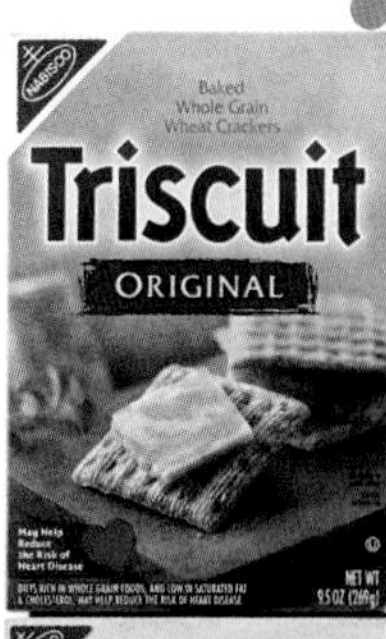

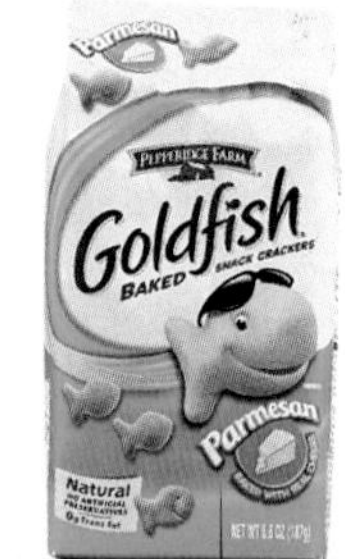

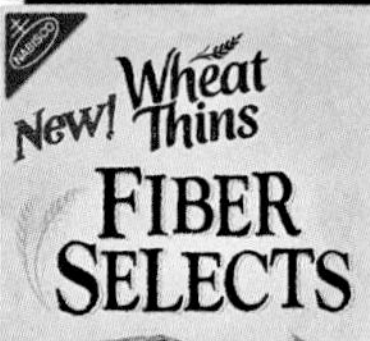

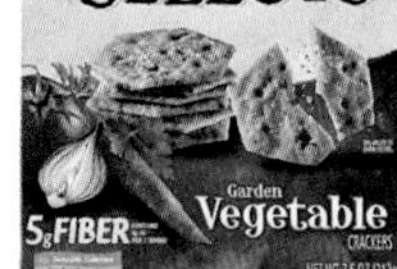

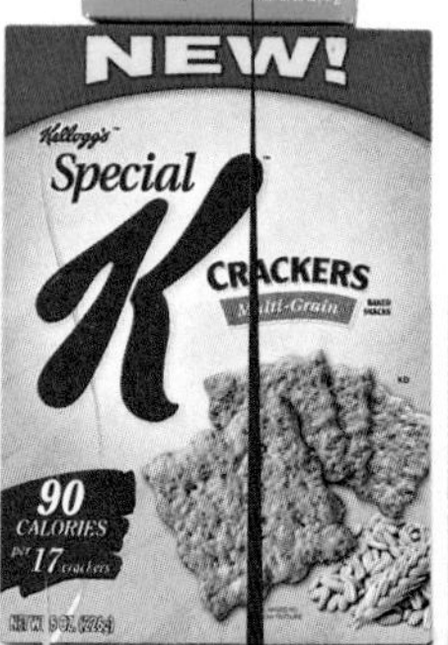

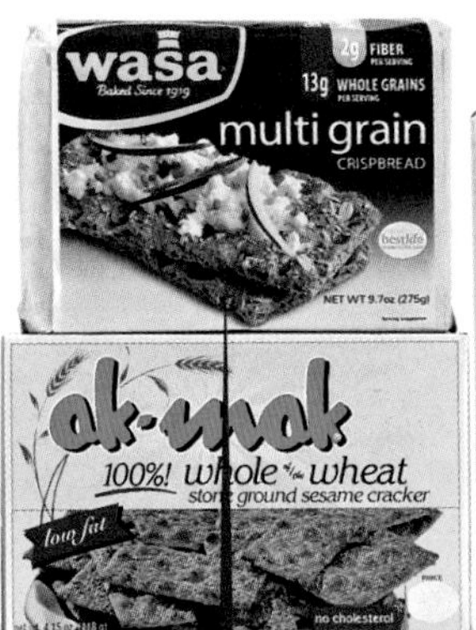

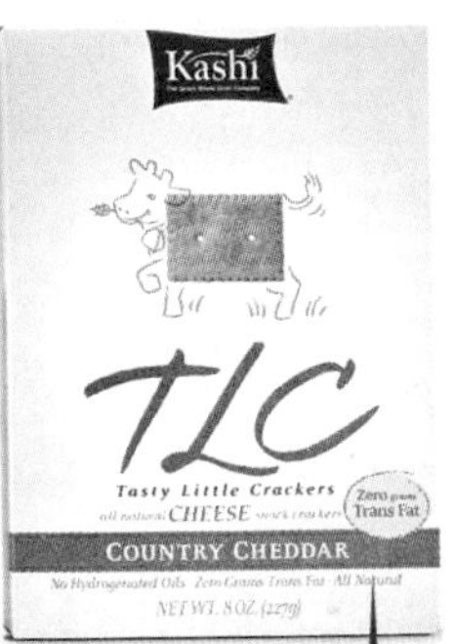

Nabisco Wheat Thins Fiber Selects Garden Vegetable
(15 crackers, 30 g)
120 calories
4 g fat
(0.5 g saturated)
5 g fiber
260 mg sodium

Special K Multi-Grain
(24 crackers, 30 g)
120 calories
3 g fat
(0 g saturated)
2 g fiber
260 mg sodium
The fiber in these crackers is their real saving grace.

Pepperidge Farm Goldfish Baked Parmesan
(60 pieces, 30 g)
130 calories
4 g fat
(1 g saturated)
<1 g fiber
280 mg sodium
Decent junk food.

Wasa Multi Grain Crispbread
(2 slices, 28 g)
90 calories
0 g fat
4 g fiber
160 mg sodium
This light cracker has four times the fiber in the Distinctives.

Ak-mak Whole of the Wheat 100% Stone Ground Sesame
(5 crackers, 28 g)
115 calories
2 g fat
(0 g saturated)
4 g fiber
220 mg sodium

Kashi TLC Country Cheddar
(18 crackers, 30 g)
130 calories
4.5 g fat
(0.5 g saturated)
<1 g fiber
220 mg sodium
Made with canola oil, so the fat here is the good stuff.

Not That!

For some reason, Wheat Thins use 15 ingredients to achieve what Triscuits does with 3. The result is a cracker with more calories and sugar and a third less fiber.

Nabisco Wheat Thins Reduced fat
(16 crackers, 31 g)
130 calories
3.5 g fat (0.5 g saturated)
1 g fiber
260 mg sodium

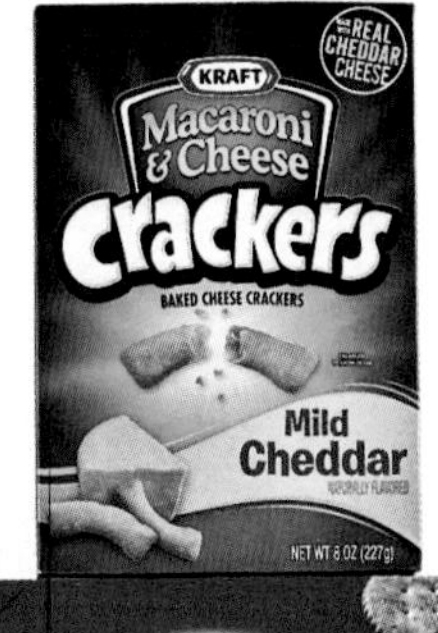

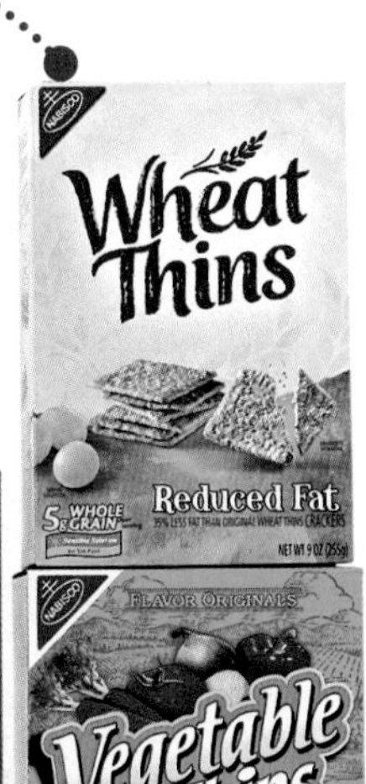

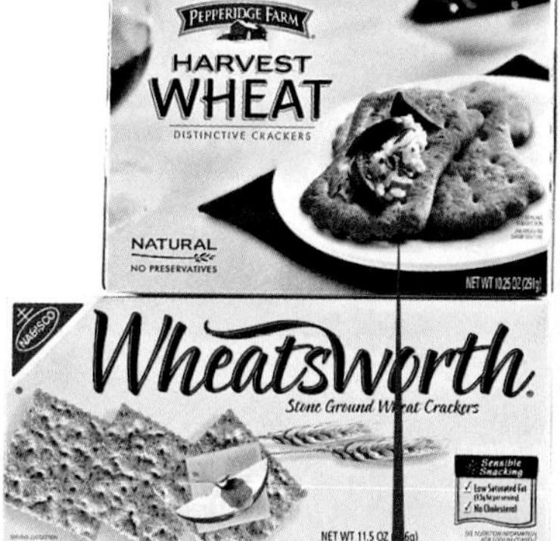

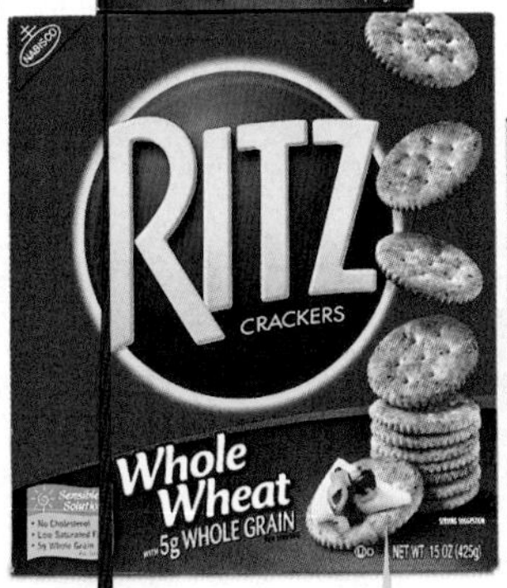

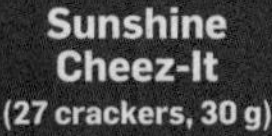

Sunshine Cheez-It
(27 crackers, 30 g)
150 calories
8 g fat
(2 g saturated)
<1 g fiber
250 mg sodium
Satisfy your cheese craving with a healthier cracker.

Nabisco Wheatsworth
(10 crackers, 32 g)
160 calories
7 g fat
(2 g saturated)
1 g fiber
360 mg sodium
Whole wheat flour should be first on the ingredients list; here it's fourth.

Pepperidge Farm Harvest Wheat Distinctive
(6 crackers, 32 g)
160 calories
7 g fat
(1 g saturated)
1 g fiber
250 mg sodium
Soaked in sugar.

Kraft Macaroni & Cheese Mild Cheddar
(45 pieces, 30 g)
150 calories
7 g fat
(2 g saturated)
<1 g fiber
310 mg sodium
True junk food.

Nabisco Ritz Whole Wheat
(10 crackers, 30 g)
140 calories
5 g fat
(1 g saturated)
1 g fiber
240 mg sodium
The main ingredient is still nutrient-stripped enriched flour.

Nabisco Vegetable Thins
(21 crackers, 30 g)
150 calories
7 g fat
(2 g saturated)
1 g fiber
320 mg sodium
The vegetable blend is listed after the oil blend.

Chips and Snacks

Eat This

Food Should Taste Good Multigrain
(~12 chips, 28 g)
140 calories
6 g fat (0.5 g saturated)
80 mg sodium

Not only do the folks at Food Should Taste Good keep the calories and sodium low, but they also boost the fiber load by sprinkling in a generous portion of corn bran.

Guiltless Gourmet All Natural Blue Corn Tortilla
(~18 chips, 28 g)
120 calories
3 g fat
(0 g saturated)
180 mg sodium
Made from exactly 4 ingredients.

Baked! Tostitos Scoops!
(~14 chips, 28 g)
120 calories
3 g fat
(0.5 g saturated)
125 mg sodium
Fill them with something wholesome like salsa or bean dip.

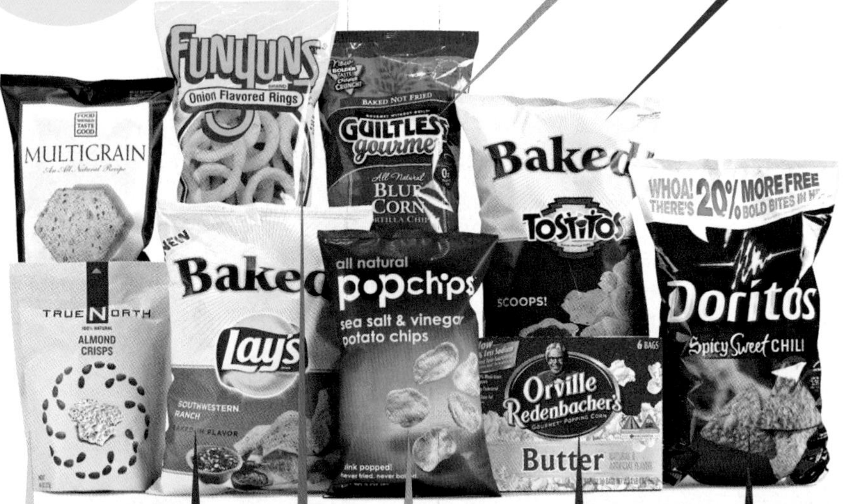

True North Almond Crisps
(12 chips, 28 g)
140 calories
7 g fat
(0.5 g saturated)
240 mg sodium
More protein, fiber, and healthy fat than normal chips.

Baked! Lay's Southwestern Ranch
(~14 chips, 28 g)
120 calories
3 g fat
(0.5 g saturated)
160 mg sodium
Baked! Lay's represents the classic potato chip at its absolute best.

Funyuns Onion Flavored Rings
(~13 pieces, 28 g)
140 calories
7 g fat
(1 g saturated)
240 mg sodium
Not bad numbers for a novelty chip.

Popchips Potato Sea Salt & Vinegar
(~20 chips, 28 g)
120 calories
4 g fat
(0 g saturated)
260 mg sodium
One of our favorite snacks. Think of these as a chip-popcorn hybrid.

Orville Redenbacher Butter Popcorn
(2 cups popped)
60 calories
4 g fat
(2 g saturated)
80 mg sodium
Boost the flavor with chili powder.

Doritos Spicy Sweet Chili
(~11 chips, 28 g)
140 calories
7 g fat
(1 g saturated)
270 mg sodium
Not a spectacular snack by any stretch, but it's one of the best chips in the spicy category.

Not That!

Fritos Scoops
(~10 chips, 28 g)

160 calories
10 g fat
(1.5 g saturated)
110 mg sodium

Yes, Fritos makes a scoopin' chip, too, but this one packs more than three times as much fat as the Tostitos.

Natural Tostitos Blue Corn Tortilla
(~6 chips, 28 g)

140 calories
6 g fat
(0.5 g saturated)
80 mg sodium

There's only one problem with these chips: too much oil.

Terra Spiced Sweet Potato Chips
(17 chips, 28 g)

160 calories
11 g fat (1 g saturated)
150 mg sodium

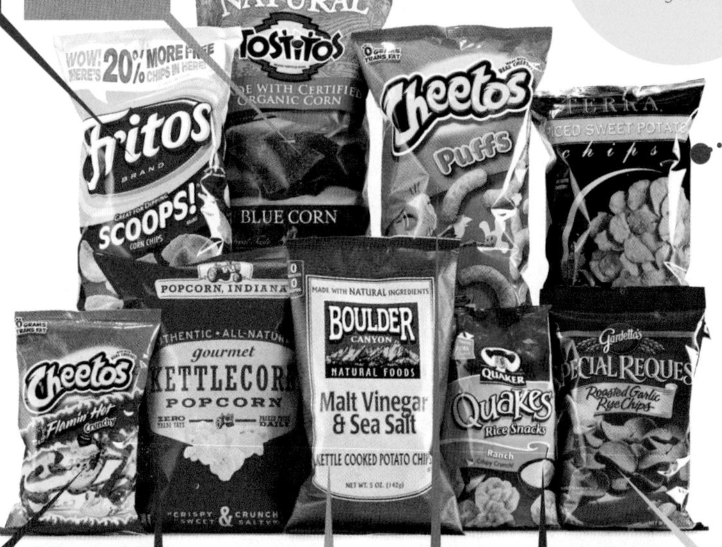

Terra's chips certainly aren't the worst decision you could make, but as long as they continue to drown their potatoes in oil, we'll have to recommend you find another chip.

Cheetos Flamin' Hot Crunchy
(~21 pieces, 28 g)

170 calories
11 g fat
(1.5 g saturated)
250 mg sodium

Cheetos are among the fattiest of all the popular crunchy snacks.

Indiana Gourmet Kettle Corn
(2 cups, 28 g)

130 calories
5 g fat
(0 g saturated)
130 mg sodium

Bagged popcorn is invariably worse than pop-it-yourself kernels.

Boulder Canyon Natural Foods Malt Vinegar & Sea Salt
(~14 chips, 28 g)

150 calories
7 g fat
(1 g saturated)
410 mg sodium

Cheetos Puffs
(~13 pieces, 28 g)

160 calories
10 g fat
(2 g saturated)
350 mg sodium

Not even a novelty snack should ask you to settle for this many calories.

Quaker Quakes Rice Snacks Ranch
(20 mini cakes, 32 g)

140 calories
5 g fat
(0 g saturated)
400 mg sodium

Made with partially hydrogenated oils.

Gardetto's Special Request Roasted Garlic Rye Chips
(½ cup, 30 g)

160 calories
10 g fat
(2 g saturated,
2.5 g trans)
400 mg sodium

Dips and Spreads

Eat This

Classico Sun-Dried Tomato Pesto
(1/4 cup, 62 g)

90 calories
5 g fat (1 g saturated)
630 mg sodium

Classico's recipe uses less oil and more tomatoes and basil, so you won't have to sprint to the gym to repent to the nutritional gods.

Ragu Pizza Sauce (2 Tbsp)

15 calories
0.5 g fat
(0 g saturated)
120 mg sodium

Try dipping vegetables and bread in marinara instead of ranch. You'll cut calories and boost your nutrient intake.

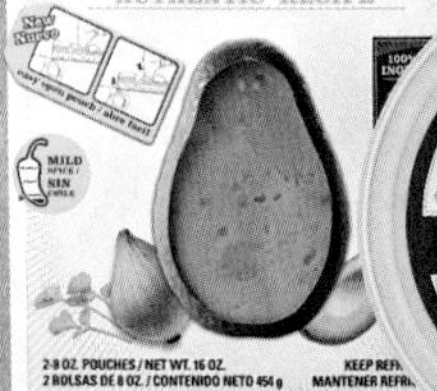

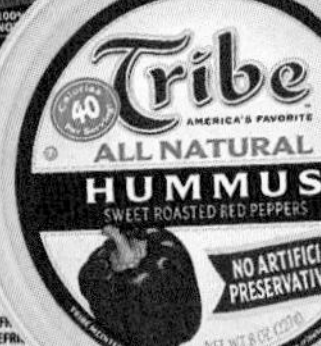

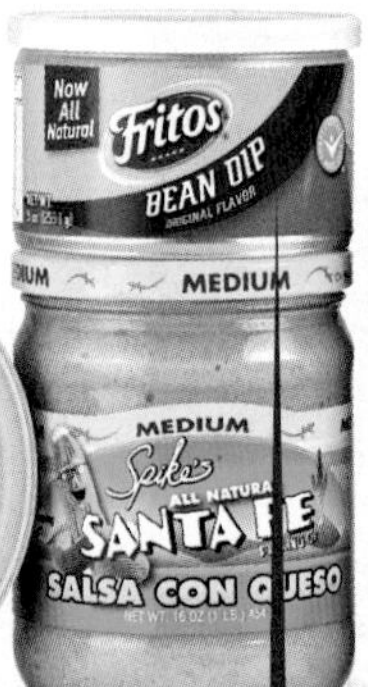

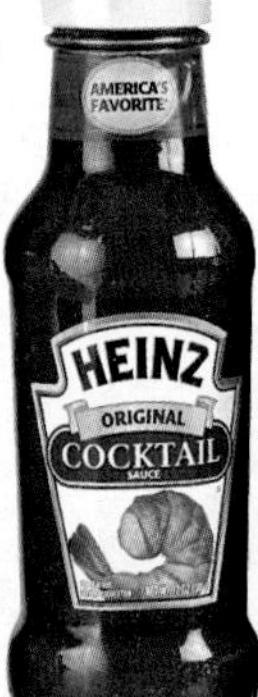

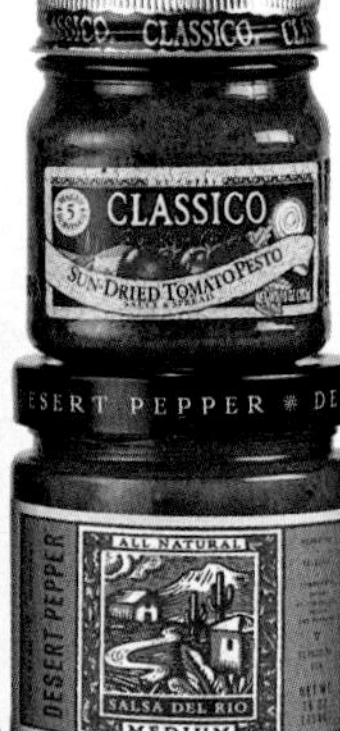

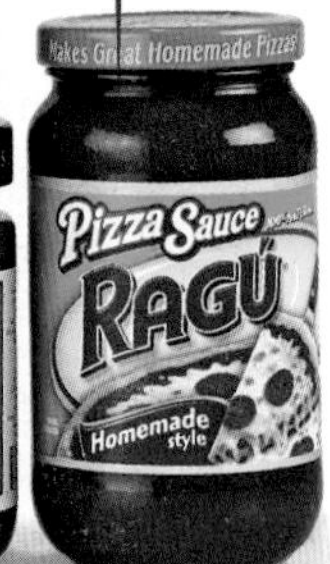

Calavo Guacamole
(2 Tbsp, 30 g)

50 calories
4.5 g fat
(1 g saturated)
95 mg sodium

Avocado is teeming with potassium, which helps your body convert sugar into energy.

Tribe Hummus Sweet Roasted Red Pepper
(2 Tbsp, 28 g)

40 calories
2.5 g fat
(0 g saturated)
125 mg sodium

Perfect for dipping and spreading.

Spike's Packing Co. Salsa Con Queso Medium
(2 Tbsp, 31 g)

50 calories
4 g fat
(0.5 g saturated)
170 mg sodium

Fritos Bean Dip
(2 Tbsp, 35 g)

35 calories
1 g fat
(0 g saturated)
190 mg sodium

Whatever you stick into this dip will emerge with a fat-fighting load of fiber and antioxidants.

Heinz Original Cocktail Sauce
(1/4 cup, 60 g)

60 calories
0 g fat
690 mg sodium

Heinz's has only 11 grams of sugar per serving, which is half as much as Del Monte's.

Desert Pepper Trading Co. Salsa del Rio
(2 Tbsp, 33 g)

10 calories
0 g fat
230 mg sodium

This tomatillo-based salsa doubles as a sauce for grilled foods.

Not That!

Marzetti Light Classic Ranch
(2 Tbsp)
80 calories
8 g fat
(1 g saturated)
250 mg sodium

Even in its lightest iteration, ranch is a truly troublesome condiment to keep in the fridge.

De Cecco Pesto Alla Genovese
(¹/₄ cup, 50 g)
260 calories
24 g fat (4 g saturated)
760 mg sodium

The main ingredient is olive oil, so even though the fats are heart-healthy, they're still responsible for an unnecessarily large load of calories.

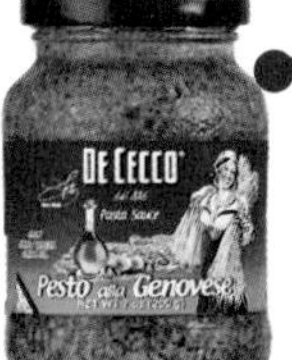

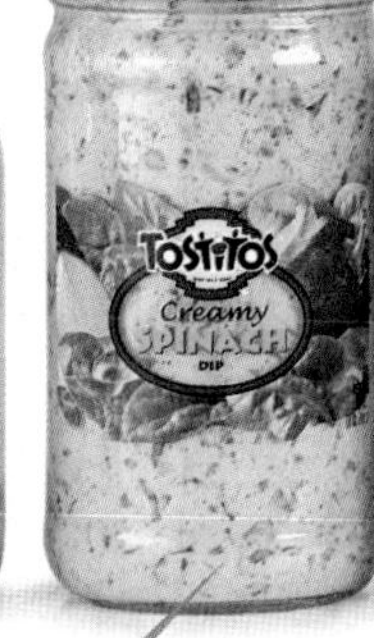

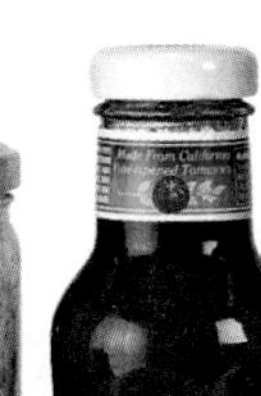

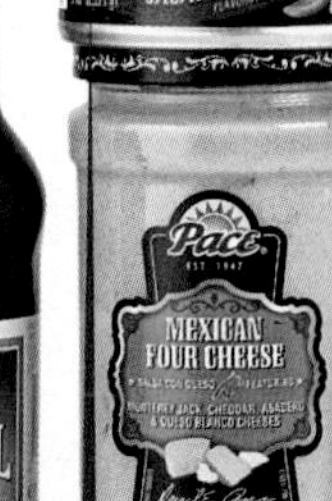

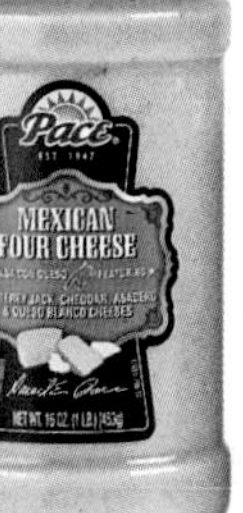

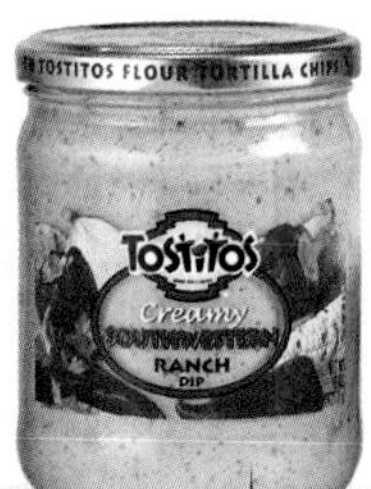

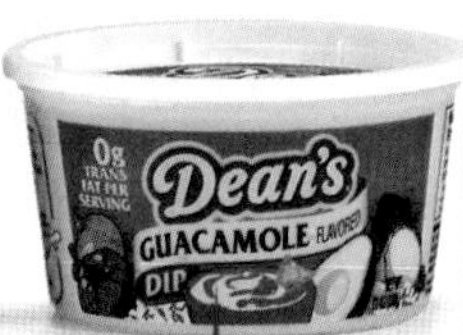

Tostitos Creamy Spinach Dip
(2 Tbsp, 32 g)
50 calories
4 g fat
200 mg sodium

Ignore the spinach in the name—the real "star" here is oil.

Del Monte Seafood Cocktail Sauce
(¹/₄ cup, 78 g)
100 calories
0 g fat
910 mg sodium

More calories, more sodium, and more sugar than Heinz.

Fritos Jalapeño Cheddar
(2 Tbsp, 34 g)
50 calories
3.5 g fat
(0.5 g saturated)
320 mg sodium

Not a shred of fiber. What it does have is MSG and partially hydrogenated oils.

Pace Mexican Four Cheese
(2 Tbsp, 30 ml)
90 calories
7 g fat
(1.5 g saturated)
430 mg sodium

The front label says "four cheese," but the back label lists water and soybean oil first.

Tostitos Creamy Southwestern Ranch Dip
(2 Tbsp, 32 g)
60 calories
5 g fat
(0.5 g saturated)
160 mg sodium

"Creamy" is always a bad sign.

Dean's Guacamole Flavored Dip
(2 Tbsp, 30 g)
90 calories
9 g fat
(2.5 g saturated)
170 mg sodium

This "guacamole dip" contains less than 2% avocado.

Salad Dressings

Eat This

Bolthouse Farms Yogurt Dressing Classic Ranch
(2 Tbsp, 30 g)

80 calories
7.5 g fat (1.5 g saturated)
290 mg sodium

As good as ranch gets. The main ingredient is yogurt, and it's sweetened with apple juice.

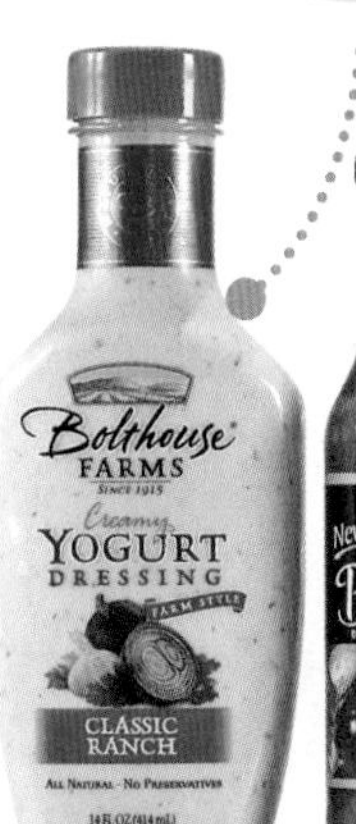

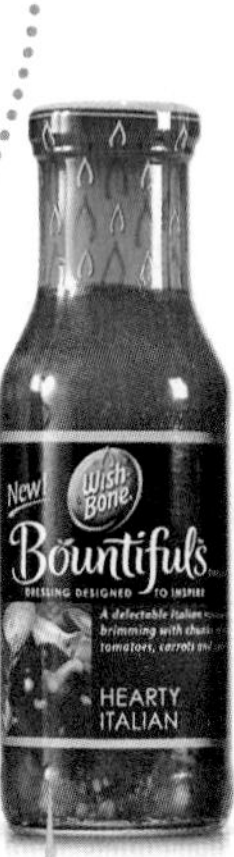

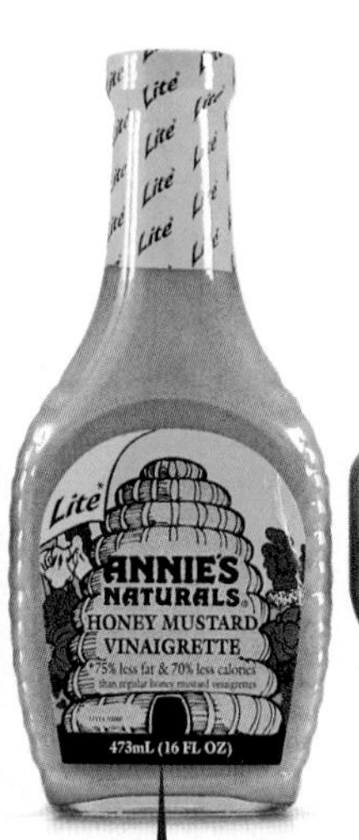

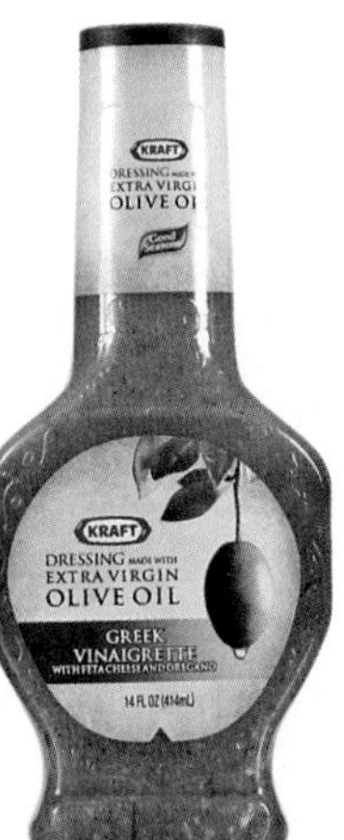

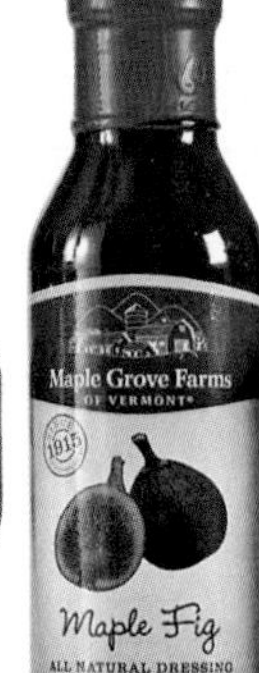

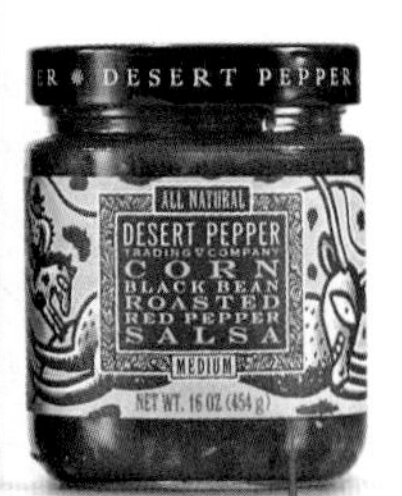

Wish-Bone Bountifuls Hearty Italian
(2 Tbsp, 30 mL)

15 calories
0 g fat
310 mg sodium

No single serving of dressing in Wish-Bone's Bountifuls line exceeds 35 calories.

Annie's Naturals Honey Mustard Vinaigrette Lite
(2 Tbsp, 31 g)

40 calories
3 g fat
(0 g saturated)
130 mg sodium

Mustard is listed before oil on the label.

Kraft Greek Vinaigrette with Feta Cheese and Oregano
(2 Tbsp, 31 g)

50 calories
5 g fat
(1 g saturated)
360 mg sodium

Always look for healthy fats in your dressings.

Maple Grove Farms Maple Fig
(2 Tbsp, 30 mL)

30 calories
0 g fat
0 mg sodium

Fruit blends can save you from the oil crutch of traditional dressings. Good luck finding a dressing with less sodium.

Desert Pepper Corn Black Bean Roasted Red Pepper Salsa
(2 Tbsp, 31 g)

15 calories
0 g fat
240 mg sodium

Salsa makes the best salad dressing imaginable.

Not That!

Nearly every single calorie in ranch comes from the fat in the soybean oil, which puts it among the worst dressings in the world.

Kraft Ranch Dressing & Dip
(2 Tbsp, 30 g)
120 calories
12 g fat (2 g saturated)
370 mg sodium

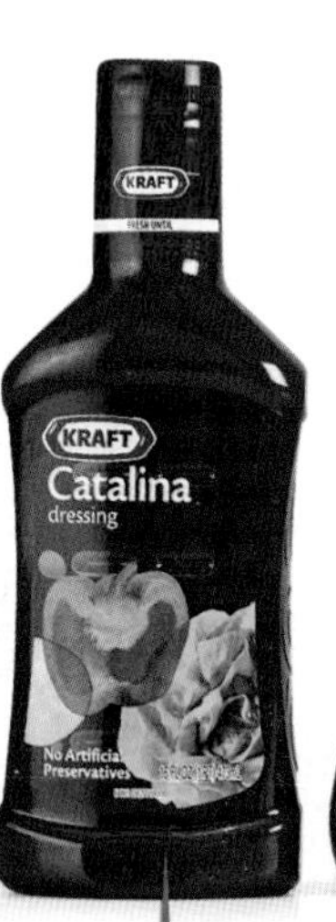

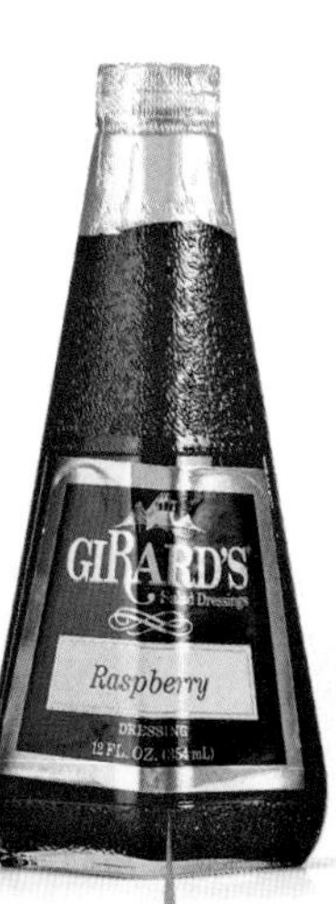

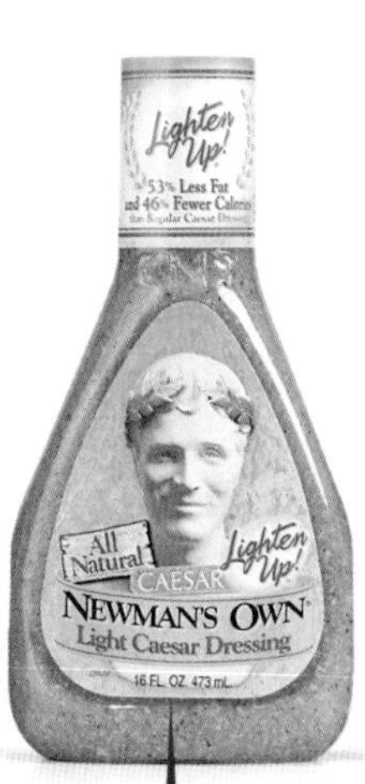

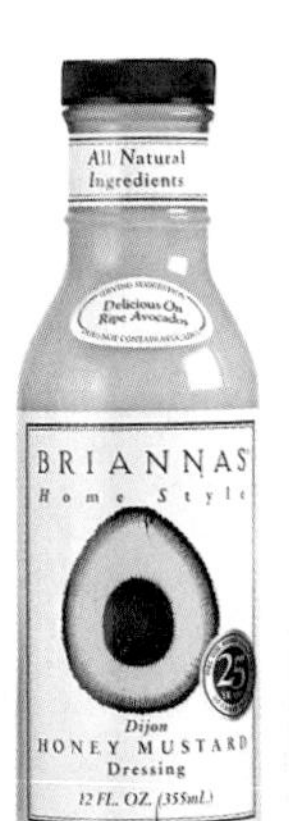

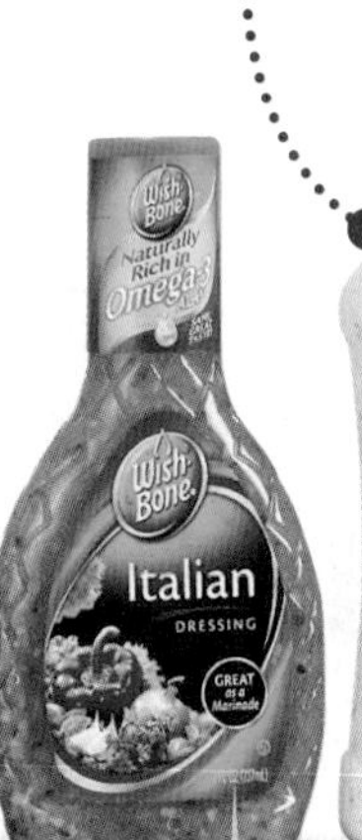

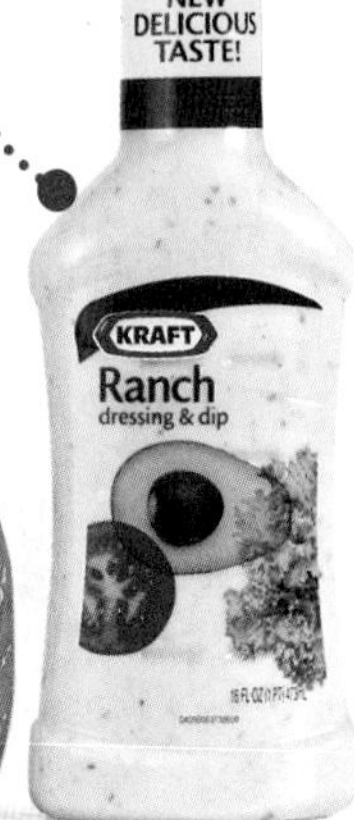

Kraft Catalina
(2 Tbsp, 31 g)
130 calories
11 g fat
(1.5 g saturated)
380 mg sodium

Adding tomato puree into the recipe was a nice touch, but it's too bad it was sandwiched between oil and sugar.

Girard's Raspberry
(2 Tbsp, 33 g)
120 calories
10 g fat
(1.5 g saturated)
65 mg sodium

Raspberry juice is the sixth ingredient. The first two are high-fructose corn syrup and soybean oil.

Newman's Own All Natural Light Caesar
(2 Tbsp, 30 g)
70 calories
6 g fat
(1 g saturated)
420 mg sodium

Even this light, watered-down version can't compete with the Greek vinaigrette.

Briannas Dijon Honey Mustard
(2 Tbsp, 30 mL)
150 calories
14 g fat
(1 g saturated)
170 mg sodium

As in a ranch dressing, oil is the first ingredient.

Wish-Bone Italian
(2 Tbsp, 30 mL)
90 calories
8 g fat
(1 g saturated)
490 mg sodium

Just 2 tablespoons packs more than 20% of your recommended daily sodium intake.

Fruits, Nuts, and Seeds

Eat This

Planters Trail Mix Berry, Nut & Chocolate
(3 Tbsp, 28 g)
120 calories
5 g fat (1 g saturated)
16 g sugars
20 mg sodium

The extra sugar comes from extra fruit. There's less chocolate in this bag than either cranberries or raisins. Make it your go-to mix.

Planters Chocolate Lovers Cashews
(10 pieces, 42 g)
230 calories
16 g fat
(7 g saturated)
15 g sugars
Think of this as a candy bar alternative, not as a healthy snack.

Sun-Maid Mixed Fruit
(1/4 cup, 40 g)
100 calories
0 g fat
17 g sugars
Look for fruit blends like this one: all fruit and no added sugar. It's a rare find, so cherish it.

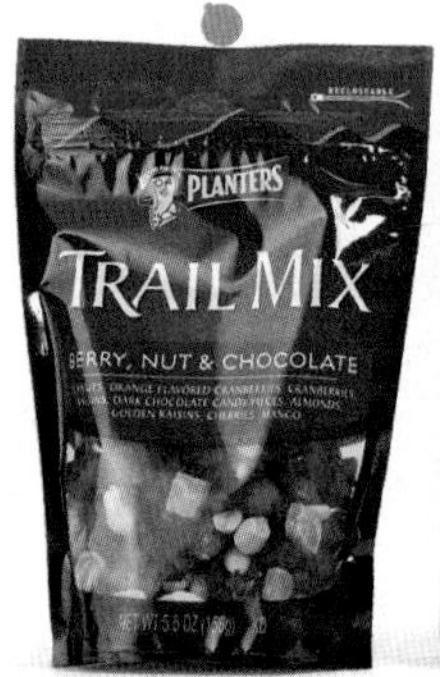

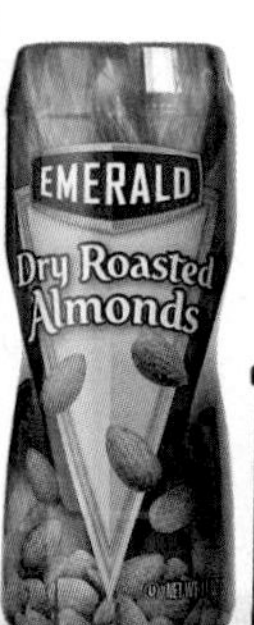

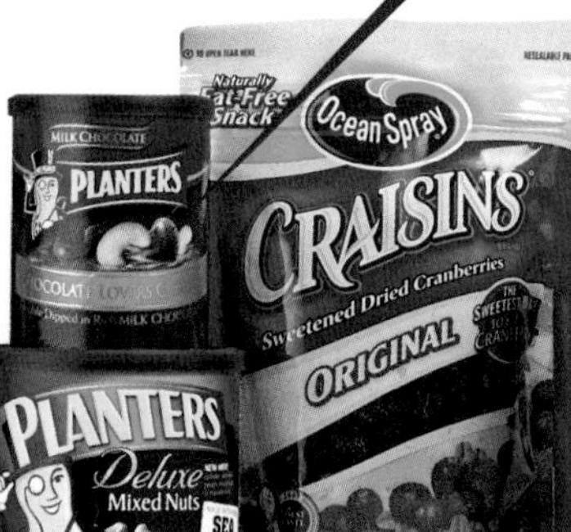

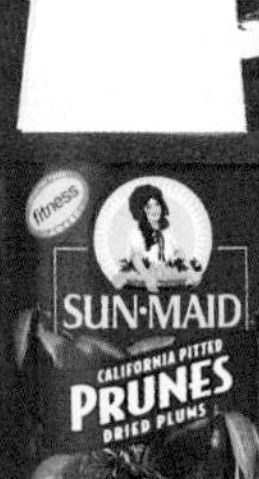

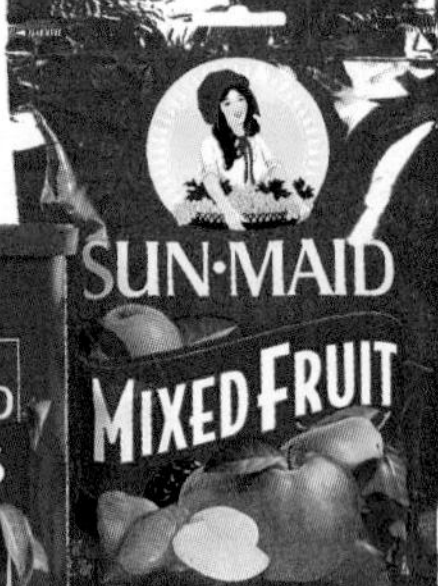

Emerald Almonds Dry Roasted
(~1/4 cup, 28 g)
150 calories
13 g fat
(1 g saturated)
230 mg sodium
"Dry roasted" means these almonds skipped the bath in vegetable oil.

Planters Deluxe Mixed Nuts
(~19 pieces, 28 g)
170 calories
15 g fat
(2.5 g saturated)
100 mg sodium
Planters Deluxe is the no-frills and no-filler can of nuts. It doesn't get any healthier.

Ocean Spray Original Craisins
(1/3 cup, 40 g)
130 calories
0 g fat
26 g sugars
Cranberries have been shown to contain more antioxidants than raspberries and strawberries combined!

Sun-Maid Pitted Prunes
(1/4 cup, 40 g)
100 calories
0 g fat
15 g sugars
Plums are loaded with fiber and score just below blueberries in the USDA's ranking of antioxidant activity.

Not That!

Planters Trail Mix Nut & Chocolate
(3 Tbsp, 33 g)
160 calories
10 g fat (2.5 g saturated)
13 g sugars
20 mg sodium

Chocolate is the first ingredient after peanuts, which makes this mix more treat than trail.

Sunsweet Berry Blend
($^1/_4$ cup, 40 g)
140 calories
0.5 g fat
(0 g saturated)
27 g sugars
These fruits are loaded with sugar and high-fructose corn syrup.

Mauna Loa Milk Chocolate Macadamias
(~10 pieces, 41 g)
250 calories
17 g fat
(7 g saturated)
19 g sugars
Macadamias have more fat and fewer antioxidants than most other nuts.

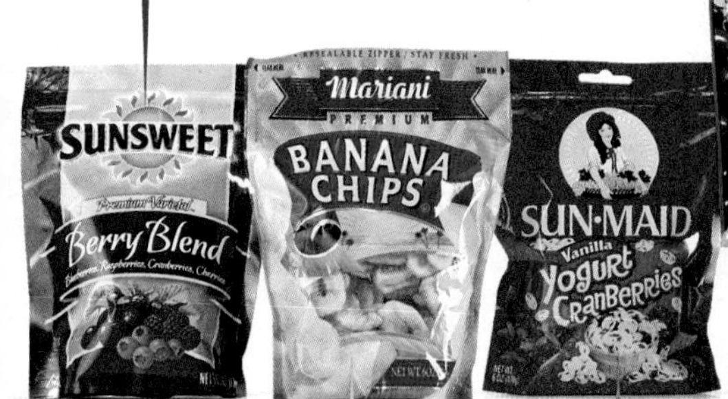

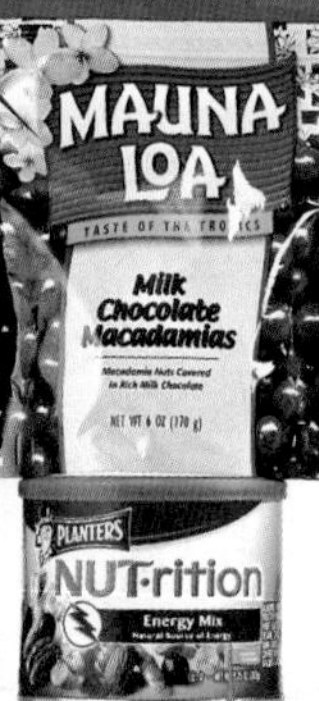

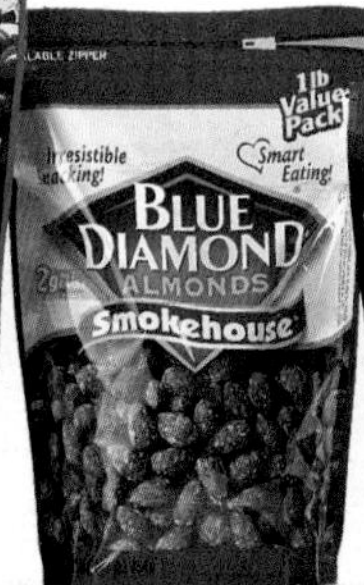

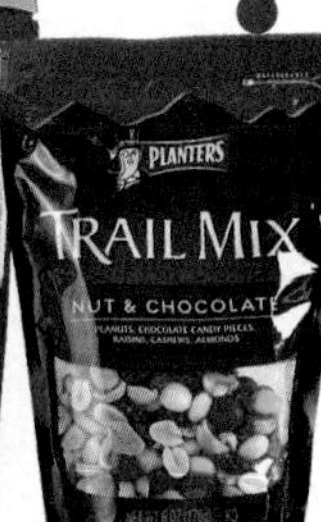

Mariani Banana Chips
($^1/_4$ cup, 28 g)
150 calories
7 g fat
(6 g saturated)
3 g sugars
Don't mistake these for "dried" fruit; like greasy potato chips, these bananas are fried in oil.

Sun-Maid Vanilla Yogurt Cranberries
(30 g)
120 calories
3.5 g fat
(3 g saturated)
20 g sugars
The "yogurt coating" is actually a blend of sugar and partially hydrogenated oils.

Planters NUTrition Energy Mix
($^1/_4$ cup, 34 g)
190 calories
15 g fat
(2 g saturated)
120 mg sodium
The NUTrition energy mix is weighed down with too many chocolate bits.

Blue Diamond Almonds Smokehouse
(~28 nuts, 28 g)
170 calories
16 g fat
(1 g saturated)
150 mg sodium
Vegetable oil is used in the smoking process, which means more fat per nut.

Cookies

Eat This

Each chewy cookie is slightly smaller than the other Chips Ahoy! cookies, and smaller cookies equate to less damage done.

Chips Ahoy! Chewy
(2 cookies, 27 g)
120 calories
6 g fat (3 g saturated)
10 g sugars

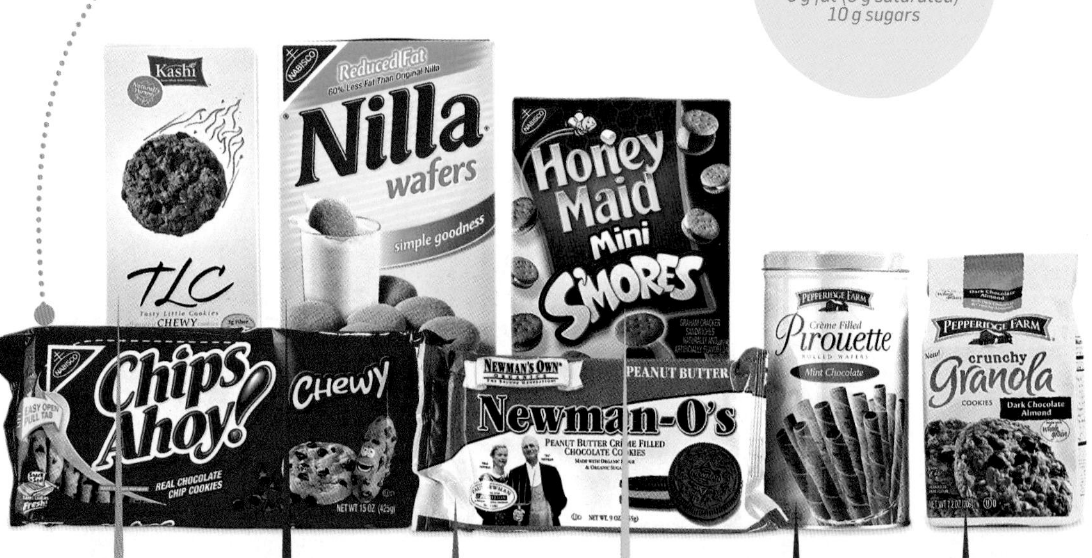

Kashi TLC Oatmeal Dark Chocolate
(1 cookie, 30 g)
130 calories
5 g fat
(1.5 g saturated)
8 g sugars
Each cookie starts with whole grains but still tastes like a splurge.

Nilla Wafers Reduced Fat
(8 wafers, 29 g)
110 calories
2 g fat
(0 g saturated)
12 g sugars
Eight wafers and a glass of milk makes for a decent after-dinner treat.

Newman-O's Peanut Butter Crème Filled Chocolate
(2 cookies, 28 g)
120 calories
5 g fat
(1.5 g saturated)
10 g sugars
Made with heart-healthy canola oil.

Honey Maid Mini S'mores Sandwiches
(8 sandwiches, 29 g)
140 calories
6 g fat
(2.5 g saturated)
10 g sugars
Not bad, as far as stuffed cookies go.

Pepperidge Farm Crème Filled Pirouette Mint Chocolate
(2 wafers, 25 g)
120 calories
4.5 g fat
(2.5 g saturated)
14 g sugars
A light indulgence.

Pepperidge Farm Crunchy Granola Dark Chocolate Almond
(1 cookie, 26 g)
130 calories
7 g fat
(2.5 g saturated)
8 g sugars
A perfect portion.

Not That!

Stick to the Chewy Chips Ahoy! You'll save 20 calories per cookie.

Chips Ahoy! Chunky
(2 cookies, 34 g)
160 calories
9 g fat (3 g saturated)
12 g sugars

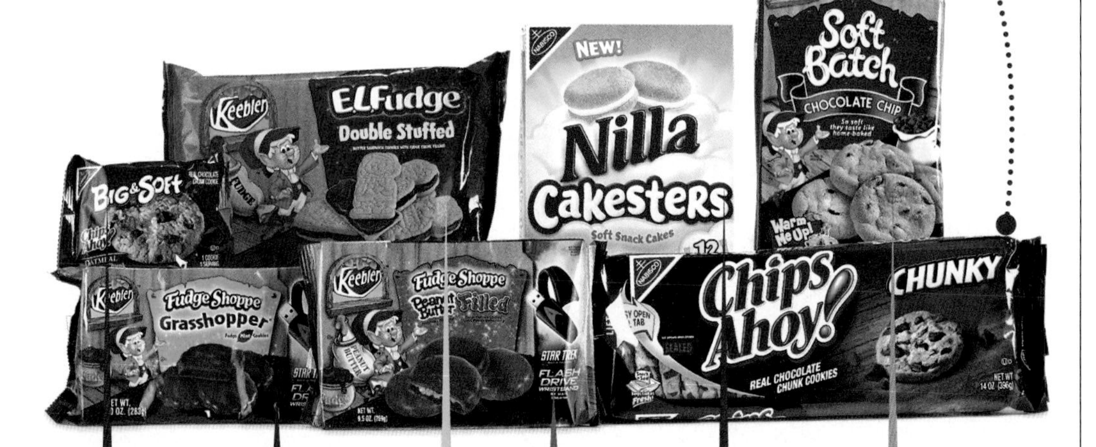

Chips Ahoy! Big & Soft Oatmeal Chocolate Chunk
(1 cookie, 39 g)
180 calories
8 g fat
(3 g saturated)
13 g sugars
Way too big.

Fudge Shoppe Grasshopper
(4 cookies, 29 g)
150 calories
7 g fat
(4.5 g saturated)
12 g sugars
Small as they are, they still pack in more than a gram of saturated fat apiece.

E.L. Fudge Double Stuffed
(2 cookies, 35 g)
180 calories
9 g fat
(3.5 g saturated)
13 g sugars
E.L. Fudge makes some of the worst cookies in the supermarket.

Keebler Fudge Shoppe Peanut Butter Filled
(2 cookies, 30 g)
170 calories
10 g fat
(5 g saturated)
9 g sugars
Made with partially hydrogenated oils.

Nilla Cakesters
(2 cakes, 50 g)
220 calories
10 g fat
(2 g saturated)
22 g sugars
A serving of these cookies has twice as much fat as a Twinkie.

Keebler Soft Batch Chocolate Chip
(2 cookies, 32 g)
160 calories
7 g fat
(3 g saturated)
12 g sugars
Mostly flour, HFCS, oil, and sugar.

Frozen Breakfast Entr

Eat This

Eggo Nutri-Grain Filled Strawberry Waffles

(1 waffle, 58 g)

130 calories
3.5 g fat (1 g saturated)
8 g sugars
300 mg sodium

For a gimmicky frozen breakfast, these waffles fare pretty well. The sugar level is moderate, there's real dehydrated fruit inside, and they're loaded with 3 grams of fiber to keep your stomach full until lunch.

Amy's Toaster Pops Apple

(1 pastry, 60 g)

150 calories
3.5 g fat
(0 g saturated)
10 g sugars
110 mg sodium

Unlike most toaster pastries, Amy's filling is made with more fruit than sugar.

Golden Blueberry Blintzes

(1 blintz, 61 g)

90 calories
1 g fat
(0 g saturated)
6 g sugars

Most of the sugar comes from the load of blueberries in the filling.

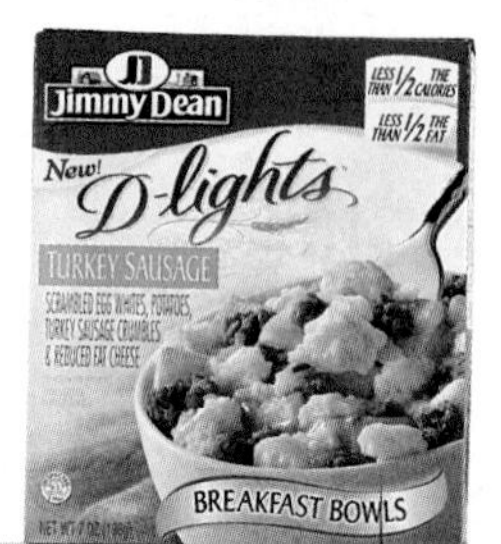

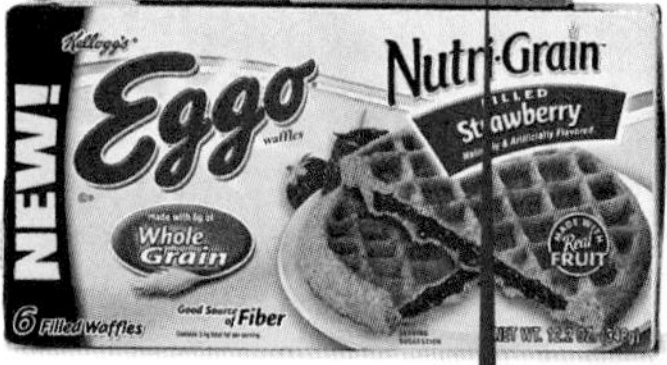

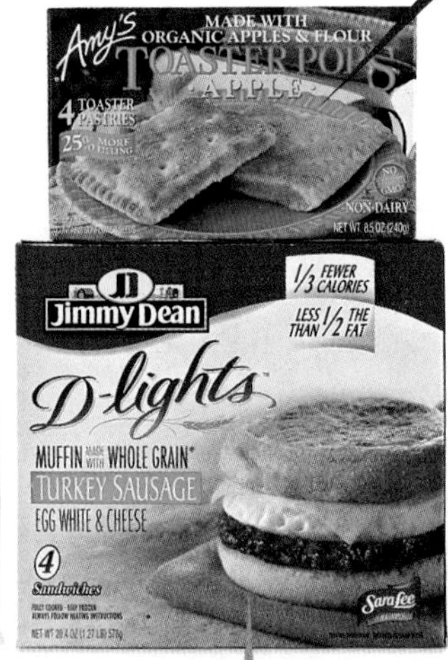

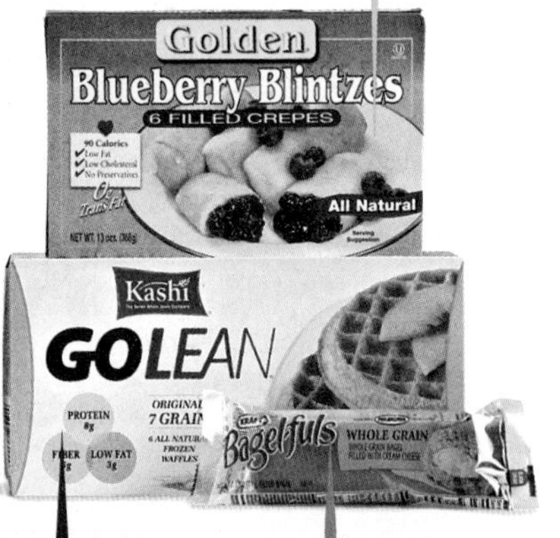

Jimmy Dean D-Lights Turkey Sausage Breakfast Bowl

(1 bowl, 198 g)

230 calories
7 g fat
(3 g saturated)
730 mg sodium

A breakfast sandwich, minus the bread.

Jimmy Dean D-Lights Turkey Sausage Muffin

(1 sandwich, 145 g)

260 calories
7 g fat
(3.5 g saturated)
790 mg sodium

Jimmy's D-Lights line is reliable for high-protein, low-calorie meals.

Kashi GoLean Waffles

(2 waffles, 84 g)

170 calories
3 g fat
(0 g saturated)
4 g sugars
330 mg sodium

Twice the protein and fiber as Eggo's Nutri-Grain.

Kraft Bagel-Fuls Whole Grain

(1 filled bagel, 71 g)

180 calories
6 g fat
(3.5 g saturated)
4 g sugars
200 mg sodium

Low in sugar, high in fiber, and easy to grab and go.

Not That!

Eggo Mini Muffin Tops Blueberry
(4 tops, 46 g)
140 calories
5 g fat
(1.5 g saturated)
9 g sugars
These muffins lose every nutritional battle to the blintzes.

Pepperidge Farm Turnovers Apple
(1 turnover, 89 g)
270 calories
15 g fat
(8 g saturated)
11 g sugars
370 mg sodium
They removed the trans fat, but there's still a long way to go.

Pillsbury Cream Cheese & Strawberry Toaster Strudel
(1 pastry, 54 g)
190 calories
9 g fat
(3.5 g saturated, 1 g trans)
9 g sugars
190 mg sodium

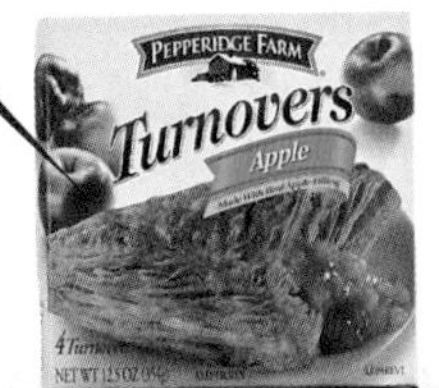

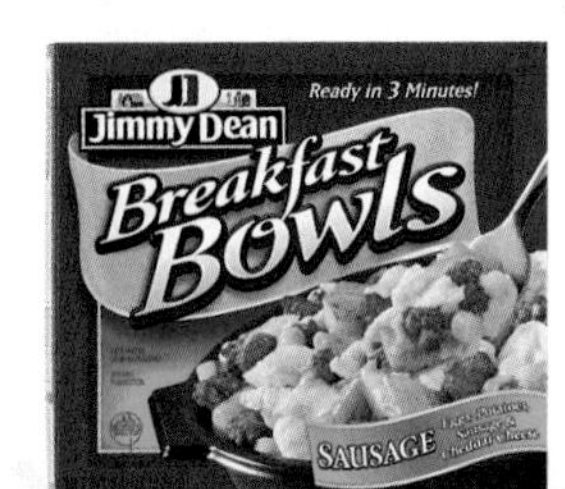

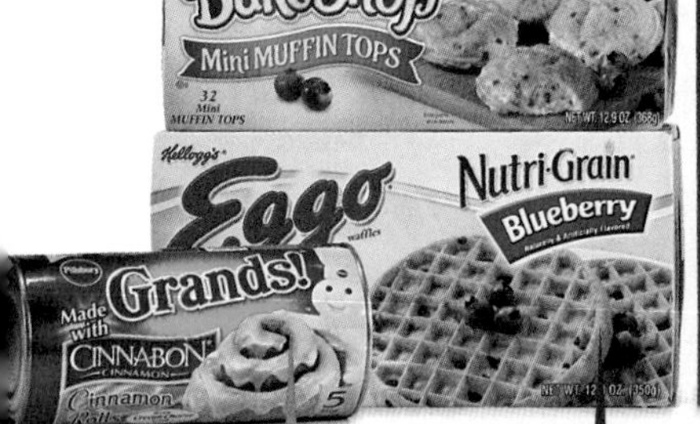

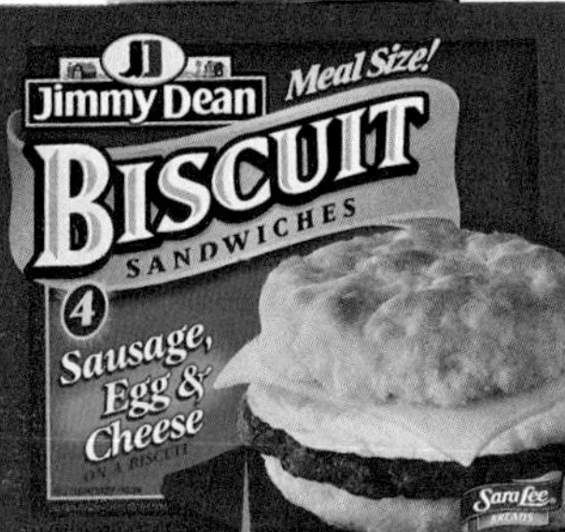

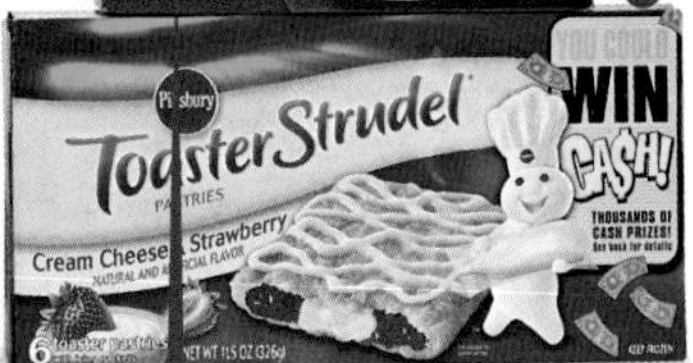

Pillsbury Grands! Cinnamon Rolls with Cream Cheese Icing
(1 roll, 99 g)
310 calories
9 g fat
(2 g saturated, 2.5 g trans)
23 g sugars
650 mg sodium

Eggo Nutri-Grain Blueberry Waffles
(2 waffles, 70 g)
180 calories
5 g fat
(1.5 g saturated)
7 g sugars
380 mg sodium
The blueberries comprise less than 2% of these waffles.

Jimmy Dean Sausage, Egg & Cheese Biscuit
(1 sandwich, 128 g)
420 calories
29 g fat
(10 g saturated, 3 g trans)
920 mg sodium
Do you really want a half day's worth of trans fat at breakfast?

Jimmy Dean Sausage Breakfast Bowl
(1 bowl, 227 g)
490 calories
34 g fat
(14 g saturated, 1.5 g trans)
1,210 mg sodium
Sausage tends to be twice as caloric as bacon.

Don't ruin your day with an early morning load of trans fat.

Frozen Pizza

Eat This

Stouffer's French Bread Cheese
(1 pizza)
360 calories
15 g fat (6 g saturated)
530 mg sodium

The more reasonable portion size helps Stouffer's cut fully half the fat and calories from DiGiorno for One pizza. One swap like this per week would save you more than 5 pounds in a year.

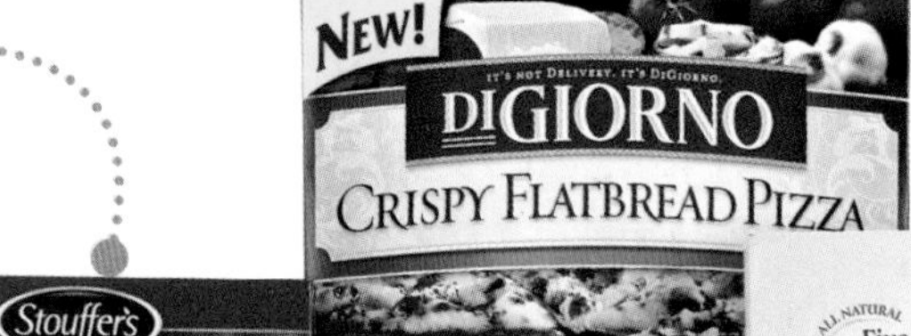

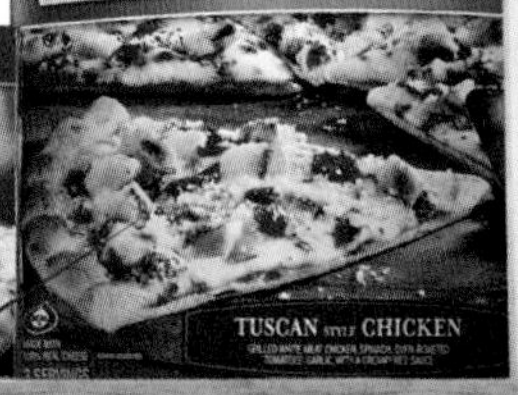

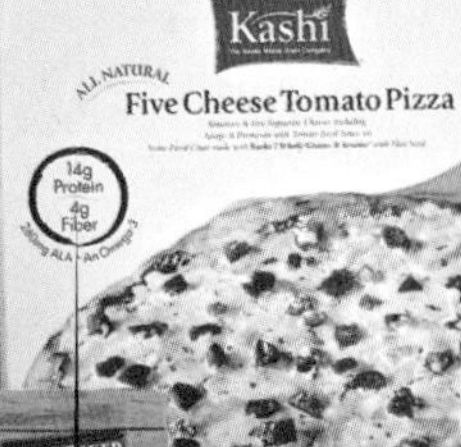

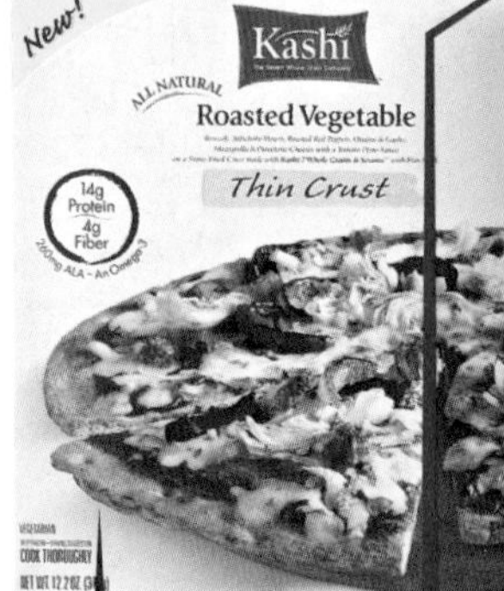

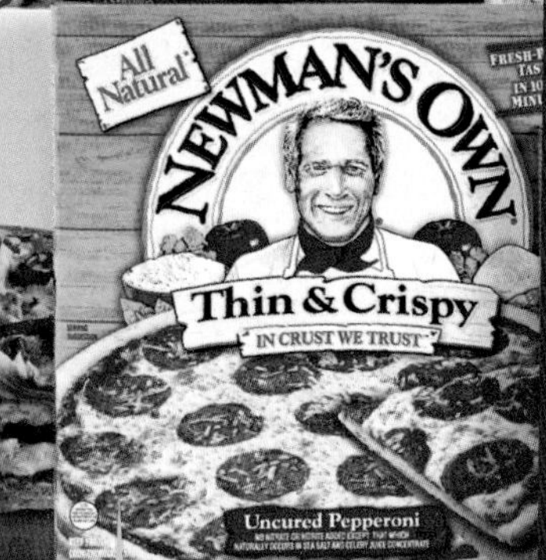

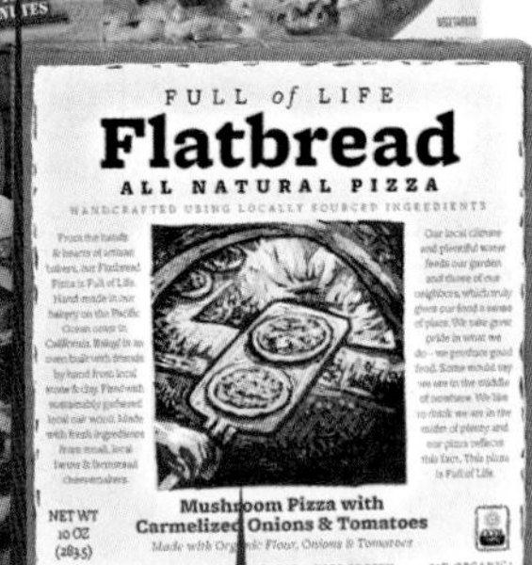

Kashi Thin Crust Roasted Vegetable
(⅓ pizza, 116 g)
250 calories
9 g fat
(4 g saturated)
630 mg sodium
Kashi makes some of the best pies around. This one is loaded with fiber and vitamin A.

DiGiorno Crispy Flatbread Tuscan Style Chicken
(⅓ pizza, 132 g)
280 calories
14 g fat
(6 g saturated)
680 mg sodium
The best DiGiorno's pizza line by far.

Newman's Own Thin & Crispy Uncured Pepperoni
(⅓ pizza, 125 g)
320 calories
16 g fat
(6 g saturated)
800 mg sodium
As good as pepperoni pizza gets.

Kashi Five Cheese Tomato
(⅓ pizza, 118 g)
290 calories
9 g fat
(3.5 g saturated)
570 mg sodium
The whole-grain–packed crust lends each serving an impressive 4 grams of fiber.

Full of Life Mushroom Pizza with Carmelized Onions & Tomatoes Flatbread
(½ pizza, 142 g)
272 calories
12 g fat
(4 g saturated)
406 mg sodium

Not That!

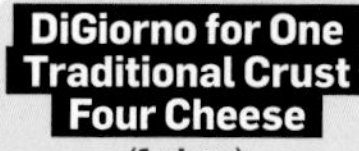

DiGiorno for One Traditional Crust Four Cheese
(1 pizza)
720 calories
30 g fat
(12 g saturated, 3 g trans)
1,190 mg sodium

DiGiorno's individual pizzas are among the most deleterious foods in the freezer aisle. This one meal has nearly half your day's sodium, more than half your day's saturated fat, and more than your day's worth of trans fat.

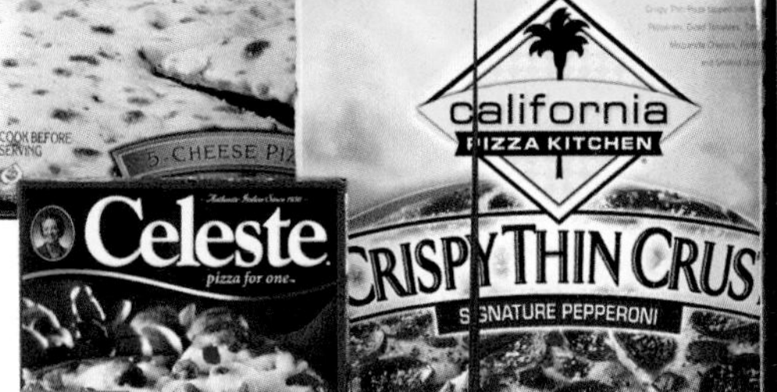

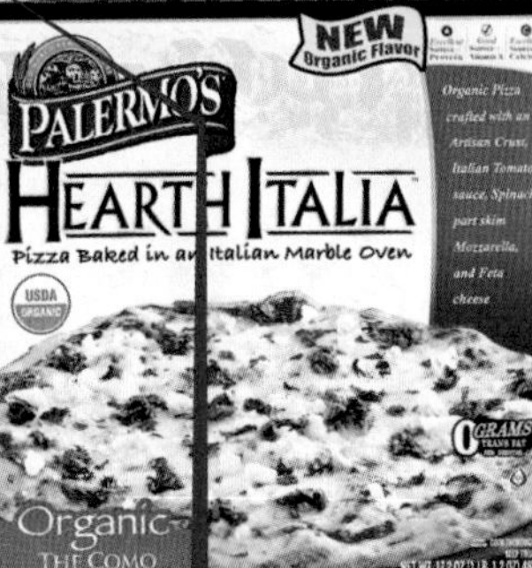

Celeste Deluxe Pizza for One
(1 pizza, 186 g)
410 calories
21 g fat
(6 g saturated, 3.5 g trans)
1,170 mg sodium
Celeste covers its pies with trans-fatty imitation cheese.

Freschetta Ultra Thin 5-Cheese
(⅓ pizza, 121 g)
330 calories
16 g fat
(8 g saturated)
680 mg sodium
Even an ultrathin pizza suffers when it's made from only refined flour and covered with an abundance of cheese.

California Pizza Kitchen Crispy Thin Crust Signature Pepperoni
(⅓ pizza, 128 g)
350 calories
18 g fat
(8 g saturated, 1 g trans)
780 mg sodium

Red Baron Thin & Crispy Tuscan Style Crust 5-Cheese
(⅓ pizza, 139 g)
360 calories
16 g fat
(8 g saturated)
790 mg sodium
Notice how half the fats are saturated?

Palermo Hearth Italia Organic The Como—Spinach& Feta
(⅓ pizza, 155 g)
340 calories
9 g fat
(5 g saturated)
1,000 mg sodium
Stick with Palermo's thin-crust pizzas.

Frozen Pasta Entrées

Eat This

Bertolli Mediterranean Style Rosemary Chicken, Linguine & Cherry Tomatoes

(½ package, 340 g)

380 calories
14 g fat (2.5 g saturated)
800 mg sodium

Bertolli's Mediterranean Style line relies on grilled meats and vegetables in olive-oil based sauces to build some of the leanest skillet entrées in the cooler.

Michelina's Ravioli Bellisio

(1 package, 227 g)

220 calories
7 g fat
(2 g saturated)
720 mg sodium

Filled with beef instead of butternut squash, they still save calories by topping the noodles in marinara.

Healthy Choice All Natural Portabella Spinach Parmesan

(1 meal, 266 g)

270 calories
7 g fat
(2.5 g saturated)
600 mg sodium

Healthy? Yes. Boring? Not even close.

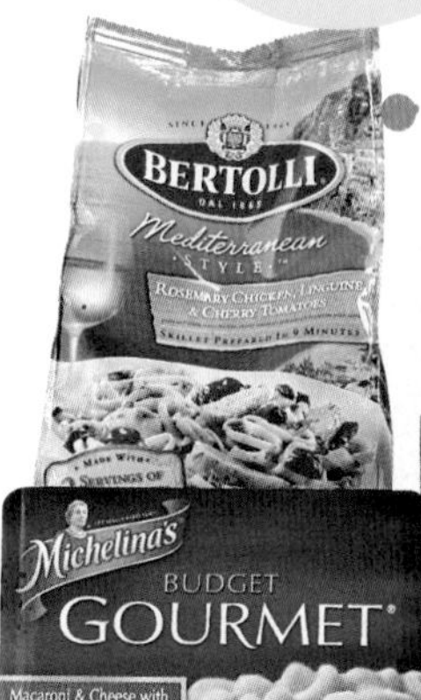

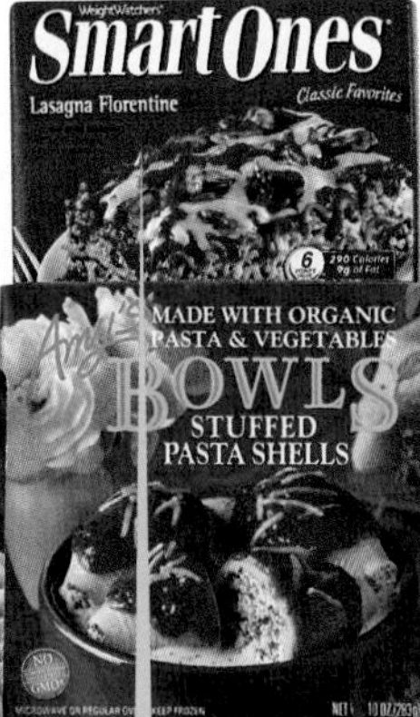

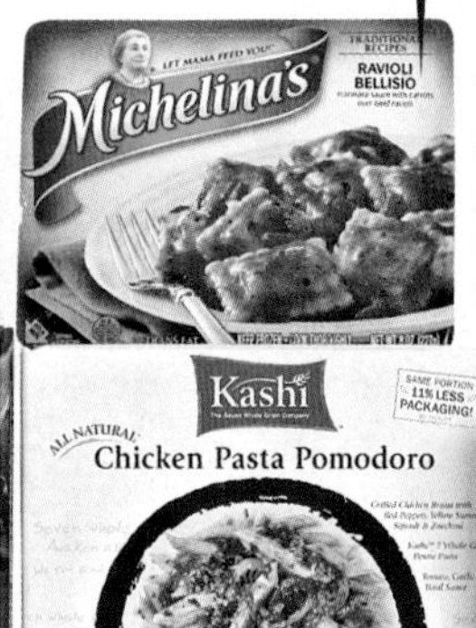

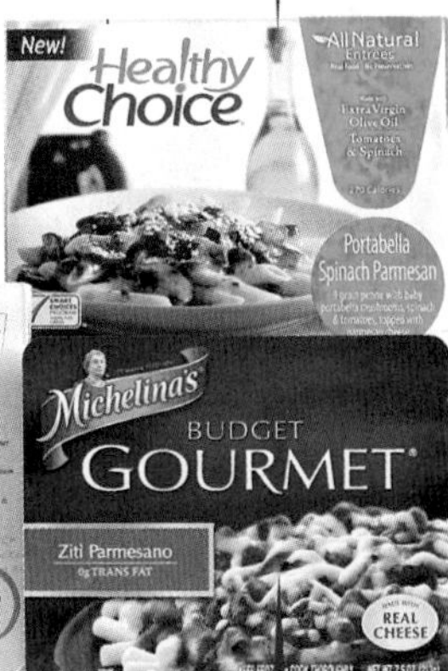

Michelina's Budget Gourmet Macaroni & Cheese with Cheddar and Romano

(1 package, 213 g)

260 calories
6 g fat
(2.5 g saturated)
460 mg sodium

Smart Ones Lasagna Florentine

(1 package, 297 g)

290 calories
9 g fat
(5 g saturated)
580 mg sodium

Loaded with zucchini, spinach, and carrots, you'll be hard-pressed to find a better lasagna.

Amy's Bowls Stuffed Pasta Shells

(1 entrée, 283 g)

310 calories
13 g fat
(7 g saturated)
740 mg sodium

Stuffed with cheese, plus organic broccoli, spinach, and onions. A great balanced dish.

Kashi Chicken Pasta Pomodoro

(1 entrée, 283 g)

280 calories
6 g fat
(1.5 g saturated)
470 mg sodium

Belly-filling calories come from 3 sources: healthy fats, protein, and fiber.

Michelina's Budget Gourmet Ziti Parmesano

(1 meal, 213 g)

240 calories
6 g fat
(2 g saturated)
480 mg sodium

The red color of the marinara sauce comes from the abundance of powerful lycopene.

Not That!

Stouffer's Fettuccini Alfredo
(1 package, 326 g)
610 calories
34 g fat
(9 g saturated)
1,030 mg sodium
Make 400 calories the upper acceptable limit for microwave-ready meals.

Lean Cuisine Butternut Squash Ravioli
(1 package, 280 g)
350 calories
9 g fat
(3 g saturated)
660 mg sodium
Too much cheese, plus 10 grams of sugar.

Bertolli Complete Skillet Meal for Two Chicken Alfredo & Fettuccine
($^1/_2$ package, 340 g)
710 calories
42 g fat (22 g saturated)
1,370 mg sodium

The glut of oil and cream in this package is massive enough to earn this meal a much-deserved spot on our list of Worst Foods in the Supermarket.

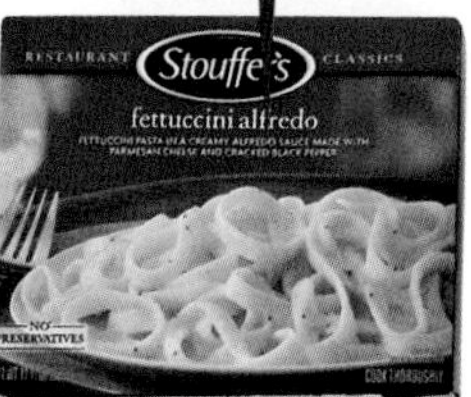

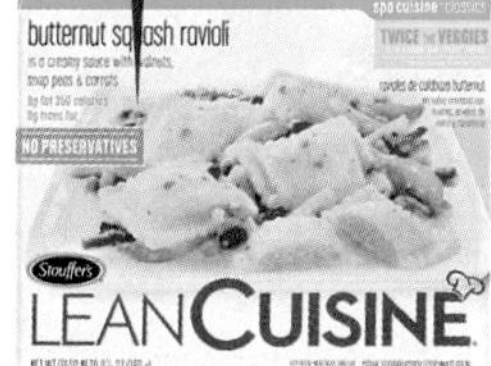

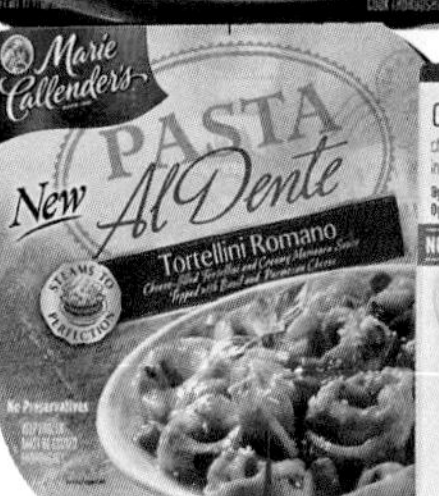

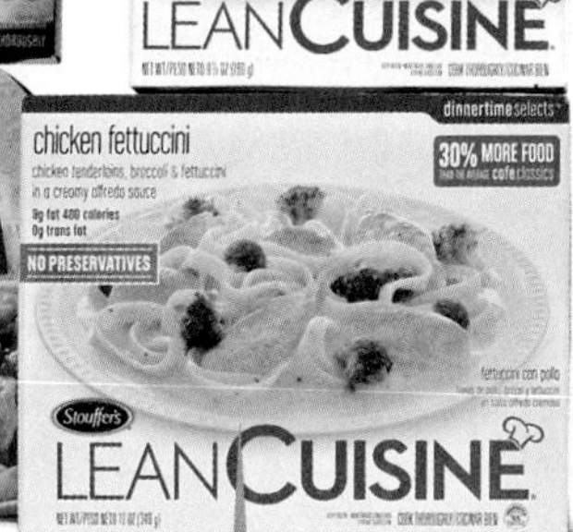

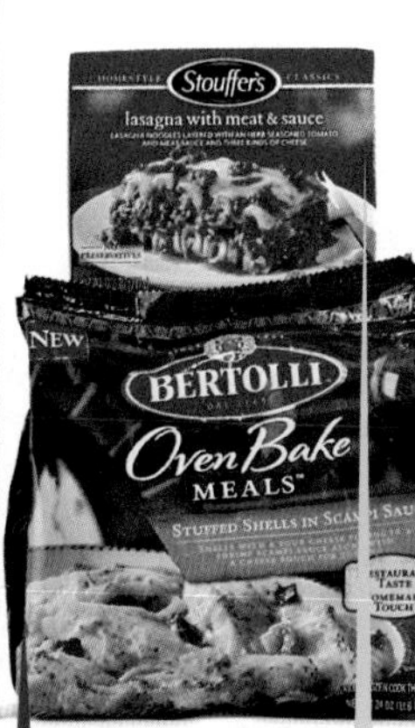

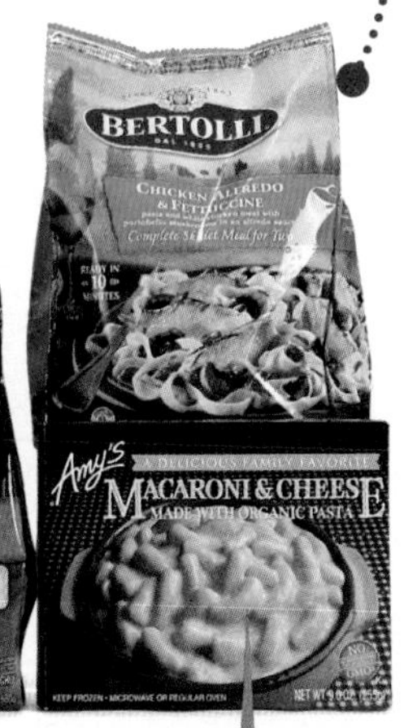

Marie Callender's Pasta Al Dente Tortellini Romano
(1 meal, 283 g)
460 calories
15 g fat
(7 g saturated)
930 mg sodium

Lean Cuisine Dinnertime Selects Chicken Fettuccini
(1 package, 340 g)
400 calories
8 g fat
(4 g saturated)
850 mg sodium
Cheese and oil can ruin even "lean" cuisine.

Bertolli Oven Bake Meals Stuffed Shells in Scampi Sauce
($^1/_2$ package, 340 g)
590 calories
33 g fat
(19 g saturated)
1,040 mg sodium
Blame the scampi sauce for the fat load.

Stouffer's Lasagna with Meat & Sauce
(1 package, 297 g)
350 calories
11 g fat
(6 g saturated)
930 mg sodium
Stouffer's lasagna subs out the veggies for ground beef—not a stellar swap.

Amy's Macaroni & Cheese
(1 package, 255 g)
410 calories
16 g fat
(10 g saturated)
590 mg sodium
The fact that the Cheddar and a heavy slab of melted butter are organic does nothing for you.

Frozen Fish Entrées

Eat This

Salmon is one of the world's best sources of omega-3 fats. Try bringing these to your next cookout.

SeaPak Salmon Burgers
(1 burger, 91 g)
110 calories
3 g fat (0.5 g saturated)
380 mg sodium

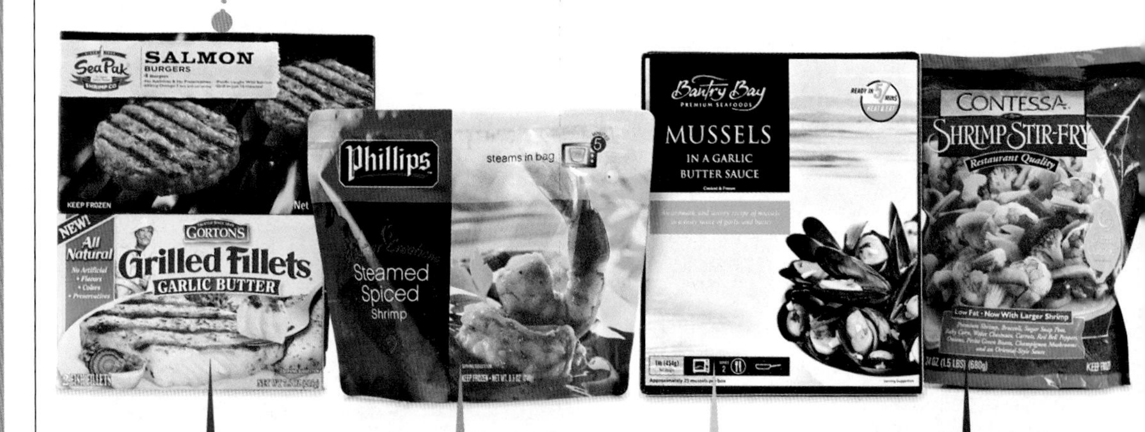

Gorton's Grilled Fillets Garlic Butter
(1 fillet, 108 g)
100 calories
3 g fat
(0.5 g saturated)
290 mg sodium
Most of the fat in this fillet actually comes from olive and canola oils.

Phillips Steamed Spiced Shrimp
(~8 shrimp, 113 g)
120 calories
2 g fat
(0 g saturated)
560 mg sodium
Each individual shrimp has more than 2 grams of protein.

Bantry Bay Mussels in a Garlic Butter Sauce
($\frac{1}{2}$ package, 8 oz.)
120 calories
8 g fat
(4 g saturated)
630 mg sodium
Mussels are a great source of lean protein, iron, and zinc, as well as energy-boosting B vitamins.

Contessa Shrimp Stir-Fry
($\frac{1}{2}$ package, 340 g)
288 calories
2.5 g fat
(0.5 g saturated)
925 mg sodium
Use only half the sauce and you'll cut an extra 50 calories and a bunch of sodium from each serving.

Not That!

SeaPak Ahi Tuna Steaks
(1 steak, 128 g)
240 calories
14 g fat (1 g saturated)
840 mg sodium

A heavy hand with the canola oil has given this otherwise lean fish as much fat as a Wendy's ¼-pound hamburger.

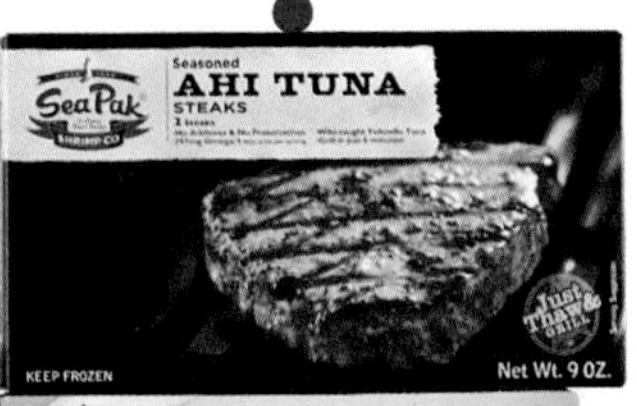

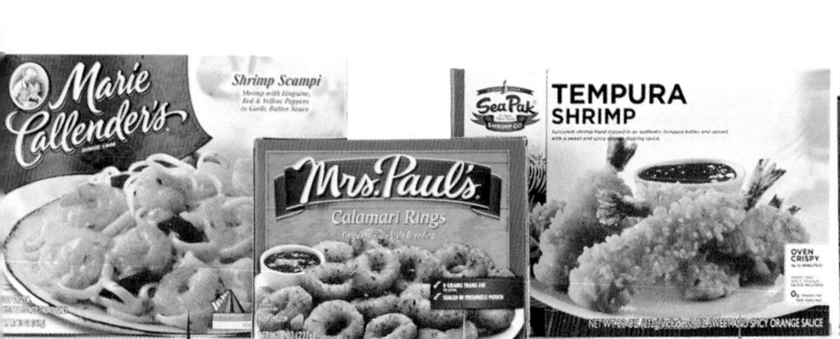

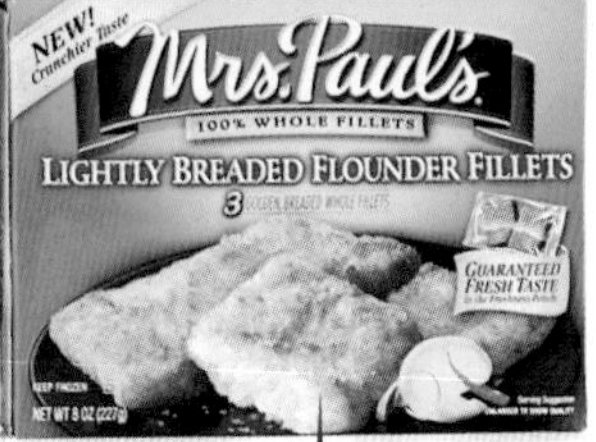

Marie Callender's Shrimp Scampi
(1 meal, 369 g)
380 calories
15 g fat
(8 g saturated)
1,200 mg sodium

Scampi means this shrimp is swimming in oil. And whereas the stir-fry is served on a bed of vegetables, these shrimp are served on a bed of carbs.

Mrs. Paul's Calamari Rings
(~15 rings, 113 g)
270 calories
13 g fat
(3.5 g saturated)
650 mg sodium

The fat absorbed into the breading drowns out any health benefit from eating the calamari.

SeaPak Tempura Shrimp with Orange Dipping Sauce
(~4 shrimp with sauce, 116 g)
240 calories
8 g fat
(2 g saturated)
570 mg sodium

Tempura is just a fancy Japanese way of saying "deep fried", which spells trouble in any language.

Mrs. Paul's Lightly Breaded Flounder Fillets
(1 fillet, 76 g)
160 calories
7 g fat
(2 g saturated)
200 mg sodium

No matter how light the breading, it will never beat a grilled fish fillet.

Frozen Chicken Entrée

Eat This

Birds Eye Steamfresh Grilled Chicken in Roasted Garlic Sauce
(½ package, 340 g)

340 calories
13 g fat (5 g saturated)
880 mg sodium

You don't have to sacrifice the creamy white sauce to save calories; you just need to pick an entrée that's not floating in a soup of the stuff.

Birds Eye Voila! Alfredo Chicken
(1½ cups, 205 g)

280 calories
12 g fat
(7 g saturated)
600 mg sodium

Voila! is one of the good guys in the freezer section. Even their more decadent dishes are decent.

Swanson Classics Boneless Fried Chicken
(1 package, 213 g)

240 calories
13 g fat
(3 g saturated)
520 mg sodium

Great stuff, as far as fried chicken goes.

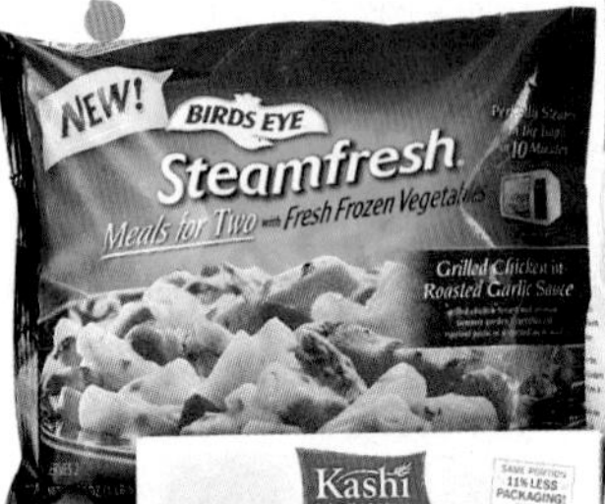

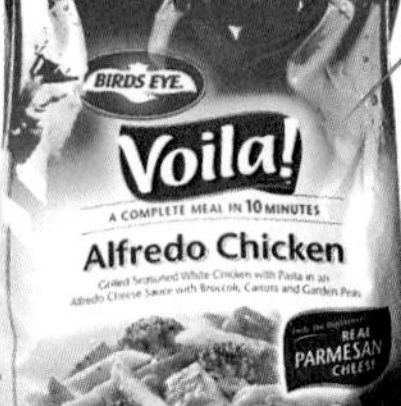

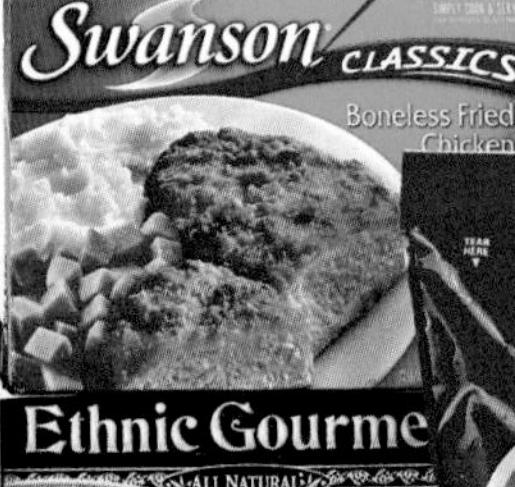

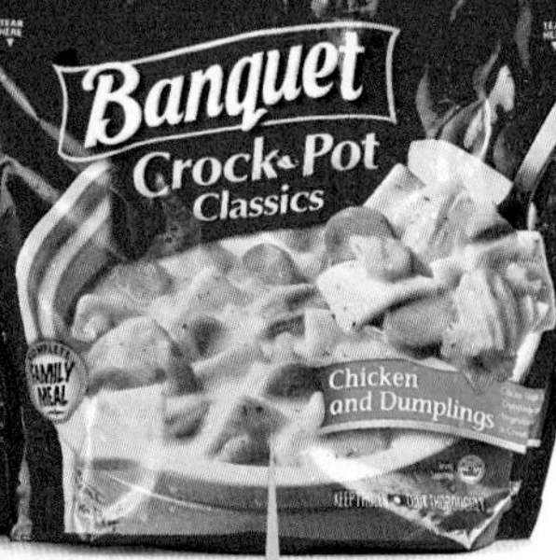

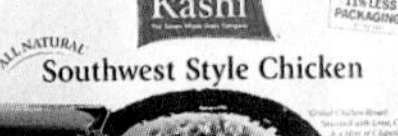

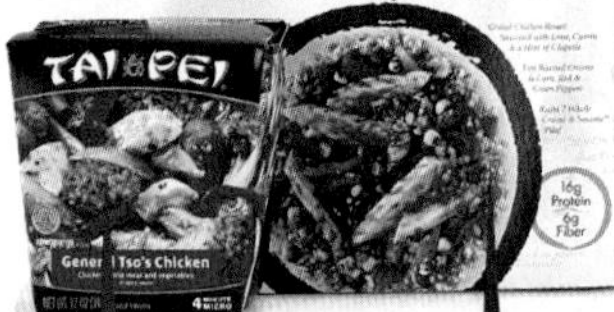

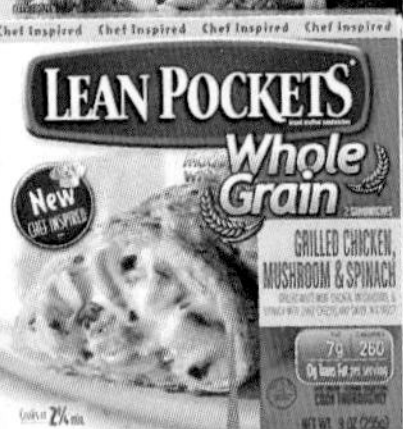

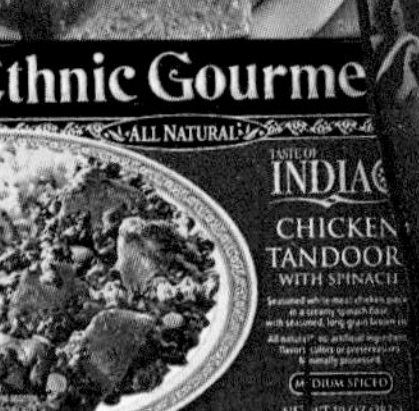

Tai Pei General Tso's Chicken
(1 container, 340 g)

175 calories
4 g fat
(0 g saturated)
725 mg sodium

This is a massive amount of food for so few calories. It's long on vegetables, short on sauce.

Kashi Southwest Style Chicken
(1 entrée, 283 g)

240 calories
5 g fat
(0 g saturated)
680 mg sodium

This is Kashi's lightest entrée, but it still packs 6 grams of fiber and 16 grams of protein.

Lean Pockets Grilled Chicken, Mushroom & Spinach
(1 piece, 127 g)

260 calories
7 g fat
(3.5 g saturated)
590 mg sodium

One of the few great pockets out there.

Ethnic Gourmet Chicken Tandoori with Spinach
(1 package, 283 g)

170 calories
4.5 g fat
(1 g saturated)
840 mg sodium

Southeast Asian cuisine relies on bold spices and healthy condiments for flavor.

Banquet Crock Pot Classics Chicken and Dumplings
([illegible])

200 calories
8 g fat
(2 g saturated)
940 mg sodium

All the ingredients of potpie, minus the fat.

Not That!

Banquet Classic Fried Chicken
(1 package, 228 g)
440 calories
26 g fat
(6 g saturated, 1.5 g trans)
1,140 mg sodium
There's no excuse for trans fat in any of our supermarket foods anymore.

T.G.I. Friday's Creamy Chicken Pasta Carbonara Skillet Meals
(1¼ cups, 270 g)
360 calories
14 g fat
(6 g saturated, 0.5 g trans)
900 mg sodium

You probably already expect Alfredo sauce to be on the indulgent side, but this is just perilous. It earns more than half your day's fat from heavy doses of whipping cream, cream cheese, soybean oil, half-and-half, and cheese.

Marie Callender's Grilled Chicken Alfredo Bake
(1 meal, 369 g)
640 calories
39 g fat
(15 g saturated, 0.5 g trans)
1,230 mg sodium

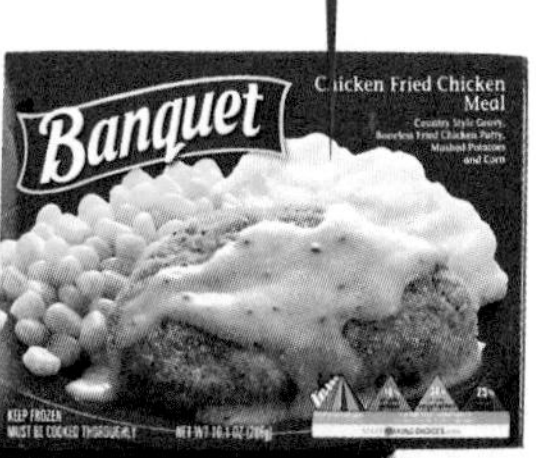

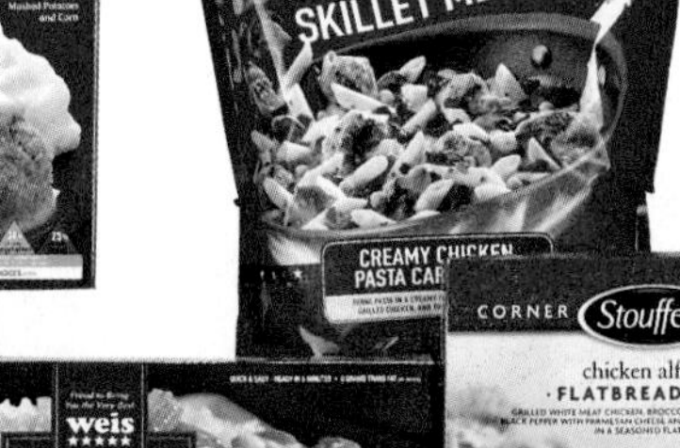

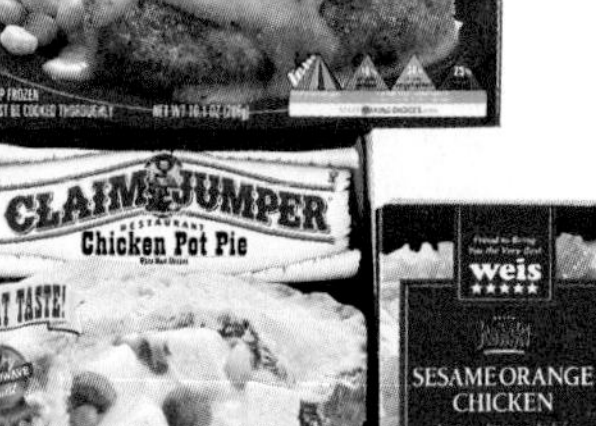

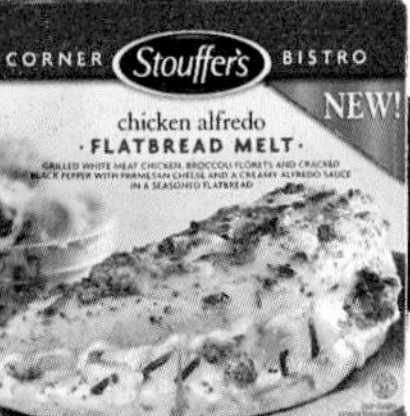

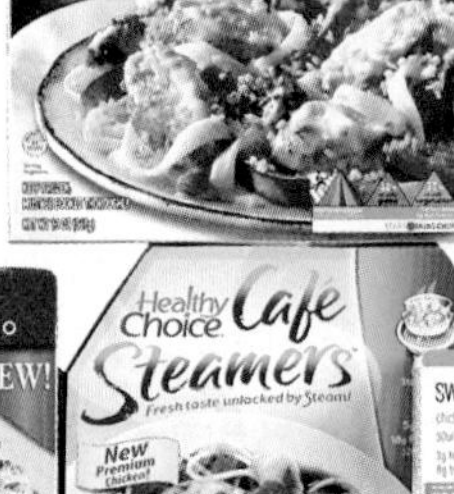

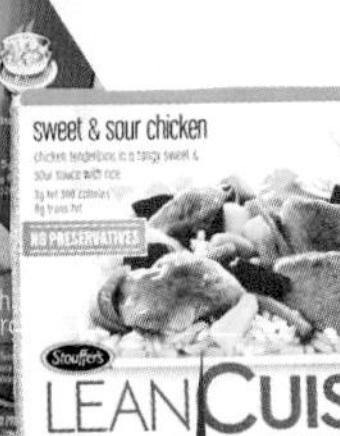

Claim Jumper Chicken Pot Pie
(½ pie, 228 g)
550 calories
37 g fat
(9 g saturated)
890 mg sodium
On top of the caloric load, the doughy base of this potpie is teeming with partially hydrogenated oils.

Kahiki Sesame Orange Chicken
(1 package, 312 g)
430 calories
5 g fat
(0.5 g saturated)
770 mg sodium
This represents the worst of Chinese food. Sugar alone accounts for 128 calories in this dish.

Stouffer's Corner Bistro Chicken Alfredo Flatbread Melt
(1 package, 170 g)
420 calories
19 g fat
(7 g saturated)
710 mg sodium
Flatbreads are far from infallible.

Healthy Choice Café Steamers Chicken Margherita
(1 entrée, 284 g)
320 calories
7 g fat
(1.5 g saturated)
580 mg sodium
Triple the sugar of the Kashi entrée.

Lean Cuisine Sweet & Sour Chicken
(1 package, 283 g)
300 calories
3 g fat
(0.5 g saturated)
560 mg sodium
There's as much sugar in this meal as in a package of Reese's Peanut Butter Cups.

Frozen Beef Entrées

Eat This

Stouffer's Stuffed Pepper
(1 package, 283 g)

210 calories
9 g fat (3 g saturated)
990 mg sodium

Healthy Choice Panini Philly Cheese Steak
(1 package, 170 g)

310 calories
4.5 g fat
(1.5 g saturated)
600 mg sodium

Paninis aren't typically considered light fare, but with 24 grams of protein, this one is both lean and substantial.

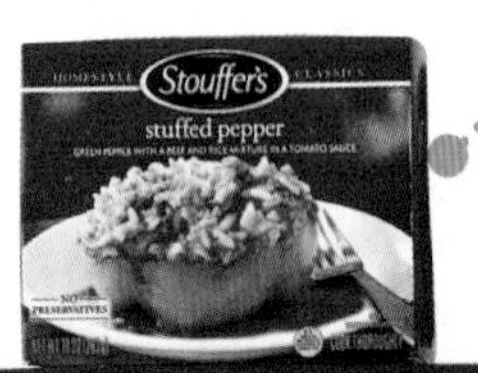

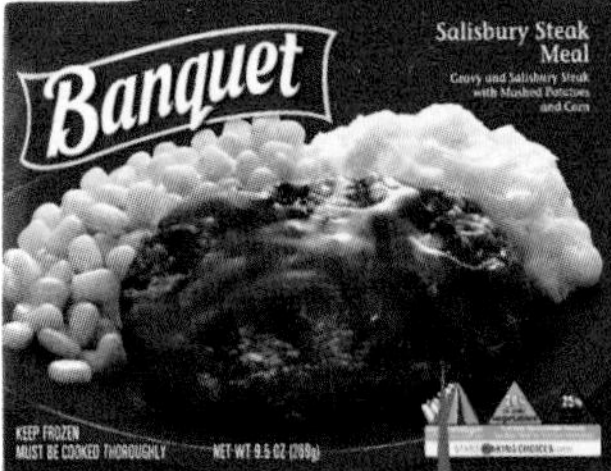

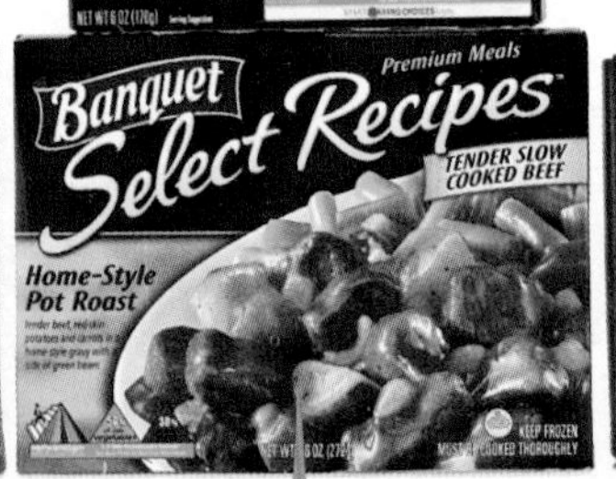

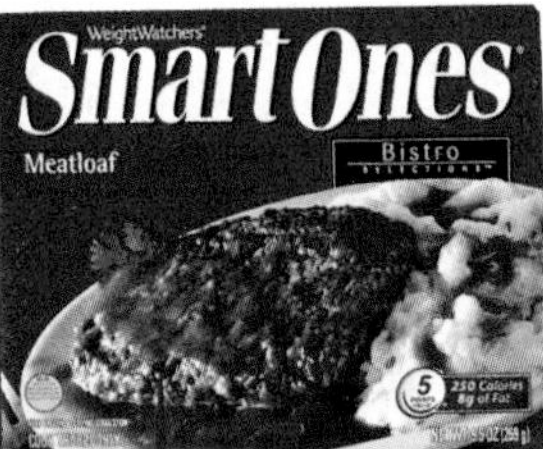

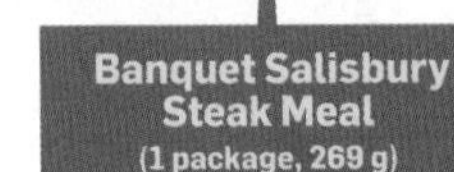

A bell pepper is the healthiest vessel for meat and veggies. Still hungry? Eat 2; you'll still save hundreds of calories over the whole potpie.

Banquet Salisbury Steak Meal
(1 package, 269 g)

290 calories
16 g fat
(7 g saturated)
1,100 mg sodium

Calorically this meal is great. Just be sure to keep the rest of the day's sodium intake to a minimum.

Banquet Select Recipes Home-Style Pot Roast
(1 meal, 272 g)

170 calories
5 g fat
(2 g saturated)
860 mg sodium

Fiber and protein contribute more than 40% of the calories in this meal (which makes up for the high sodium count).

Smart Ones Meatloaf with Gravy and Garlic-Herb Mashed Potatoes
(1 package, 269 g)

250 calories
8 g fat
(3 g saturated)
880 mg sodium

You would have to eat more than 6 of these meals to equal the amount of fat in Hungry-Man's problematic patties.

Not That!

Hot Pockets Panini Steak & Cheddar
(1 piece, 212 g)

440 calories
16 g fat
(9 g saturated)
1,000 mg sodium

The nutrition label lists a serving as half a piece. Don't be duped; once the box is open, you'll eat the whole panini.

Marie Callender's Beef Pot Pie
(½ pie, 234 g)

510 calories
29 g fat (11 g saturated)
780 mg sodium

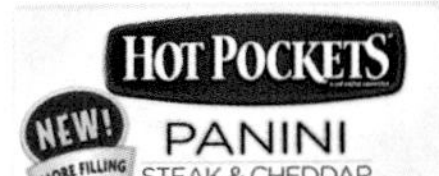

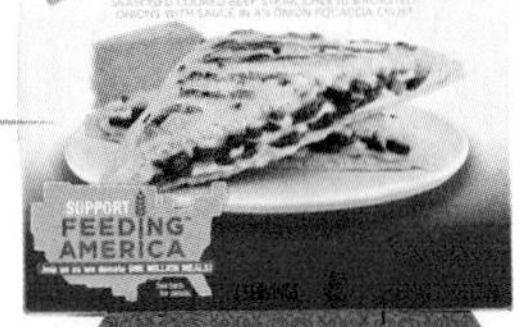

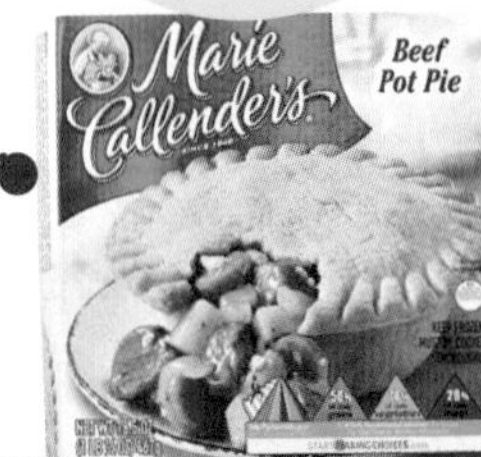

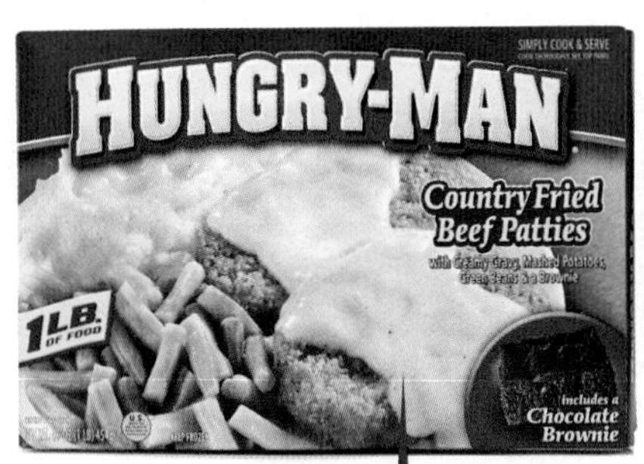

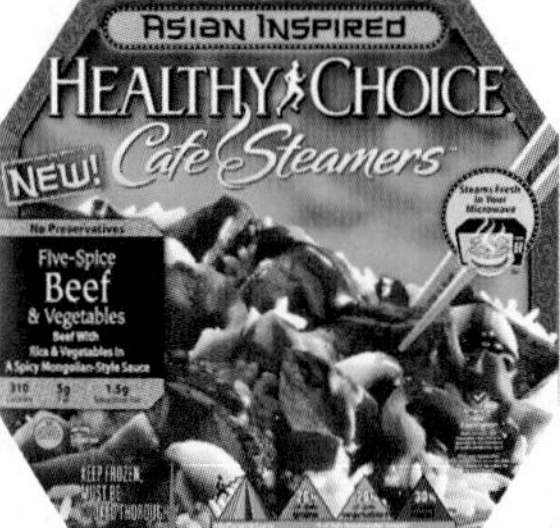

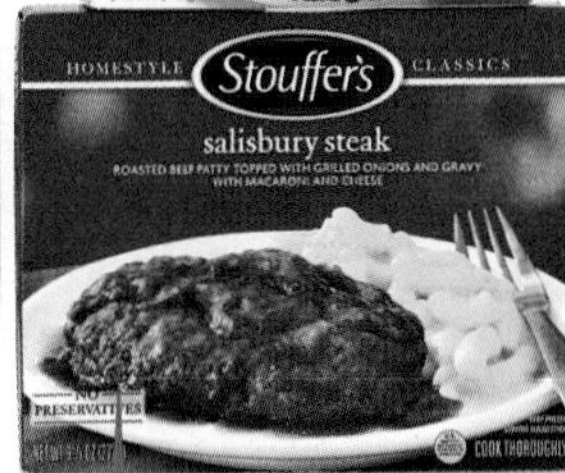

Hungry-Man Country Fried Beef Patties
(1 package, 454 g)

810 calories
50 g fat
(16 g saturated)
1,850 mg sodium

Trans fat is conveniently left off the packaging, but partially hydrogenated oils show up no fewer than seven times on the ingredients list.

Healthy Choice Café Steamers Five-Spice Beef & Vegetables
(1 meal, 289 g)

310 calories
5 g fat
(1.5 g saturated)
600 mg sodium

The white rice gives this meal a load of fast-burning calories, so you'll be hungry again in 2 hours.

Stouffer's Salisbury Steak
(1 package, 272 g)

410 calories
22 g fat
(10 g saturated, 1 g trans)
1,090 mg sodium

With so many light options in the cooler, why would you ever eat a frozen meal with more than 400 calories?

Next to the deep-fried Mars bar, potpies are the biggest nutritional crime ever perpetrated. This whole entrée has more calories than 5 glazed doughnuts.

Frozen Sides, Snacks,

Eat This

Applegate Farms Chicken Nuggets
(7 nuggets, 88 g)

180 calories
9 g fat (1.5 g saturated)
210 mg sodium

The light breading on these nuggets makes up less than 2% of the total weight, making them the lightest nuggets we've ever come across.

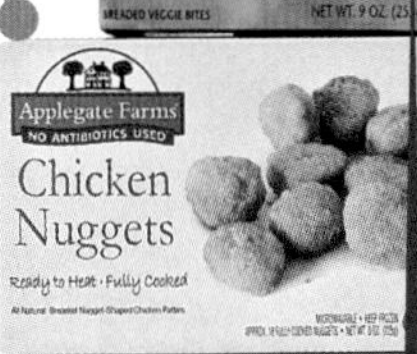

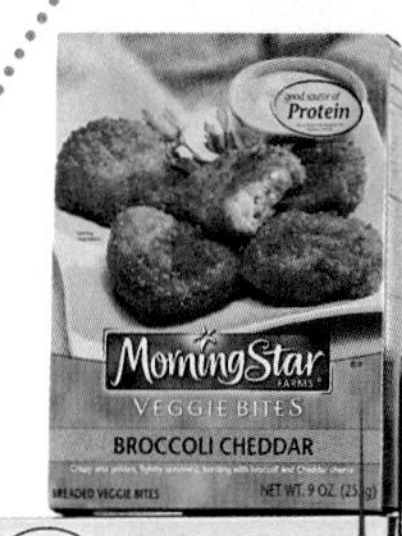

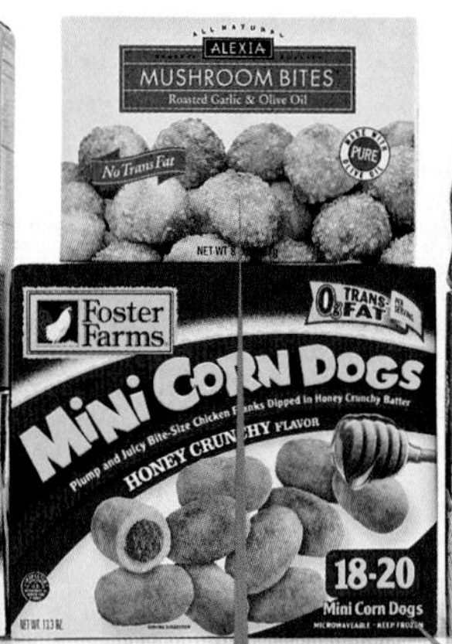

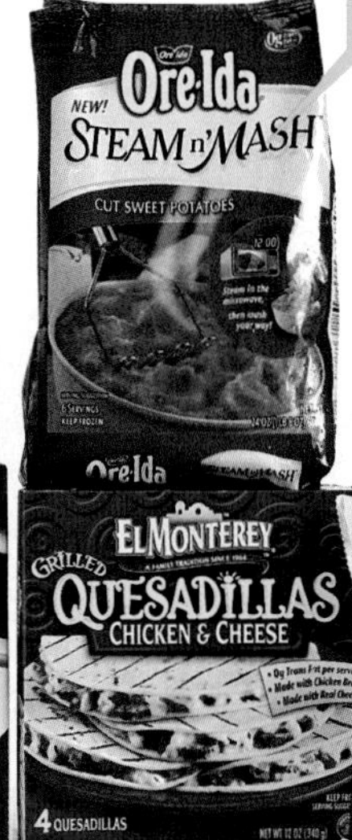

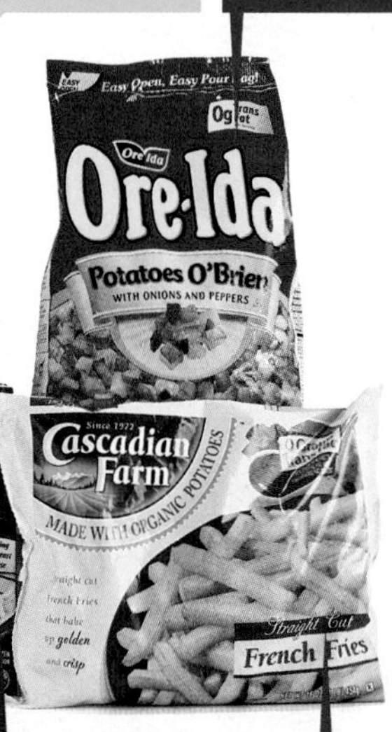

Ore-Ida Steam n' Mash Cut Sweet Potatoes
(1 cup, 123 g)

90 calories
0 g fat
30 mg sodium

This sweet mash brings a ton of vitamin A to the dinner table.

Ore-Ida Potatoes O'Brien with Onions and Peppers
(¾ cup, 85 g)

60 calories
0 g fat
40 mg sodium

The best of the bagged potatoes.

Morningstar Farms Veggie Bites Broccoli Cheddar
(3 pieces, 85 g)

180 calories
10 g fat
(2.5 g saturated)
550 mg sodium

Less fat, more fiber and protein.

Alexia Mushroom Bites
(~5 pieces, 60 g)

110 calories
4 g fat
(0.5 g saturated)
280 mg sodium

Mushrooms are packed with energy-boosting vitamins.

Foster Farms Mini Corn Dogs, Honey Crunchy
(4 dogs, 76 g)

220 calories
13 g fat
(3.5 g saturated)
510 mg sodium

A meager 55 calories per dog.

El Monterey Grilled Quesadillas Chicken & Cheese
(1 quesadilla, 85 g)

190 calories
7 g fat
(3 g saturated)
460 mg sodium

Cascadian Farm Straight Cut French Fries (85 g)

100 calories
4 g fat
(1 g saturated)
10 mg sodium

Just potatoes, a dash of oil, and apple juice to help them brown.

and Appetizers

Not That!

Tyson Chicken Nuggets
(4 nuggets, 90 g)
230 calories
16 g fat (4 g saturated)
360 mg sodium

The thicker breading on Tyson's nuggets soaks up twice as much oil as the Applegate Farms nuggets.

Ore-Ida Original Roasted Potatoes
(3/4 cup, 75 g)
130 calories
4.5 g fat
(1 g saturated)
310 mg sodium
Weighed down with vegetable oil.

Ori-Ida Steam n' Mash Garlic Seasoned Potatoes
(1 cup, 127 g)
145 calories
5.5 g fat
(3.5 g saturated)
440 mg sodium
Too much cream.

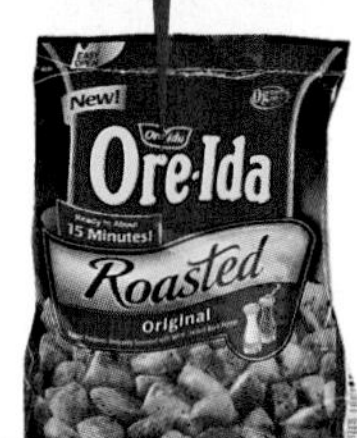

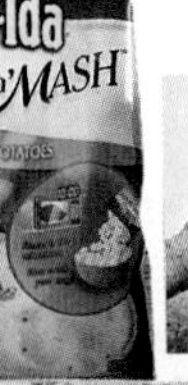

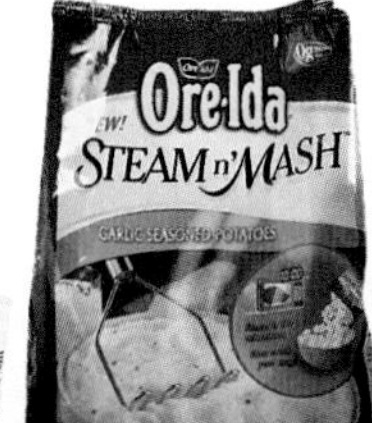

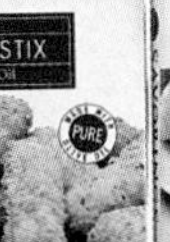

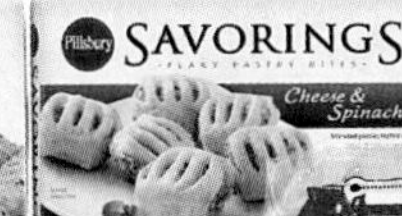

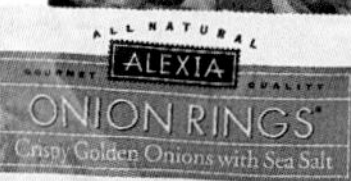

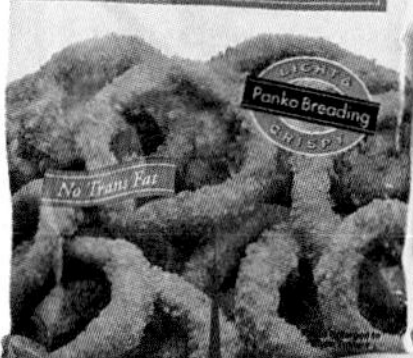

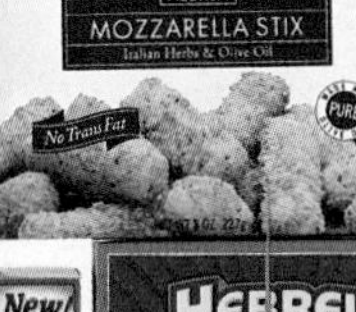

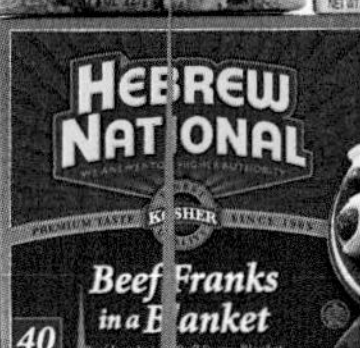

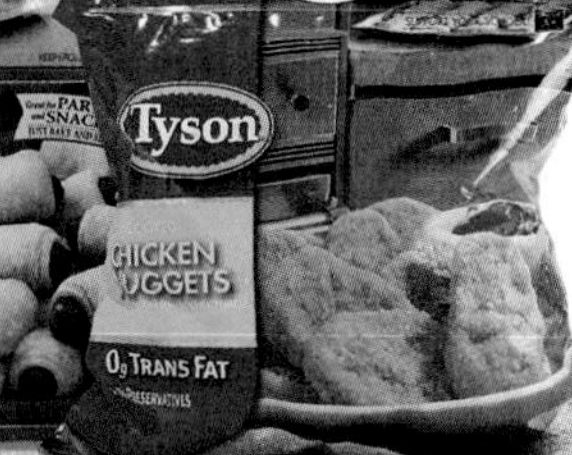

Alexia Onion Rings
(6 rings, 85 g)
230 calories
12 g fat
(1 g saturated)
230 mg sodium
Each ring packs 2 grams of fat. Fries nearly always trump rings.

José Olé Quesadillas Grilled Chicken & 3 Cheese
(1 quesadilla, 113 g)
270 calories
9 g fat
(4 g saturated, 1 g trans)
770 mg sodium

Hebrew National Beef Franks in a Blanket
(5 pieces, 81 g)
300 calories
24 g fat
(8 g saturated, 3 g trans)
680 mg sodium
A trans-fatty mess.

Alexia Mozzarella Stix
(4 sticks, 74 g)
240 calories
14 g fat
(2 g saturated)
440 mg sodium
Deep-fried cheese is about as safe as BASE jumping. Live a less perilous life.

Pillsbury Savorings Pastry Bites Cheese & Spinach
(4 pastry bites, 80 g)
260 calories
17 g fat
(8 g saturated)
430 mg sodium

Ice Cream

Eat This

Breyers All Natural Mint Chocolate Chip (½ cup)

150 calories
8 g fat (5 g saturated)
17 g sugars

Stonyfield Farm Frozen Yogurt Minty Chocolate Chip (½ cup)

140 calories
2.5 g fat
(1.5 g saturated)
21 g sugars

The milk is antibiotic- and hormone-free.

Häagen-Dazs Five Vanilla Bean (½ cup)

220 calories
11 g fat
(7 g saturated)
22 g sugars

Made with just 5 ingredients. Still, this should be eaten in small quantities only.

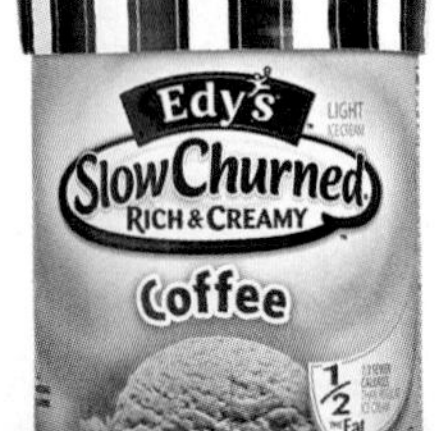

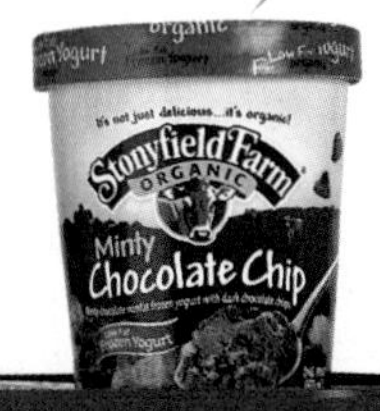

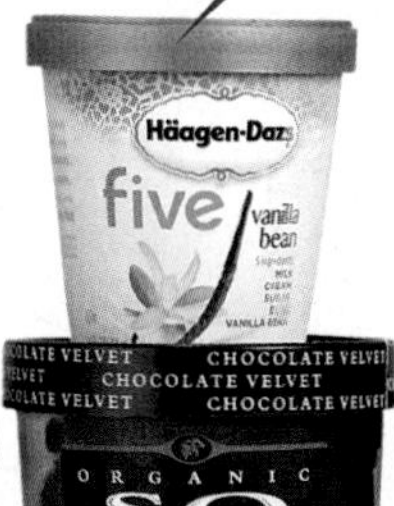

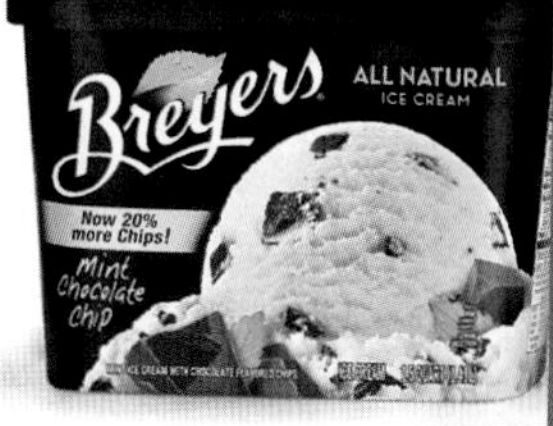

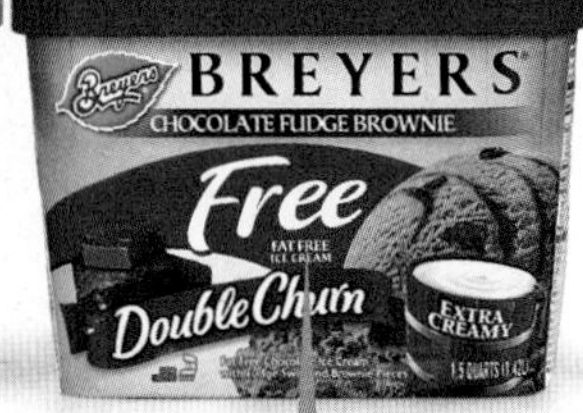

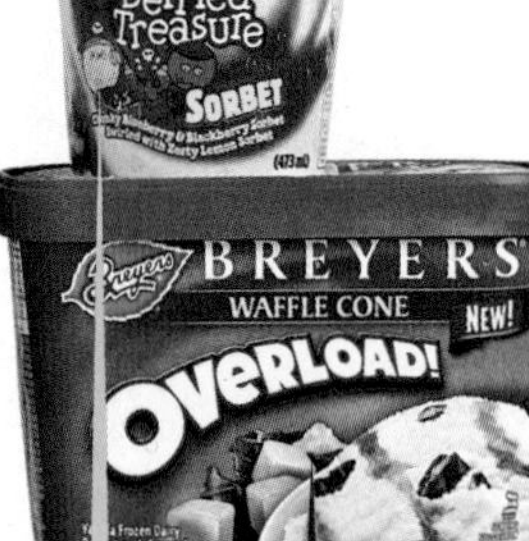

Make this simple swap three times a week and you'll save more than 6 pounds in a year.

Edy's Slow Churned Rich & Creamy Coffee (½ cup)

105 calories
3.5 g fat
(2 g saturated)
11 g sugars

Edy's Slow Churned line is as low-calorie as you'll find.

Breyers Fat Free Double Churn Chocolate Fudge Brownie (½ cup)

110 calories
0 g fat
(0 g saturated)
15 g sugars

SO Delicious Chocolate Velvet (½ cup)

130 calories
3.5 g fat
(0.5 g saturated)
14 g sugars

SO Delicious makes some of the best dairy-free desserts in the cooler.

Ben & Jerry's Berried Treasure Sorbet (½ cup, 97 g)

110 calories
0 g fat
24 g sugars

Loaded with a potent class of antioxidants called anthocyanins.

Breyers Waffle Cone Overload! (½ cup)

130 calories
3 g fat
(2 g saturated)
16 g sugars

Only Breyers is capable of making a decadent ice cream so light.

Not That!

Häagen-Dazs Mint Chip
(½ cup)

300 calories
19 g fat (12 g saturated)
23 g sugars

Thanks to an excessive amount of cream, each scoop of this ice cream has more than half your day's saturated fat allotment.

Häagen-Dazs Vanilla Bean
(½ cup)

270 calories
17 g fat
(10 g saturated)
23 g sugars

You know you're in trouble when the first ingredient is cream. Look for skim milk instead.

Dove Give in to Mint
(½ cup)

300 calories
18 g fat
(12 g saturated)
24 g sugars

One scoop has more fat than 2 slices of pepperoni pizza from Domino's.

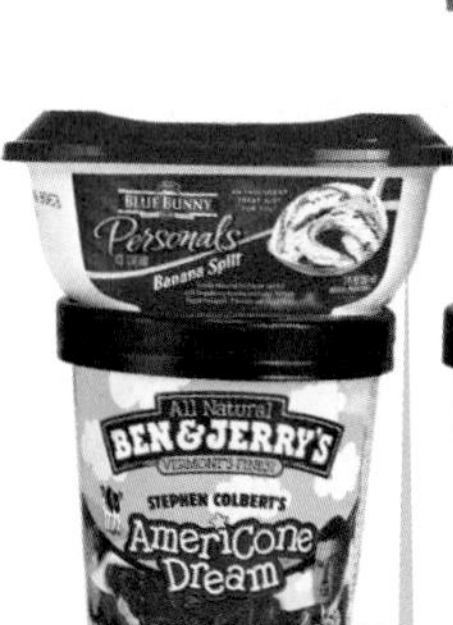

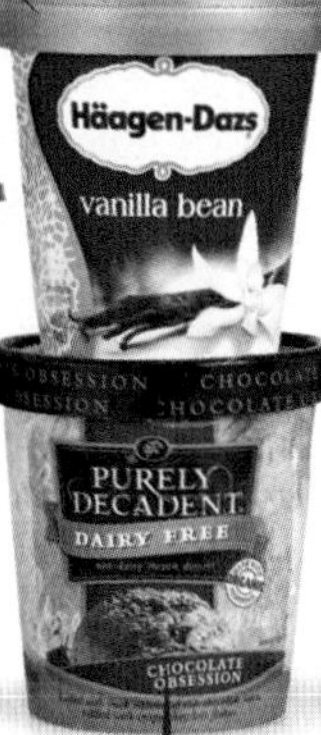

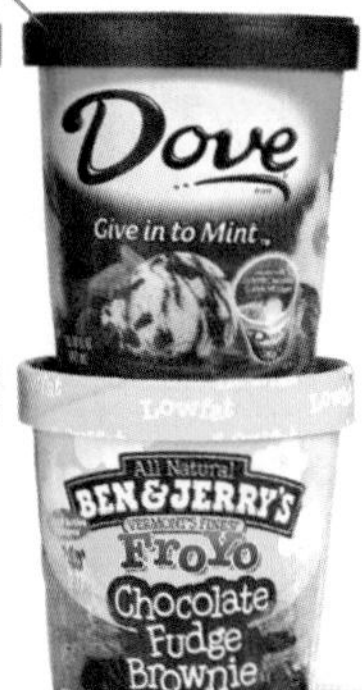

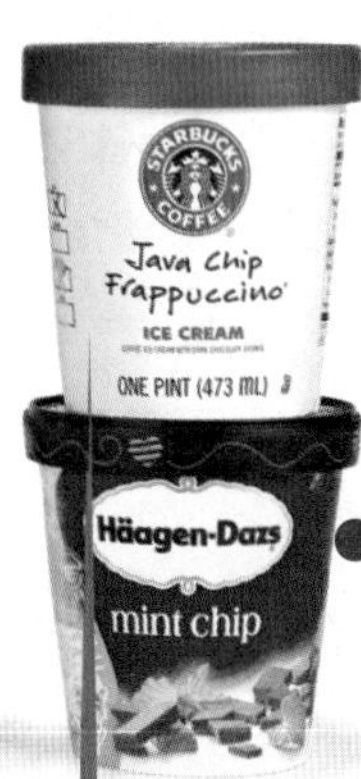

Ben & Jerry's Stephen Colbert's Americone Dream (½ cup)

280 calories
15 g fat
(10 g saturated)
24 g sugars

Colbert should stick to jokes.

Blue Bunny Banana Split
(½ cup)

170 calories
8 g fat
(4 g saturated)
18 g sugars

If it's real fruit you're after, look no further than sorbet.

Purely Decadent Dairy Free Chocolate Obsession
(½ cup)

180 calories
7 g fat
(3 g saturated)
20 g sugars

Ben & Jerry's FroYo Chocolate Fudge Brownie
(½ cup)

170 calories
2.5 g fat
(0.5 g saturated)
23 g sugars

Swimming in sugar.

Starbucks Coffee Java Chip Frappuccino
(½ cup)

250 calories
15 g fat
(10 g saturated)
22 g sugars

As bad as most of their frozen drinks.

Frozen Treats

Eat This

Breyers Ice Cream Sandwiches Oreo

(1 sandwich, 55 g)

170 calories
6 g fat (2.5 g saturated)
13 g sugars

Like most Breyers products, these Oreo sandwiches deliver serious sweet-tooth satisfaction for minimal caloric investment.

Fudgsicle No Sugar Added Fudge Bar

(1 bar, 41 g)

40 calories
1 g fat
(0 g saturated)
2 g sugars

Good luck finding better. A full 40% of the calories come from protein and fiber.

Soy Dream Lil' Dreamers Vanilla

(1 sandwich, 40 g)

100 calories
4 g fat
(0.5 g saturated)
7 g sugars

Made from mostly organic ingredients and nothing hydrogenated.

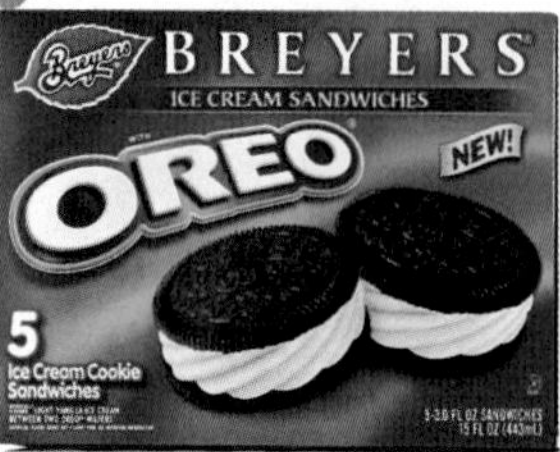

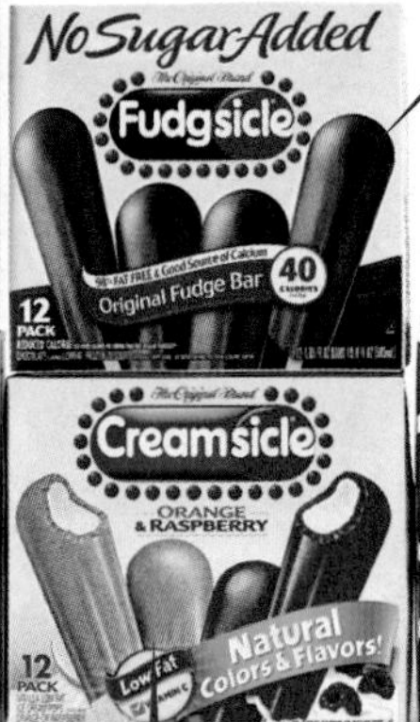

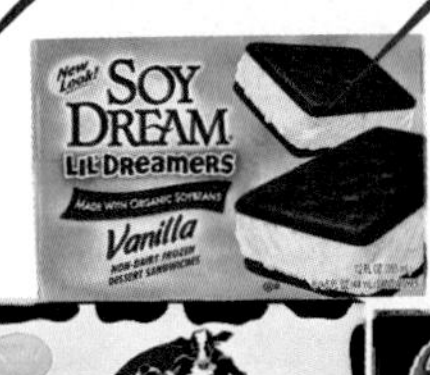

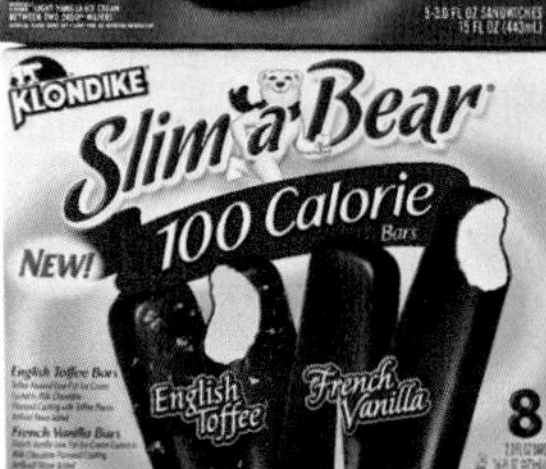

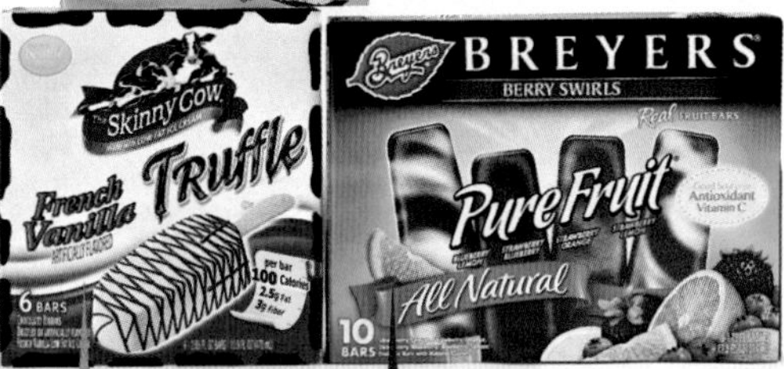

Slim a Bear 100 Calorie Bars (English Toffee/ French Vanilla)

(1 bar, 38 g)

100 calories
6 g fat
(4.5 g saturated)
8.5 g sugars

Slim a Bear are the only decent Klondikes.

Creamsicle Orange & Raspberry

(1 pop, 43 g)

70 calories
1 g fat
(0.5 g saturated)
8 g sugars

Creamsicle combines sherbet and low-fat ice cream to make an innocent indulgence.

The Skinny Cow Truffle Bar French Vanilla

(1 bar, 63 g)

100 calories
2.5 g fat
(1.5 g saturated)
12 g sugars

Skinny Cow fortifies its Truffles with inulin fiber, which keeps blood sugar from spiking.

Breyers Pure Fruit Berry Swirls

(1 bar, 51 g)

40 calories
0 g fat
9 g sugars

This bar is loaded with real fruit purees, pulps, and juices. Make this a go-to treat.

Not That!

Tofutti Cuties Vanilla
(1 sandwich, 38 g)
130 calories
6 g fat
(1 g saturated)
9 g sugars
Tofutti is the worst choice among the nondairy treats.

Weight Watchers Giant Chocolate Fudge Ice Cream Bar
(1 bar, 76 g)
110 calories
1 g fat
(0.5 g saturated)
16 g sugars
You could do worse, but why not do better?

Nearly 100 calories more than the Breyers take on the classic cookie.

Klondike Oreo
(1 bar, 73 g)
260 calories
17 g fat (11 g saturated)
19 g sugars

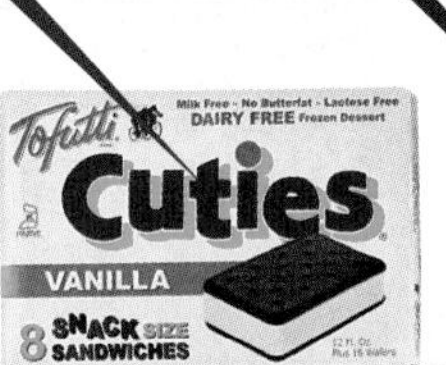

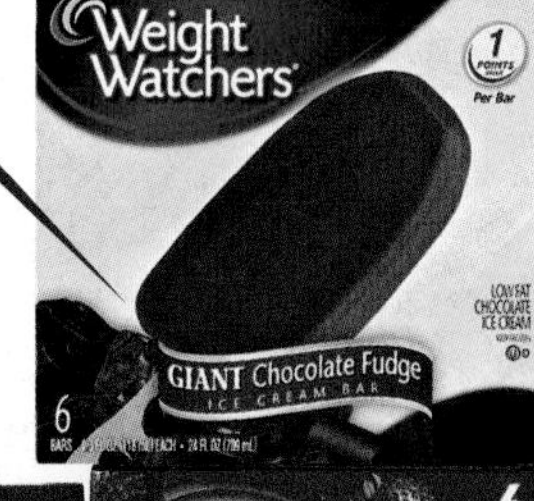

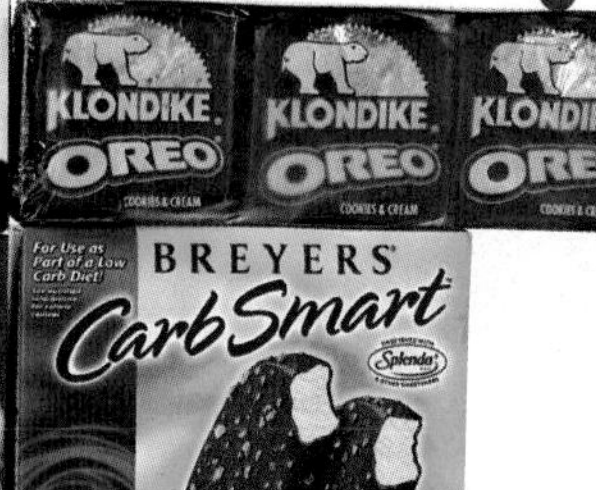

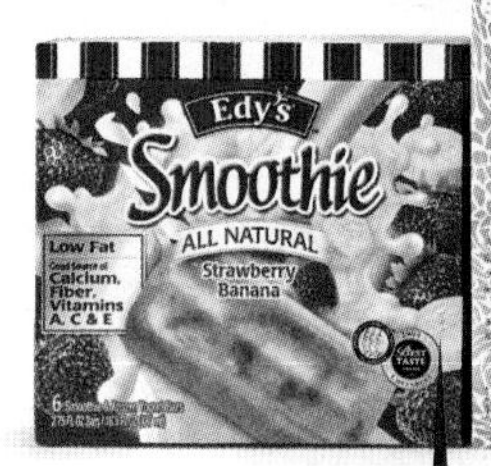

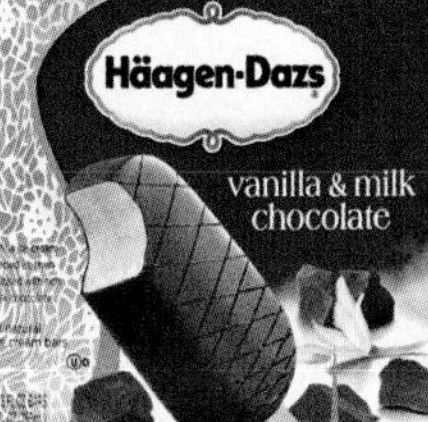

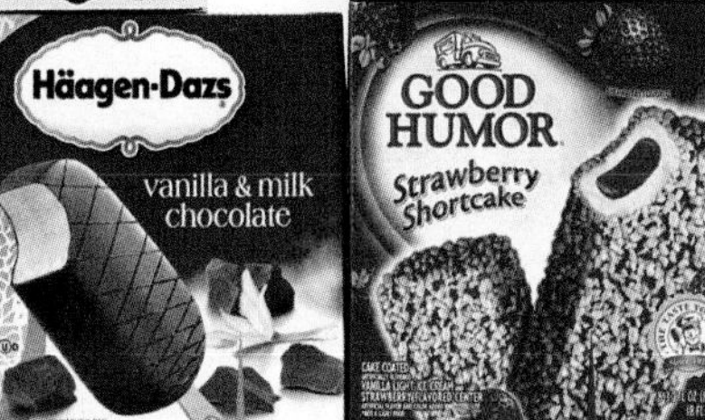

Edy's All Natural Smoothie Strawberry Banana
(1 bar, 64 g)
100 calories
2 g fat
(1 g saturated)
13 g sugars
Contains a staggering 31 ingredients.

Häagen-Dazs Vanilla & Milk Chocolate
(1 bar, 83 g)
280 calories
20 g fat
(13 g saturated)
20 g sugars
This bar has more saturated fat than a dozen strips of bacon.

Good Humor Strawberry Shortcake
(1 bar, 60 g)
160 calories
7 g fat
(2.5 g saturated)
13 g sugars
That "cake coating" is really just sweetened gobs of wheat flour and palm oil.

Breyers CarbSmart Almond Bar
(1 bar, 56 g)
180 calories
15 g fat
(10 g saturated)
5 g sugars
There's nothing smart about it; Breyers really missed the mark with this bar.

Juice

Eat This

R.W. Knudsen Just Cranberry
(8 fl oz)
70 calories
0 g fat
9 g sugars

Here's the litmus test for any juice worth its weight in fruit: It must have no sugar added to the bottle. This one passes. Beyond that, this one is made from 100% cranberries, a rarity in the juice section.

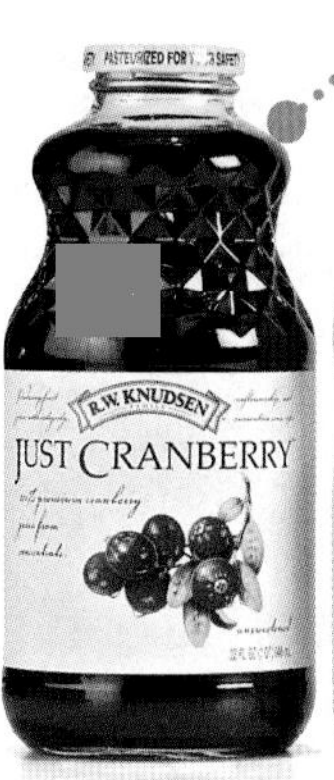

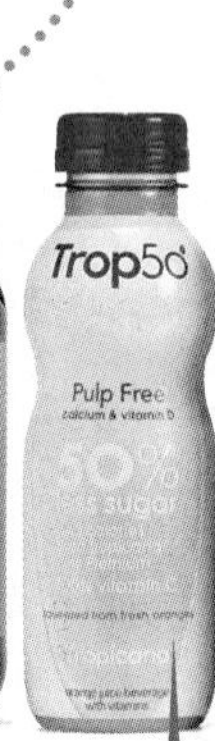

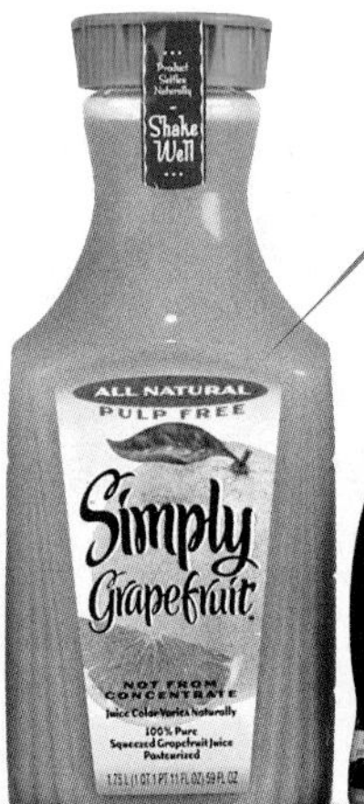

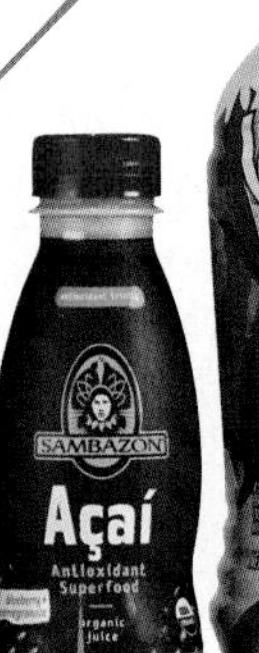

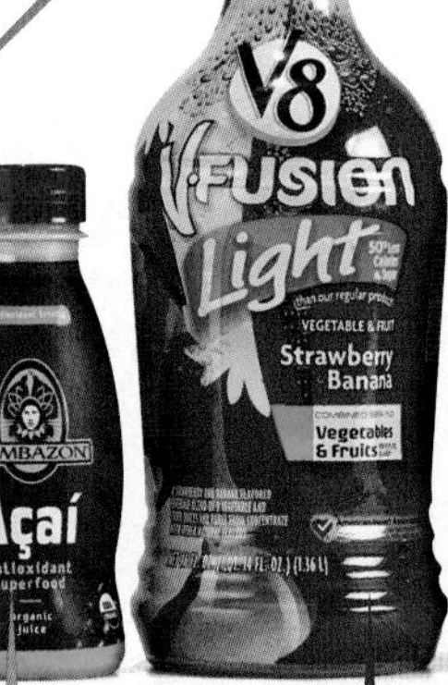

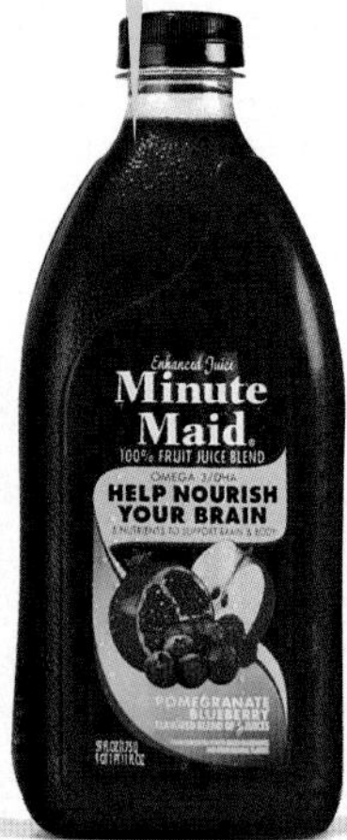

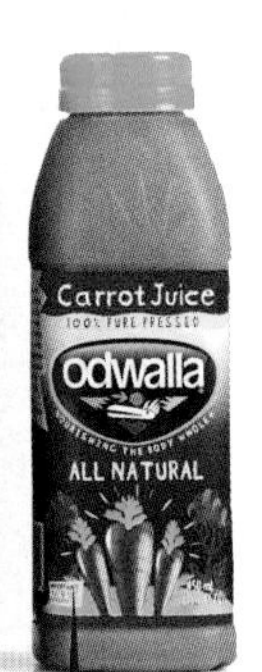

Simply Grapefruit 100% Pure Squeezed Grapefruit
(8 fl oz)
90 calories
0 g fat
18 g sugars
Low in sugar, high in nutrients. A great mixer to have at the bar, too.

Minute Maid Pomegranate Blueberry Enhanced Juice
(8 fl oz)
120 calories
0.5 g fat
29 g sugars
Fortified with a big dose of brain-boosting omega-3s.

Tropicana Trop50
(1 bottle, 12 fl oz)
80 calories
0 g fat
15 g sugars
Trop50's water-and-OJ blend has half the sugar of regular OJ, plus it's fortified with vitamins A, D, and E.

Sambazon Açai Blueberry Pomegranate Antioxidant Trinity
(1 bottle, 10.5 fl oz)
145 calories
2.5 g fat
(0 g saturated)
28 g sugars

V8 V-Fusion Light Strawberry Banana (8 fl oz)
50 calories
0 g fat
10 g sugars
This vegetable-fruit blend packs a serving of produce into every glass.

Odwalla Carrot Juice
(1 bottle, 15.2 fl oz)
133 calories
0 g fat
25 g sugars
It has 400% of your vitamin A and is surprisingly tasty. Mix with a splash of OJ, if you like.

Not That!

Welch's Berry Pineapple Passion Fruit
(8 fl oz)
140 calories
0 g fat
33 g sugars
This juice blend is actually only 25% real juice.

Newman's Own Virgin Lemonade
(8 fl oz)
110 calories
0 g fat
27 g sugars
Lemonade is trouble. Even Newman's has more corn syrup than lemon.

OceanSpray Cran-Pomegranate
(8 fl oz)
120 calories
0 g fat
30 g sugars

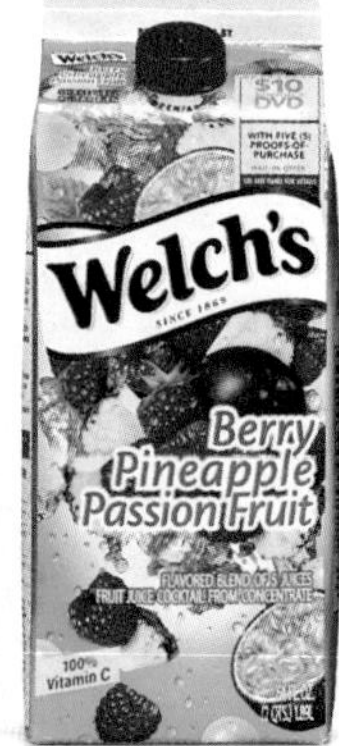

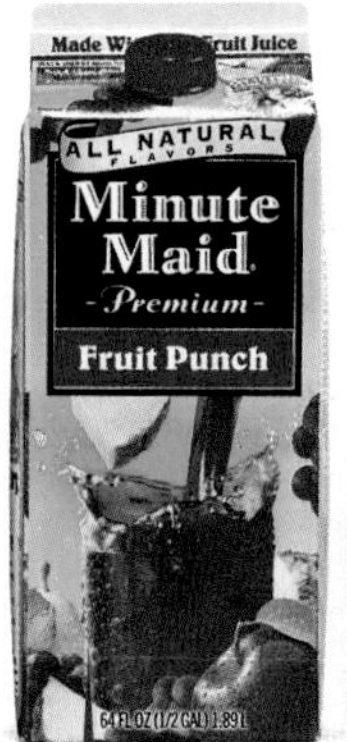

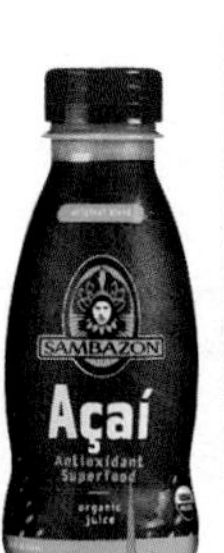

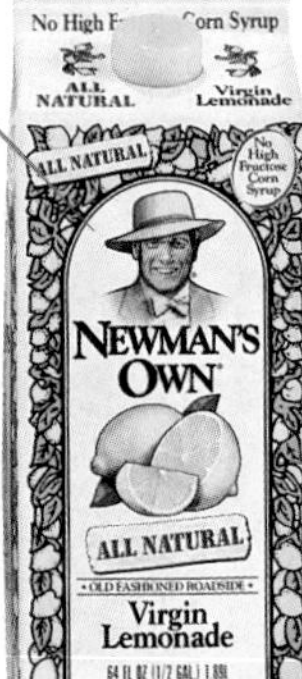

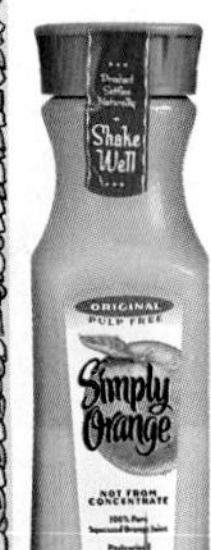

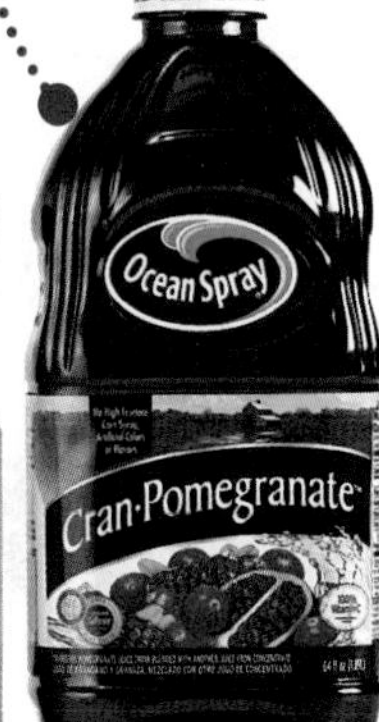

Kern's Peach Nectar
(1 can, 11.5 fl oz)
200 calories
0 g fat
42 g sugars
Two-thirds of the calories in every Kern's can come from high-fructose corn syrup.

Minute Maid Premium Fruit Punch
(8 fl oz)
120 calories
0 g fat
31 g sugars
"Punch," "drink," "-ade," and "cocktail" are industry terms for sugar water.

Sambazon Açai Original Blend
(1 bottle, 10.5 fl oz)
200 calories
3.5 g fat
(1.5 g saturated)
33 g sugars
This Sambazon has 38% more calories and 84% less vitamin C.

Simply Orange Original Pulp Free Orange Juice
(1 bottle, 13.5 fl oz)
190 calories
0 g fat
41 g sugars
Even the pure stuff has more sugar than a candy bar.

OceanSpray's cranberry fusions don't typically earn much more than a quarter of their calories from juice. This one earns only 15%; the rest is from added sugar.

Eat This

Java Monster Lo-Ball
(1 can, 15 fl oz)

100 calories
3 g fat (2 g saturated)
8 g sugars

A lighter dose of sugar makes this can much more manageable than most of the alternatives.

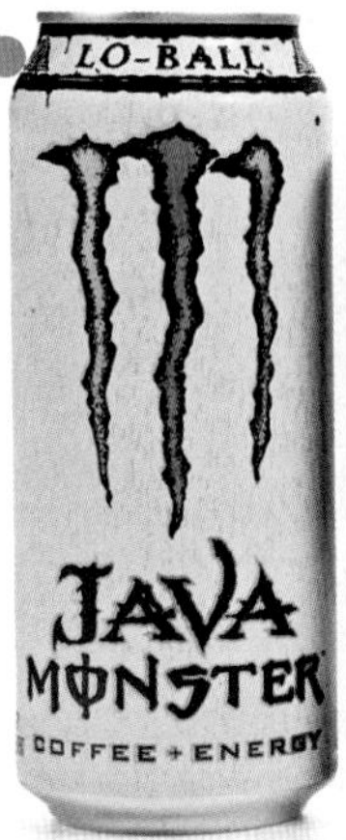

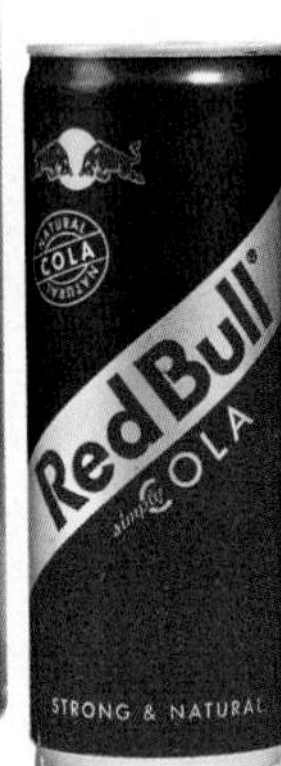

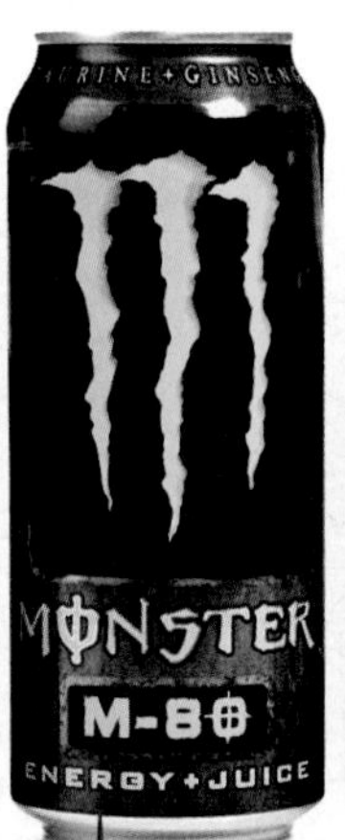

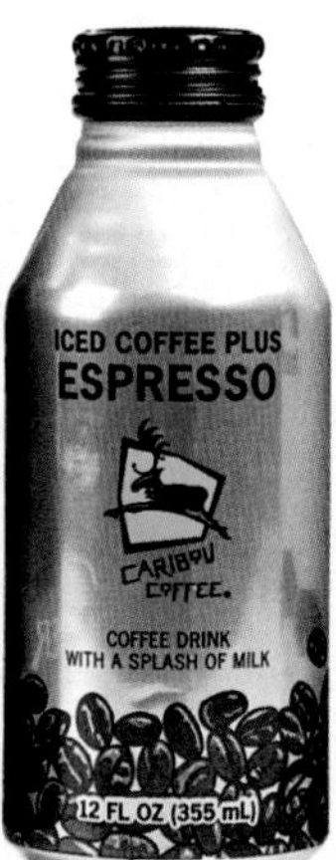

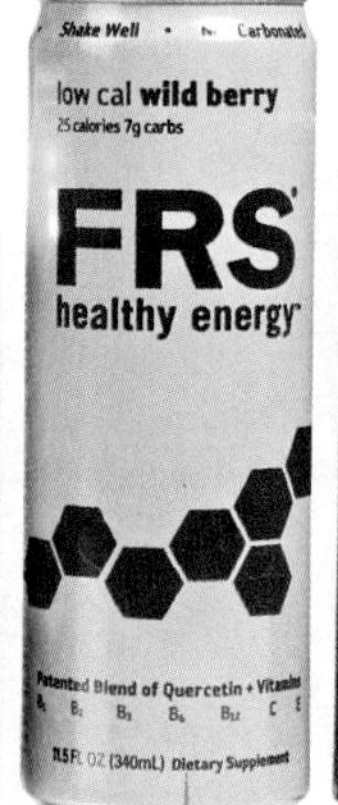

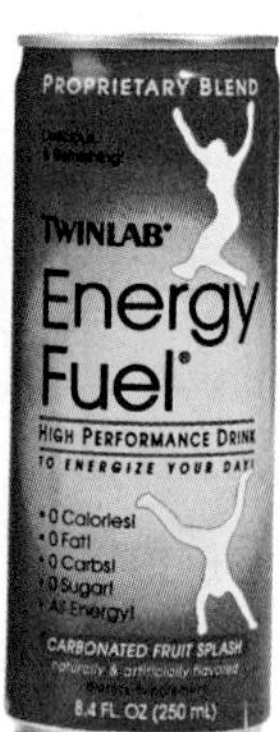

Red Bull Cola
(1 can, 8.4 fl oz)

90 calories
0 g fat
22 g sugars

Red Bull Cola has slightly less sugar than other colas even after adjusting for size, but it's the small can that makes it more drinkable. Still, don't make it a habit.

Monster M-80
(1 can, 16 fl oz)

180 calories
0 g fat
46 g sugars

If you must suck down a high-calorie energy drink, make it this one. The sugars come from an 80% juice mix, and it still has all the taurine, ginseng, and B vitamins you want.

Caribou Iced Coffee Plus Espresso
(1 bottle, 12 fl oz)

100 calories
0.5 g fat
(0 g saturated)
20 g sugars

Swap daily for Starbucks Frapp and you'll lose more than 10 pounds in a year.

FRS Healthy Energy Low Cal Wild Berry
(1 can, 11.5 fl oz)

25 calories
0 g fat
5 g sugars

FRS is made with real juice, has fiber (2 grams), and is fortified with antioxidants from green tea.

TwinLab Energy Fuel
(1 can, 8.4 fl oz)

0 calories
0 g fat
0 g sugars

This can is sweetened with sucralose, one of the most trusted members of the artificial sweetener family.

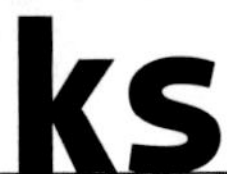

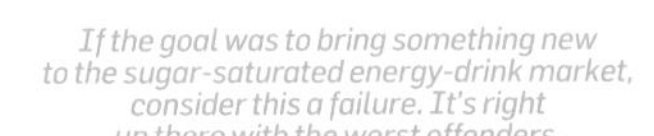

Not That!

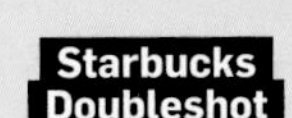

Starbucks Doubleshot
(1 can, 16 fl oz)
210 calories
3 g fat (2 g saturated)
28 g sugars

If the goal was to bring something new to the sugar-saturated energy-drink market, consider this a failure. It's right up there with the worst offenders.

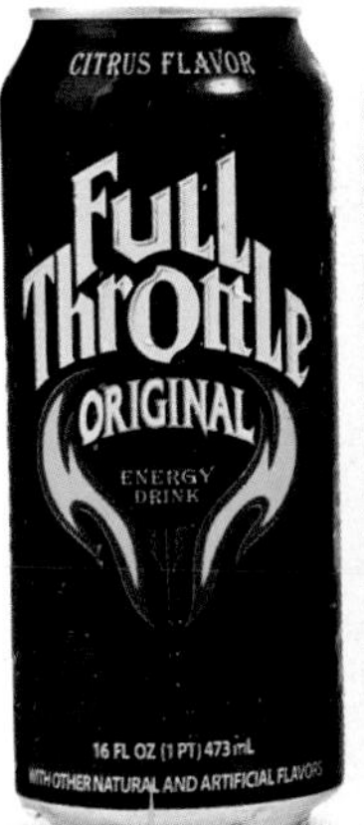

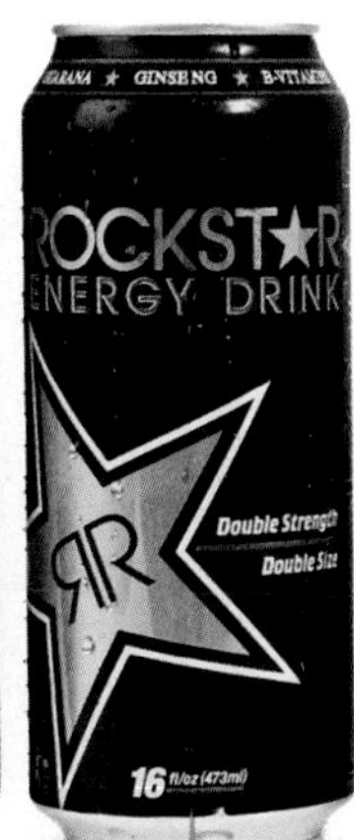

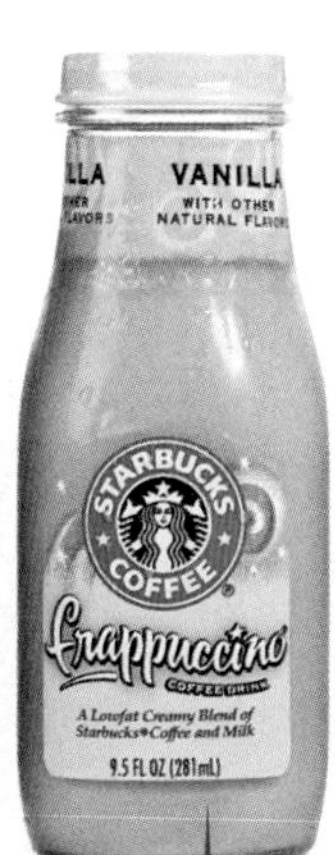

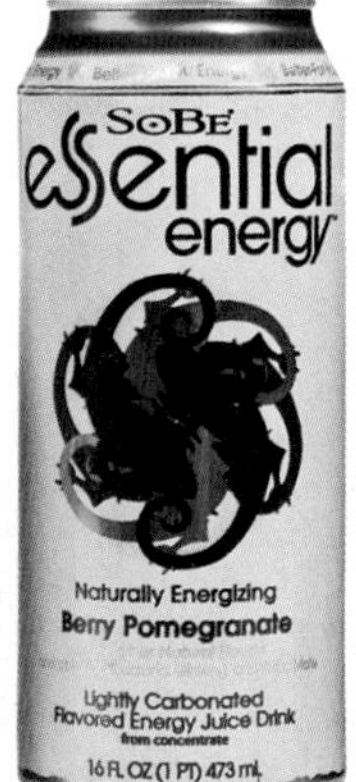

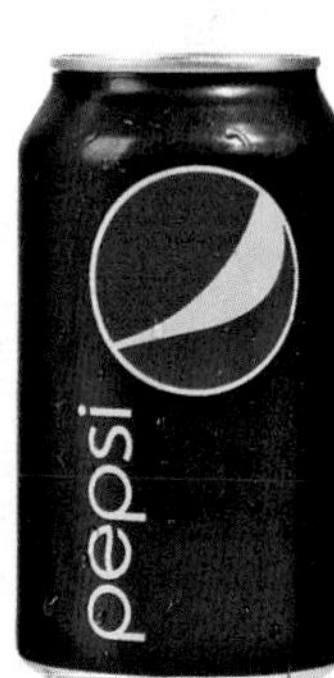

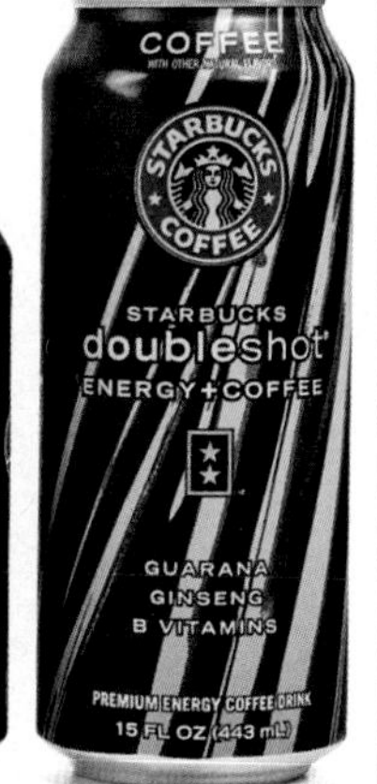

Full Throttle Original
(1 can, 16 oz)
220 calories
0 g fat
57 g sugars
This massive can has more sugar than two full-size Butterfinger bars.

Rockstar Original
(1 can, 16 oz)
280 calories
0 g fat
62 g sugars
Drinking 3 of these a week for a year will result in 10 pounds of additional body fat.

Starbucks Coffee Frappuccino Vanilla
(1 bottle, 9.5 fl oz)
200 calories
3 g fat
(2 g saturated)
31 g sugars
Bottled Starbucks drinks are perilous.

Sobe Essential Energy Naturally Energizing Berry Pomegranate
(1 can, 16 fl oz)
240 calories
0 g fat
56 g sugars
For an extra 60 calories you get 50% less juice. Not exactly a stellar swap.

Pepsi
(1 can, 12 oz)
150 calories
0 g fat
41 g sugars
Soda is among the top causes of obesity and diabetes in this country. If you need caffeine, find a (much) better fix.

Mixers

Eat This

Canada Dry Club Soda (8 fl oz)

0 calories
0 g fat
0 g sugars

Club soda is nothing but unsweetened carbonated water, so it won't spike your booze with a sugary punch. Look for it also under its other name: seltzer water.

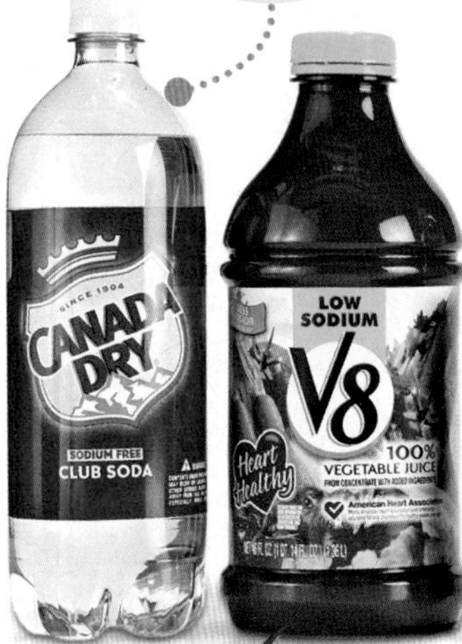

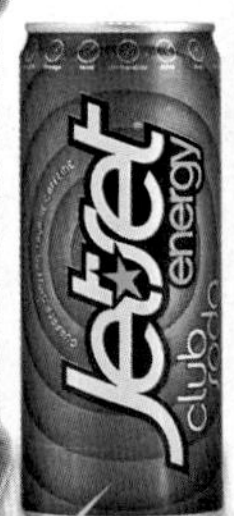

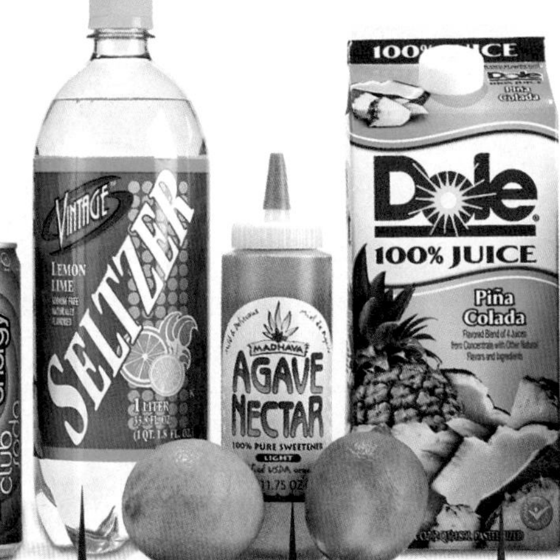

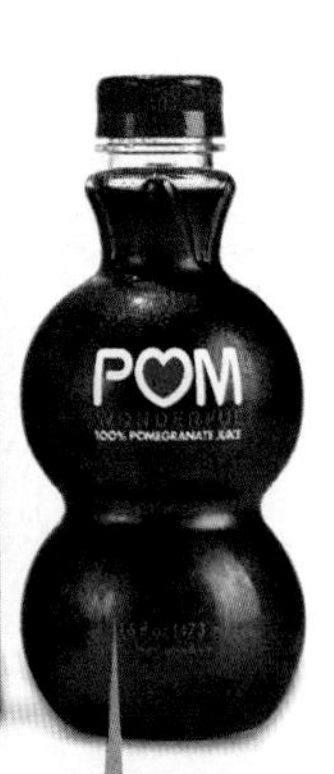

V8 Vegetable Juice Low Sodium (8 fl oz)

50 calories
0 g fat
8 g sugars
140 mg sodium

Like it hot? Skip the V8 Spicy and add hot sauce yourself. You'll save 480 mg of sodium per glass.

JetSet Club Soda Energy Mixer (1 can, 10.5 fl oz)

0 calories
0 g fat
0 g sugars

This club soda has an energy profile nearly identical to Red Bull's, minus the sugar.

Vintage Seltzer Lemon Lime (8 fl oz)

0 calories
0 g fat
0 g sugars

Flavored seltzers make for great mixers with clear spirits.

Juice of two limes and 1 Tbsp Agave Nectar

60 calories
0 g fat
15 g sugars

How the best margaritas are made. Agave nectar has a gentle effect on blood sugar.

Dole 100% Juice Piña Colada (4 fl oz)

60 calories
0 g fat
12 g sugars

This 100% juice blend is loaded with hangover-fighting vitamin C.

Pom Wonderful 100% Pomegranate Juice (8 fl oz)

150 calories
0 g fat
32 g sugars

Pomegranate juice is loaded with heart-healthy antioxidants.

Not That!

Think of tonic water as glorified Sprite. It's made from carbonated water, high-fructose corn syrup, and flavoring and contains nearly as much sugar.

Canada Dry Tonic Water
(8 fl oz)

90 calories
0 g fat
23 g sugars

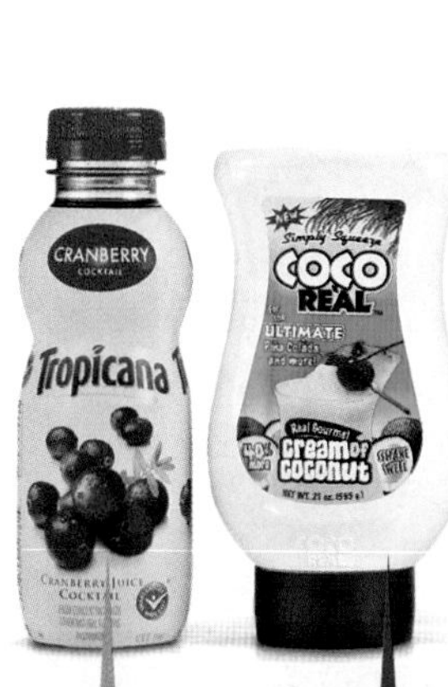

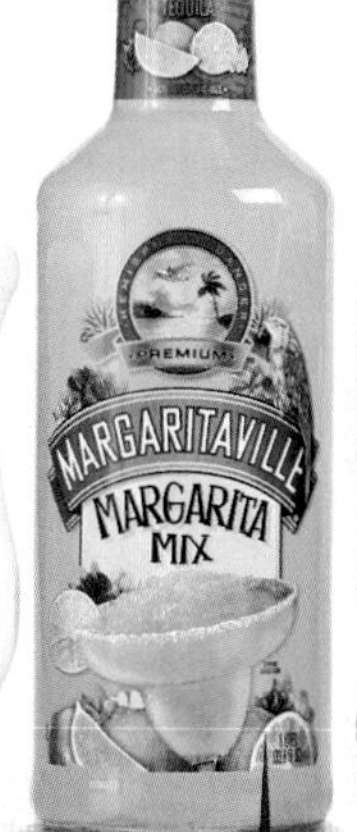

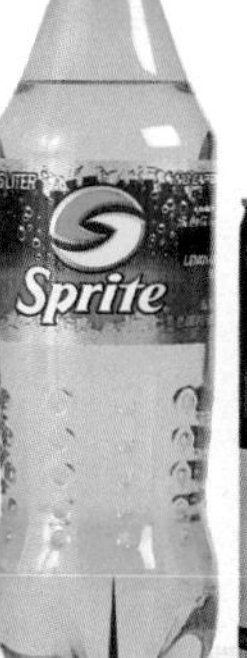

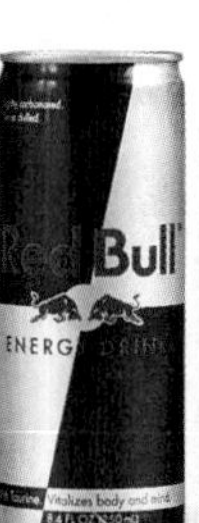

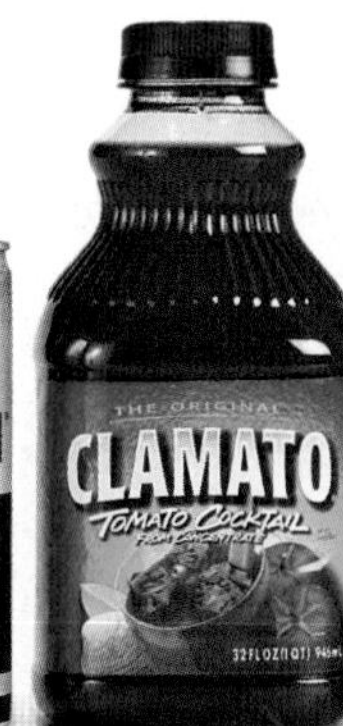

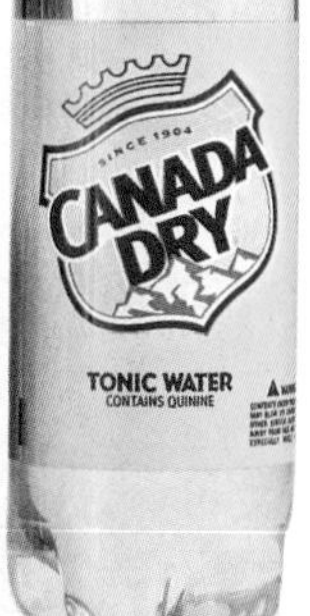

Tropicana Cranberry Cocktail
(12 fl oz)

140 calories
0 g fat
34 g sugars

Just 27% real juice. If you're going to use high-sugar mixers, they need to be 100% juice.

Coco Real Cream of Coconut
(2 fl oz)

248 calories
8 g fat
(8 g saturated)
42 g sugars

One drink made with this can blast away 20% of your day's calories.

Margaritaville Margarita Mix
(4 fl oz)

110 calories
0 g fat
26 g sugars

There's not even a drop of lime in this bottle, but there's no shortage of artificial coloring and corn syrup.

Sprite Lemon-Lime Soda
(8 fl oz)

100 calories
0 g fat
26 g sugars

Don't do diet, either. Research found that diet soda may increase the effect of alcohol by 50%.

Red Bull
(1 can, 8.4 fl oz)

110 calories
0 g fat
27 g sugars

Keep in mind that the calories are going to double when you add in a shot of vodka.

Clamato Tomato Cocktail
(8 fl oz)

60 calories
0 g fat
8 g sugars
880 mg sodium

Just 34% juice, but 37% of your daily sodium allotment.

Eat This

Guinness Draught
(12 fl oz)
125 calories
10 g carbs
4% alcohol

For our money, Guinness Draught has the best flavor-to-calorie ratio in the cooler.

Keystone Premium
108 calories
6 g carbs
4.4% alcohol

Amstel Light
95 calories
6 g carbs
3.5% alcohol

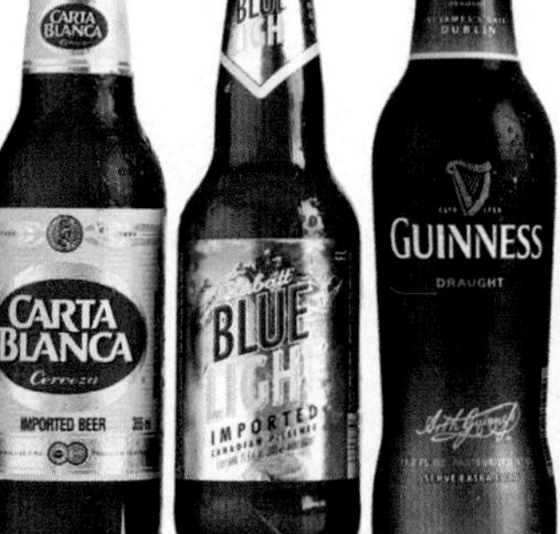
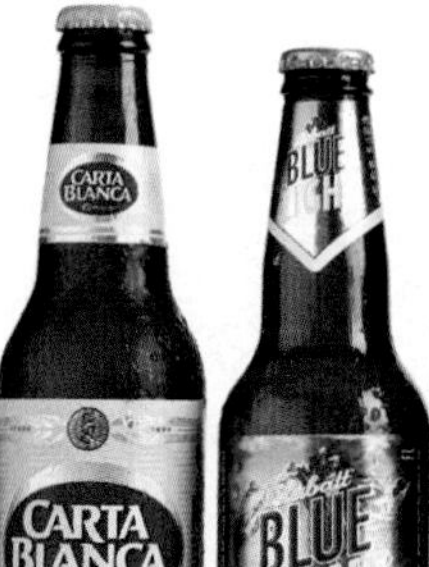
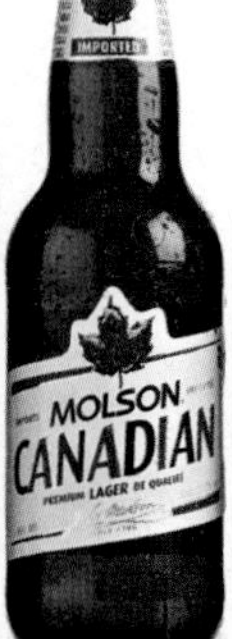
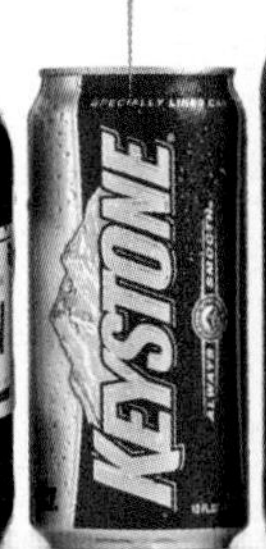
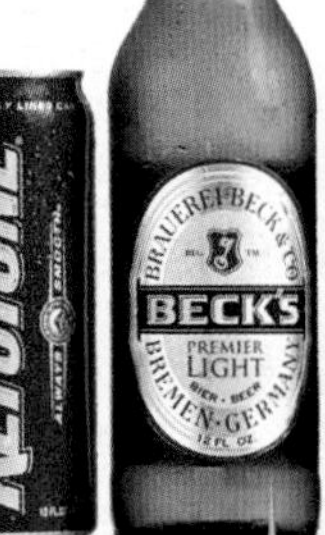
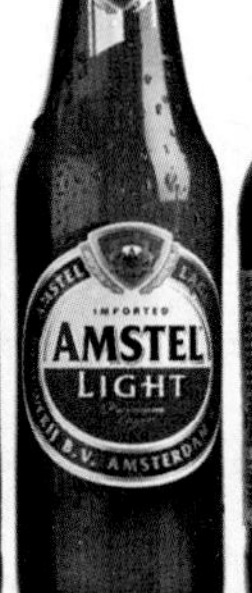
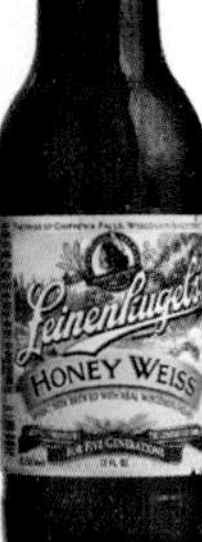

Rolling Rock
120 calories
7 g carbs
4.5% alcohol

Carta Blanca
128 calories
11 g carbs
4% alcohol

Labatt Blue Light
108 calories
8 g carbs
4% alcohol

Molson Canadian
143 calories
11 carbs
5% alcohol

Beck's Premier Light
64 calories
4 g carbs
3.8% alcohol

Leinenkugel's Honey Weiss
149 calories
12 g carbs
4.9% alcohol

Not That!

Guinness Extra Stout
(12 fl oz)
176 calories
14 g carbs
6% alcohol

Make sure you never get these two popular Guinness varities mixed up. If you do, it could cost you 10 or more pounds over the course of a year.

Bass
156 calories
13 g carbs
5.1% alcohol

Pabst Blue Ribbon
144 calories
13 g carbs
4.7% alcohol

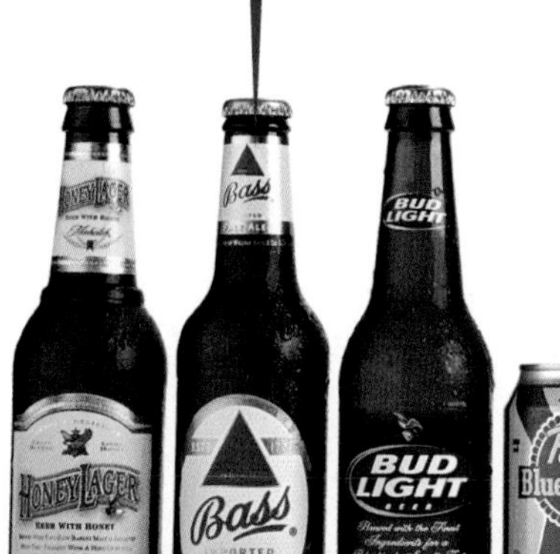
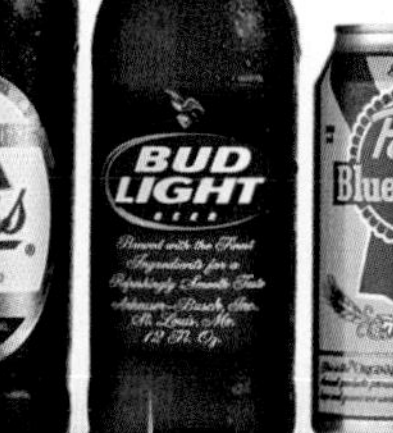
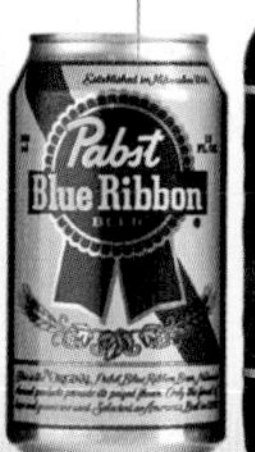
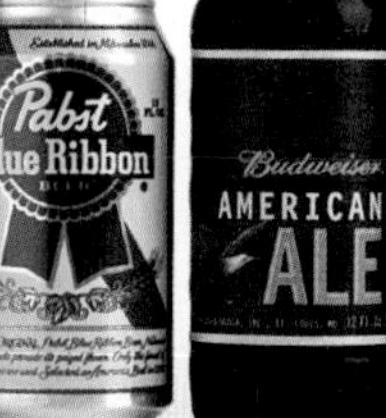
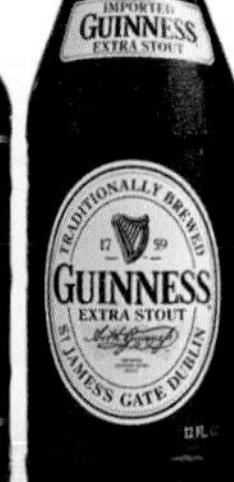
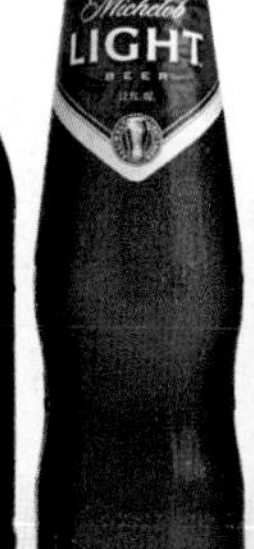
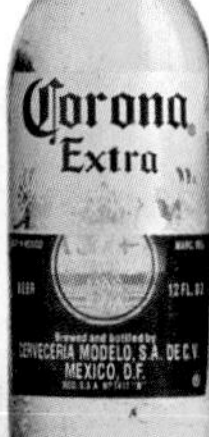
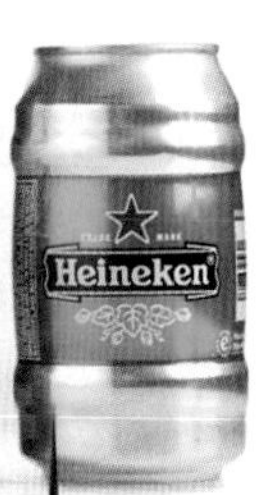

Michelob Honey Lager
178 calories
19 g carbs
4.9% alcohol

Bud Light
110 calories
7 g carbs
4.2% alcohol

Budweiser American Ale
182 calories
18 g carbs
5.3% alcohol

Michelob Light
123 calories
9 g carbs
4.3% alcohol

Corona Extra
148 calories
14 g carbs
4.6% alcohol

Heineken
166 calories
10 g carbs
5.4% alcohol

5

Eat This, Not That!

HOLIDAYS & SPECIAL OCCASIONS

There's an old joke that says...

every Jewish holiday celebrates the same idea: "They tried to kill us, we won, let's eat."

Sadly, too many holiday traditions in too many cultures today focus only on those last two words: "Let's eat." Whether you're cooking up a ham for Christmas, turkey for Thanksgiving, jerked chicken for Kwanzaa, or flanken for Passover, every holiday on the American calendar seems to carry an egregious caloric load. And that's before the Thanksgiving wine, the Christmas egg nog, the Easter brunch mimosas, and the brewskis on the Fourth of July.

Consider that most astronomically caloric, gastronomically uneconomic of holidays, Thanksgiving. According to the Calorie Control Council, the average American will consume 4,500 calories and 229 grams of fat on Thanksgiving day, a feat worthy of competitive eating accolades on any other day. But that doesn't mean you can't stuff your face without testing the fortitude of your new designer jeans. We imagine you'll want turkey. Cranberry sauce. Potatoes, sure. Gravy. Maybe some veggies on the side. Oh, and pie? Yeah, go for it! But just by making a couple of smart at-the-table swaps (like choosing pumpkin over pecan pie, or white meat over the drumstick), you could eat to your heart's content and still take in 700 fewer calories than you did last year.

Now imagine if you could do that at every holiday: whack off 700 calories from Christmas, New Year's, Fourth of July, and Halloween and you've just shaved an entire pound off your body. And the sacrifice? Well, there is none. You can still raid the kids' stockings and trick-or-treat bags, feast on grilled goodies and all the fixings at the summer barbecue, and drink champagne toasts a plenty to welcome in the new year.

You'll just look leaner and fitter while you do it.

Thanksgiving

Eat This

White Meat Turkey Dinner
895 calories
37 g fat (11.5 g saturated)
1,115 mg sodium

Turkey is the least of your concerns on Turkey Day. Pick smart sides and a reasonable dessert and you can save 500 calories or more.

Pumpkin pie with low-fat whipped cream
(1 medium slice; ⅙ pie)
335 calories
15 g fat
(6.5 g saturated)
38 g sugars
Want portion control? Cut the slice yourself.

Green bean casserole
(½ c)
100 calories
6 g fat
(1 g saturated)
300 mg sodium
Can the cream of mushroom and fried onions and make it with fresh green beans and sautéed onions.

Mashed potatoes (½ c) with turkey gravy (¼ c)
140 calories
7 g fat
(2 g saturated)
340 mg sodium
Don't nix the mash—just go easy with the butter and use low-fat milk to prepare them.

Turkey breast (4 oz) with homemade cranberry sauce (2 Tbsp)
195 calories
4 g fat
265 mg sodium
White meat turkey is as lean as meat gets. Homemade cranberry sauce cuts the sugar.

Dinner roll with butter
130 calories
5 g fat
(2 g saturated)
210 mg sodium
A small pat of butter helps lower the glycemic index of the roll, meaning the carbs will have less of an effect on blood sugar.

Not That!

Dark Meat Turkey Dinner

1,475 calories
62 g fat (23 g saturated)
1,370 mg sodium

Stuffing, sweet potatoes, and cornbread are among the worst of the Thanksgiving staples. Combined, they bring 615 calories to this plate.

Cornbread with butter

190 calories
9 g fat
(4 g saturated)
360 mg sodium

Sweeter, saltier, and fattier than a regular roll.

Dark turkey meat (4 oz) with jellied cranberry sauce (½" slice)

410 calories
10 g fat
(4 g saturated)
320 mg sodium

More fat and sugar. Any other questions?

Candied sweet potatoes with marshmallow topping (½ c)

250 calories
8 g fat
(5 g saturated)
270 mg sodium

Sweet potatoes lose their nututitional edge once they're covered in marshmallows.

Stuffing (½ c)

175 calories
14 g fat
(6 g saturated)
420 mg sodium

True stuffing is nothing more than a pile of croutons moistened with fat and loaded with sodium.

Pecan pie (1 medium slice; ⅙ pie)

450 calories
21 g fat
(4 g saturated)
70 g sugars

The healthy fat from the pecans is not enough to justify the extra load of corn syrup calories.

Christmas

Eat This

Beef Tenderloin Dinner

815 calories
30 g fat (11 g saturated)
665 mg sodium

Medium-rare beef, crispy potatoes, red wine, and chocolate: What more could you ask for from a Christmas feast?

Glass of red wine (5 oz)

125 calories
5.3 g carbohydrates

Research shows that pinot noir has the highest concentration of the flavonoids in wine that may protect your cardiovascular system.

Roasted red potatoes (½ c)

100 calories
5 g fat
(1 g saturated)
170 mg sodium

Any roasted vegetable will be a welcome addition to a holiday feast.

Peas and pearl onions (½ c)

90 calories
2 g fat
95 mg sodium

Fend off the food coma: The fiber in the peas and the chromium in the onions both help to regulate blood sugar levels.

Beef tenderloin (6 oz)

300 calories
15 g fat
(6 g saturated)
400 mg sodium

Save cash by purchasing a whole tenderloin. Rub the lean hunk of beef with olive oil, garlic and rosemary, and roast at 450°F.

Chocolate fondue (1 oz) **with fruit** (½ c)

200 calories
8 g fat
(4 g saturated)
18 g sugars

Go with dark instead of milk chocolate and you'll get a deeper-flavored fondue with more antioxidants.

Not That!

Prime Rib Dinner

1,865 calories
77 g fat (35 g saturated)
1,850 mg sodium

There's a big difference between splurging and gorging. Here, that difference amounts to more than 1,000 calories and 47 grams of excess fat.

Cheesecake
(1 slice; 1/8 cake)

470 calories
26 g fat
(13 g saturated)
39 g sugars

Even a modest slice of cheesecake will account for more than half your day's recommended intake of saturated fat.

Prime rib
(6 oz)

600 calories
25 g fat
(12 g saturated)
870 mg sodium

The rib roasts used to make prime rib are among the most caloric cuts of beef, teeming with surface and intramuscular fat.

Salad with croutons and Italian dressing

240 calories
12 g fat
(4 g saturated)
390 mg sodium

It's a noble gesture to serve a salad with dinner, but first ditch the croutons and go easy on the dressing.

Baked potato with butter and sour cream

400 calories
14 g fat
(6 g saturated)
590 mg sodium

This baby's barely dressed; add bacon and cheese to the mix and tack on an extra 150 calories.

Glass of beer
(12 oz)

155 calories
0 g fat
12.8 g carbohydrates

Choose an India Pale Ale if you want your beer to deliver a higher dose of antioxidants.

Fourth Of July

Eat This

Pork tenderloin is one of the most underrated cuts in the meat case. Not just lean, but loaded with thiamin, a B vitamin that converts sugar into energy.

Pork tenderloin
(6 oz)
328 calories
11.5 g fat (4 g saturated)
95 mg sodium

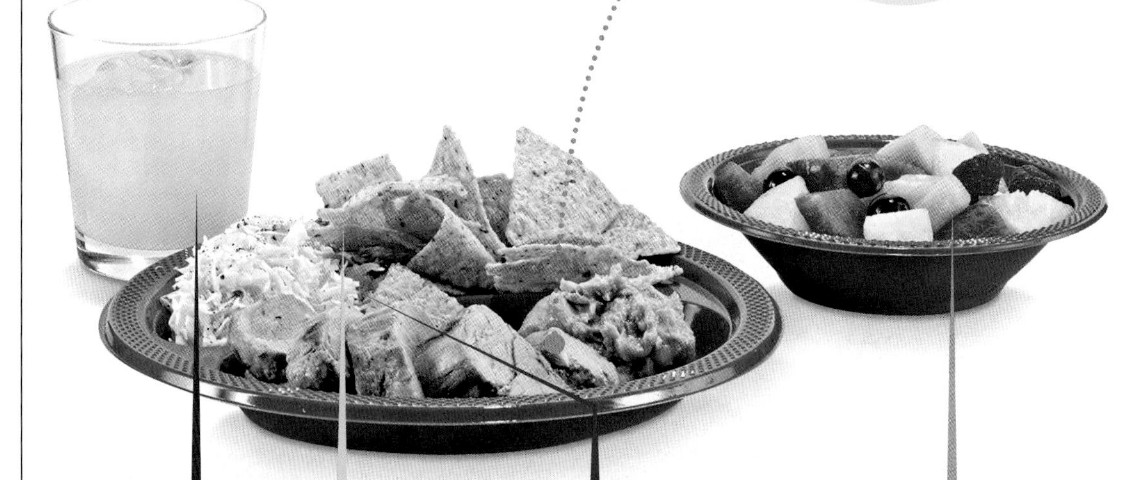

Grapefruit and vodka
(6 oz)
160 calories
0 g fat
10 g sugars

Use Simply Grapefruit's 100% pure juice, with its relatively low levels of natural sugars, to make this cocktail (called a Greyhound). You'll knock out 90% of your day's vitamin C requirements while you celebrate.

Tortilla chips and guacamole
(about 10 chips)
160 calories
11 g fat (3 g saturated)
280 mg sodium

Choose a whole-grain chip like those made by Garden of Eatin' and you'll get a boost of fiber to go along with guacamole's good monounsaturated fats.

Coleslaw
(½ c)
150 calories
8 g fat (1 g saturated)
350 mg sodium

Both coleslaw and potato salad are vehicles for the same fatty passenger, mayo. So it all comes down to which one makes a healthier vehicle.

Fruit salad
(½ c)
55 calories
0 g fat
5 mg sodium
13 g sugars

Dice up some melons, kiwi, and pineapple and then toss in a few grapes for good measure. Naturally sweet and loaded with fiber and antioxidants.

Not That!

Cheeseburger
(5 oz)

630 calories
41 g fat (15 g saturated)
735 mg sodium

A sucker for a burger? Try switching to grass-fed beef. You'll get a leaner chuck with a higher concentration of omega-3s.

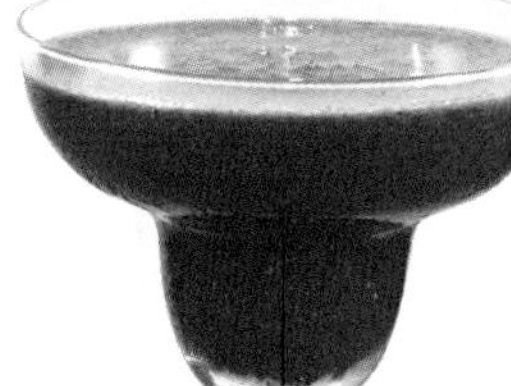

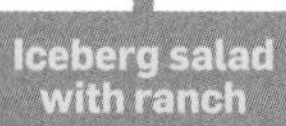

Iceberg salad with ranch

175 calories
11 g fat (2 g saturated)
240 mg sodium

Along with mayonnaise, ranch is responsible for turning more healthy foods unhealthy than any other condiment.

Potato salad
(½ c)

190 calories
12 g fat (3 g saturated)
430 mg sodium

If you want to do potato salad, do it German-style: mustard-based potato salad instead. It will cut close to 100 calories from each serving.

Corn on the cob with butter

200 calories
7 g fat (4 g saturated)
190 mg sodium

It's an American birthright to eat corn, but truthfully, it offers little nutritionally compared to a powerhouse like avocado. Fix that by sprinkling it with chili powder and lime juice.

Strawberry daiquiri
(8 oz)

325 calories
0 g fat
68 g sugars

Unless you personally blended the strawberries, you can assume this is a cup full of high-fructose corn syrup. You can also assume you're going to have a pounding headache in the morning.

Cocktail Party

Eat This

Jumbo shrimp
(12) with cocktail sauce (2 Tbsp)

165 calories
<1 g fat
480 mg sodium

Shrimp are essentially fat free and protein packed, which makes them one of the few foods you can gorge on without paying the price. But limit yourself on the cocktail sauce—it's mostly tomatoes, but it's heavy on sodium.

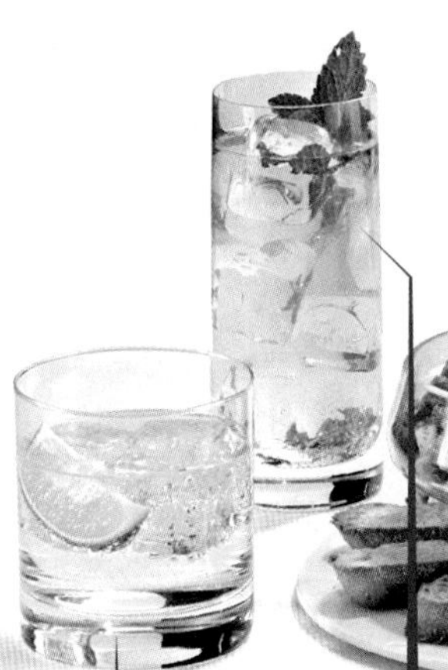

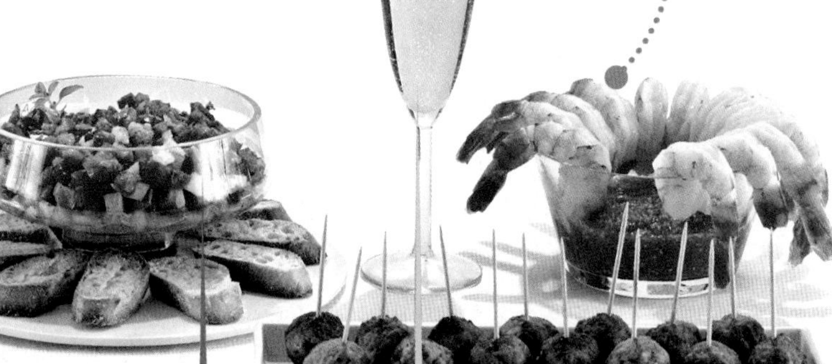

Vodka soda
(8 oz)

120 calories
0 g fat
0 g carbohydrates

All clear spirits pack around the same amount of calories and carbs, so the only variable with cocktails is mixers. Here, soda trumps tonic for one reason: It's calorie free.

Mojito
(8 oz)

180 calories
0 g fat
15 g carbohydrates

Made with a bevy of healthy components, including lime juice, fresh mint, and sugar-free club soda.

Tomato bruschetta
(2 pieces)

200 calories
4 g fat
(1 g saturated)
230 mg sodium

Other than the bread, it's a bunch of A-list players: tomatoes, garlic, basil, and extra-virgin olive oil.

Glass of champagne
(6 oz)

130 calories
6 g carbohydrates

Turns out the perfect New Year's drink can also help reduce heart-threatening inflammation.

Meatballs
(3)

240 calories
12 g fat
(4.5 g saturated)
650 mg sodium

Start off with protein-based bites and you'll fill your belly quickly, saving you from senseless snacking the rest of the night.

Not That!

Crab cake with aioli

400 calories
27 fat (6g saturated)
620 mg sodium

The crab lumps are bound in mayo, then rolled in breadcrumbs and fried, which is why only one of these does more damage than a dozen shrimp.

Pigs in a blanket
(3)

400 calories
25 g fat
(9 g saturated)
1,200 mg sodium

Hot dogs in a bun are one thing, but dogs wrapped in a buttery pastry blanket are a waistline-expanding combination.

Corona Extra
(12 oz)

148 calories
14 g carbohydrates

Corona, despite its light taste, ranks in the middle of the pack when it comes to beers and calories. If you want suds, try an Amstel Light for 95 calories.

Spinach artichoke dip
(¼ cup dip and 8 chips)

325 calories
19 g fat
(9 g saturated)
625 mg sodium

If you want an acceptable version of this ubiquitous dip, try our suped-up version on page 304.

Margarita
(8 oz)

450 calories
0 g fat
65 g carbohydrates

If you really want a margarita, ditch the sugar-spiked neon mix and shake them up with fresh lime juice and a bit of agave syrup.

Gin and tonic
(8 oz)

240 calories
0 g fat
16 g carbohydrates

An 8-ounce splash of tonic water has nearly as much sugar as some regular soft drinks. Opt for diet, if available: It's sugar free.

At the Ballpark

Eat This

Not only will a hot dog save you calories over a plate of nachos, but it will also give a bellyful of protein to help ward off late-game munchies.

Hot dog with relish, ketchup, and mustard

320 calories
18 g fat (8 g saturated)
960 mg sodium

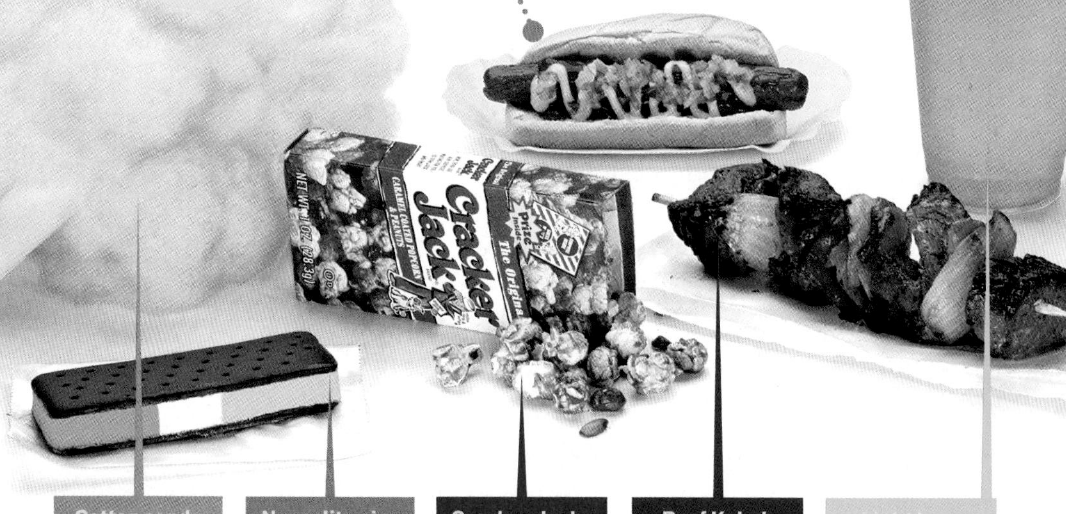

Cotton candy (1 serving)

220 calories
0 g fat
56 g sugars

We're not going to pretend this is healthy; it is, after all, pure sugar. But in terms of weight, it's ultra light, helping minimize the overall calorie count.

Neapolitan ice cream sandwich

190 calories
7 g fat
(3.5 g saturated)
15 g sugars

Ice cream sandwiches all come in the same small portion, so you know you're getting less than 200 calories, regardless of brand.

Cracker Jacks

420 calories
7 g fat
(0 g saturated)
245 mg sodium

See that regular fat to saturated fat ratio? That's because the fat in this classic box is the healthy monounsaturated variety found in peanuts.

Beef Kabob

220 calories
9 g fat
(4.5 g saturated)
120 mg sodium

Most kabobs are made with lean sirloin. Find one with vegetables on the skewer and you've located the best meal in the ballpark.

Light beer (20 oz)

174 calories
0 g fat
9.6 g carbohydrates

When it comes to stadium-size cups, you'd be wise to stick to light beer.

Not That!

This is a nutritionist's nightmare. It's loaded with sodium, has close to a day's worth of saturated fat, and offers nothing by way of redeeming nutrients.

Nachos
(40 chips and 4 oz cheese)
1,101 calories
59 g fat (18.5 g saturated)
1,580 mg sodium

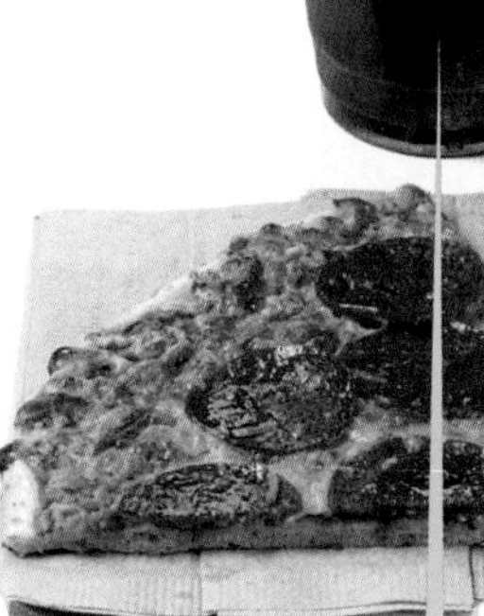

Cola
(20 oz)
243 calories
0 g fat
67.5 g carbohydrates

Once again soda proves to be the nutritional loser. It's just a cupful of carbonated water and high-fructose corn syrup.

Pepperoni Pizza
(1 slice)
425 calories
19 g fat
(7 g saturated)
820 mg sodium

There's certainly no higher standard at the amusement park. If it's bad for you in the outside world, it's bad for you at Disney Land.

French Fries
600 calories
32 g fat
(10 g saturated)
890 mg sodium

Make this your regular ballpark snack and you'll need to turn the seventh inning stretch into a full-game workout to keep the pounds off.

Chocolate ice cream in a helmet
(1½ cups)
429 calories
21 g fat
(12 g saturated)
51 g sugar

Mini helmets house about a cup and a half of cream, i.e., three times too much for you.

French vanilla soft-serve ice cream
(1 cup)
380 calories
22 g fat
(13 g saturated)
36 g sugars

Malts and soft serve come in huge portion sizes, making them a dangerous choice.

At the Mall

Eat This

Auntie Anne's Cinnamon Sugar Pretzel without butter

380 calories
1 g fat
29 g sugars

Ask for your pretzel with no butter and you'll save 90 calories of pure fat.

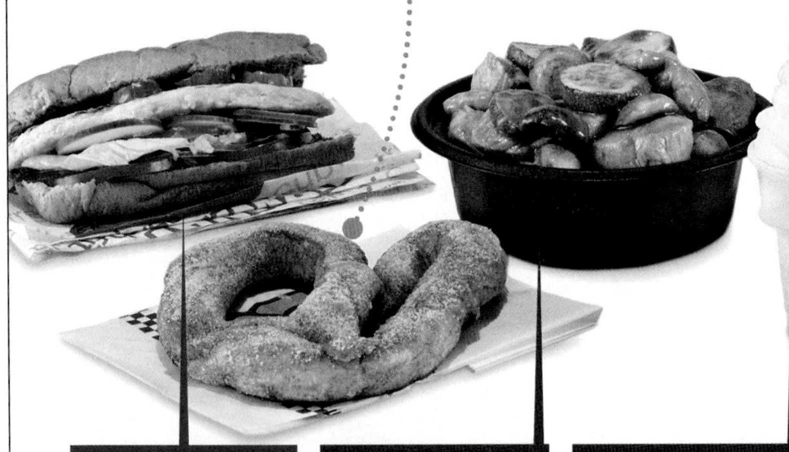

Subway 6" Oven Roasted Chicken Breast

320 calories
5 g fat (1.5 g saturated)
880 mg sodium

Who says you can't eat light at the mall? If you're fortunate enough to find a Subway in the food court, make a beeline for it.

Panda Express Mushroom Chicken with Mixed Vegetables

280 calories
16 g fat (3 g saturated)
940 mg sodium

As long as you skip the orange chicken (and the rice and noodles), Panda Express can be a solid spot to squash a growing hunger.

McDonald's Vanilla Ice Cream Cone

150 calories
3.5 g fat (2.5 g saturated)
18 g sugars

Slice the saturated fat from the chocolate chip treat in half with Mickey D's well-portioned cone.

Orange Julius (20 oz)

160 calories
0.5 g fat
38 g sugars

Short of unsweetened iced tea and H_2O, this is the best beverage you'll find in the food court.

Not That!

Cinnabon Classic Cinnamon Roll

730 calories
24 g fat
(8 g saturated, 5 g trans)
49 g sugars

Cinnabon reps say this roll's big size makes it ideal for taking home leftovers. But why would you want to bring all that trans fat into your house?

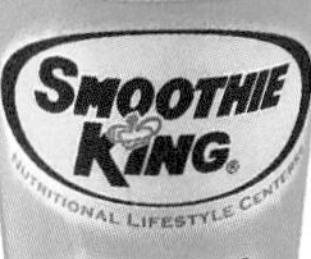

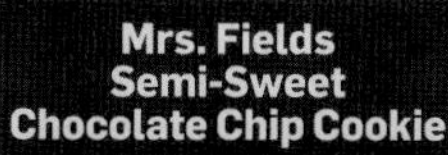

Smoothie King Orange Ka-Bam
(20 oz)

465 calories
0 g fat
108 g sugars

Sounds healthy enough, but the numbers tell a different story. Ounce for ounce, this sweetener-spiked drink has more sugar than a Mountain Dew.

Mrs. Fields Semi-Sweet Chocolate Chip Cookie

210 calories
10 g fat (5 g saturated)
19 g sugars

It beats out most of the other specialty sweets in the mall but the cone reigns supreme in the classic dessert showdown.

Sbarro New York Style Thin Crust Chicken and Vegetable Pizza
(1 slice)

530 calories
17 g fat (8 g saturated)
1,260 mg sodium

This one slice of pizza will eat up about a quarter of your day's calories.

Quiznos Chicken Carbonara
(Small)

520 calories
25 g fat (7 g saturated)
1,230 mg sodium

There are very few sandwich battles Quizno's wins—that is, unless you opt for a Sammie or two.

At the Movie Theater

Eat This

As long as you're not dipping it into molten cheese, a large soft pretzel makes a reasonable movie theater or street corner snack. Be really good and ask them to skip the salt—mustard packs plenty of sodium as it is.

Soft pretzel with mustard

290 calories
0 g fat
850 mg sodium

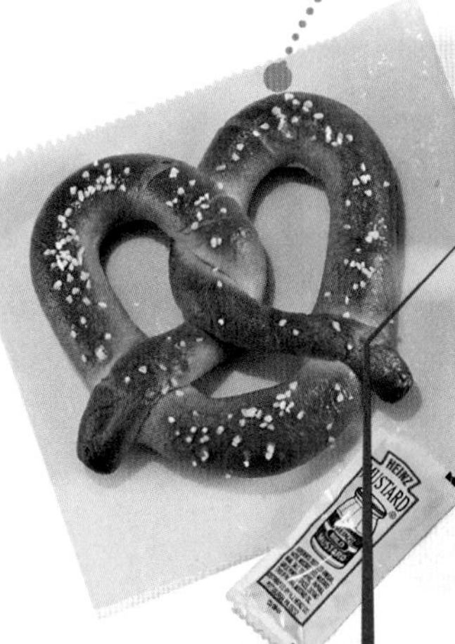

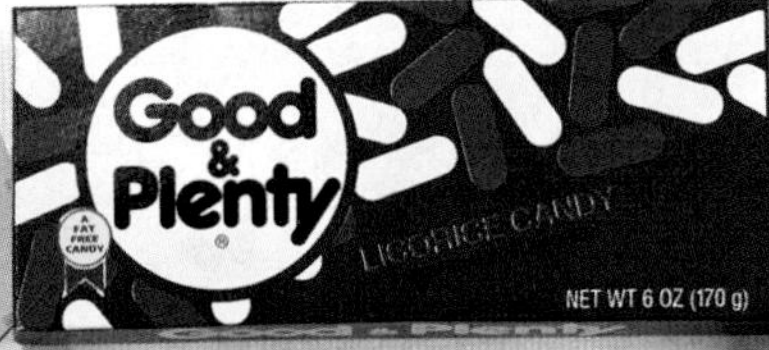

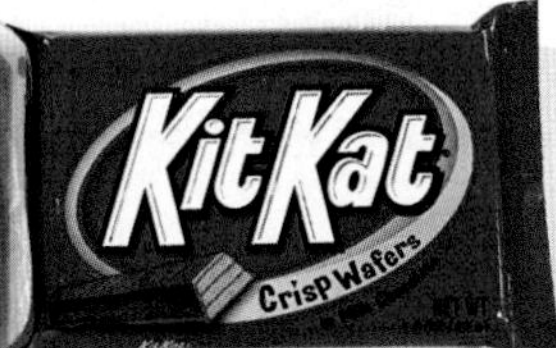

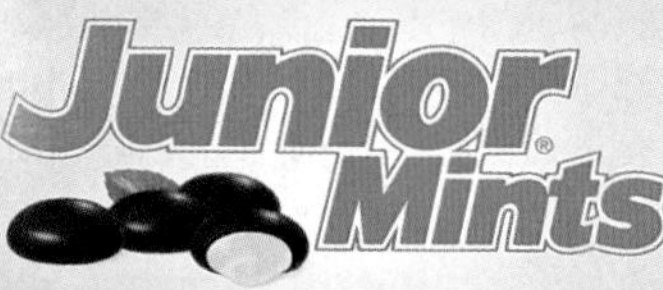

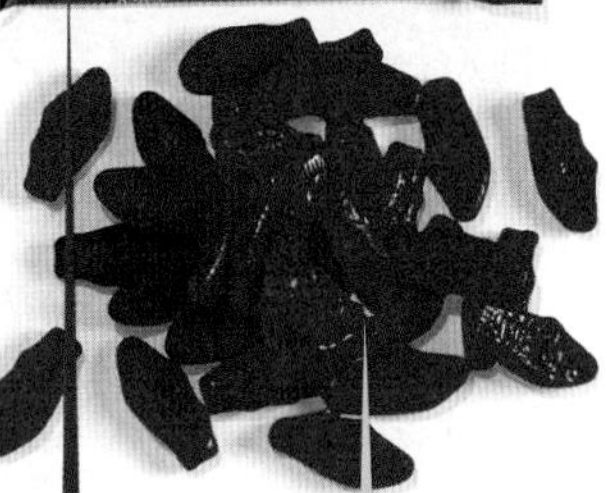

Good & Plenty
(33 pieces)

130 calories
0 g fat
21 g sugars

Many cultures have viewed licorice as a healing herb for centuries, with anti-inflammatory properties. But we're just thankful they have less sugar and fewer calories than traditional chewy fruit candies.

Junior Mints
(½ box)

170 calories
3 g fat
(2.5 g saturated)
32 g sugars

Minty candies like Junior Mints and Peppermint Patties tend to be the best of the chocolate choices.

Kit Kat Bar

200 calories
11 g fat
(7 g saturated)
20 g sugars

Have some friends nearby? Break this bar up and dole out the pieces. Just because there are four in a package doesn't mean you need to eat them all yourself.

Swedish Fish
(2 oz)

200 calories
0 g fat
28 g sugars

In the world of pure sugar candies, few are better than the fish from Sweden.

Not That!

Buttered popcorn
(medium; 10–12 cups)

600 calories
39 g fat (12 g saturated)
1,120 mg sodium

Popcorn can be a great, fiber-rich snack, as long as you stay away from the dreaded butter pump. Besides tripling the calories of a bag of popcorn, many movie theater "butters" are teeming with trans fat. Instead, seek flavor from the spice mixes many theaters carry now.

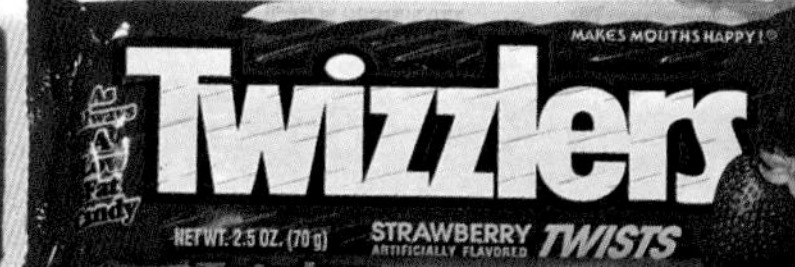

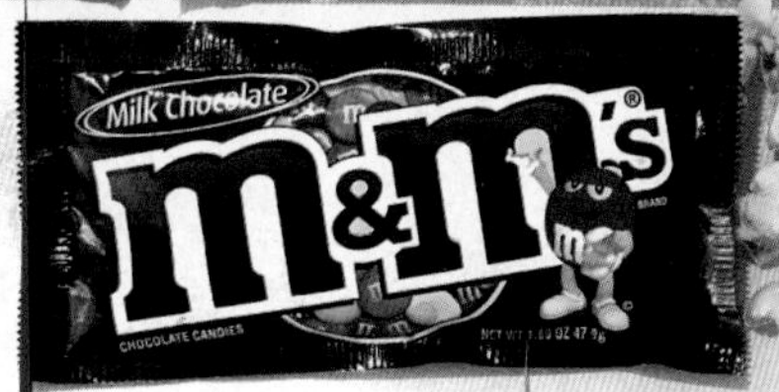

Dots
(22 pieces)

260 calories
0 g fat
42 g sugars

They stick to your teeth just like they stick to your waistline. You're better off going for nearly any other gummy product besides these.

Hershey's Milk Chocolate Bar

210 calories
13 g fat
(8 g saturated)
24 g sugars

If you're going to eat pure chocolate, you're better off picking up a bar with at least 65% cacao. That way, you lower your sugar intake while maximizing antioxidants.

M&M's
(1 bag)

240 calories
10 g fat
(6 g saturated)
31 g sugars

They may seem harmless and fun in their tiny candy-coated vessels, but a few generous handfuls of M&M's can wipe out a meal's worth of calories before you know it.

Twizzlers
(½ 6-oz package)

240 calories
1 g fat
32 g sugars

Ignore the "low fat" claims on the side of the package—these are nothing more than ropes of high-fructose corn syrup.

Vending Machine

Eat This

100 Grand

190 calories
8 g fat (5 g saturated)
22 g sugars

The "best" (we use that term loosely) candy bar in America. This is the only full-size chocolate bar we've ever seen under 200 calories.

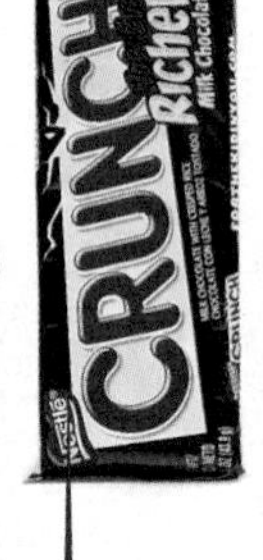

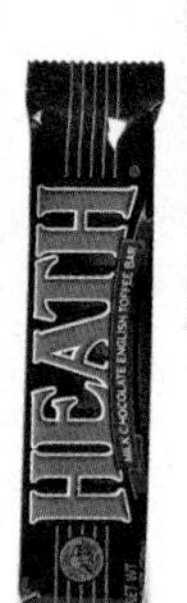

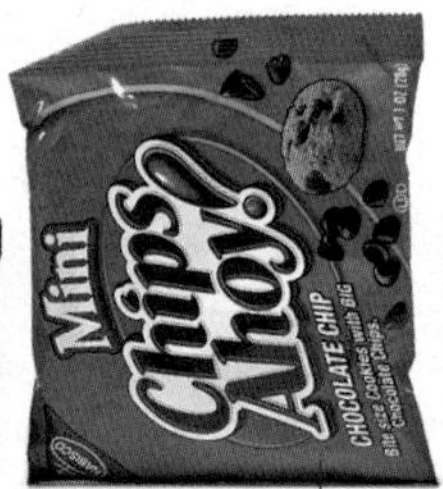

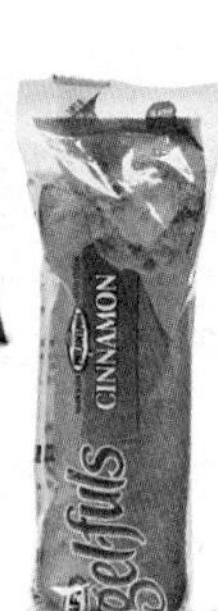

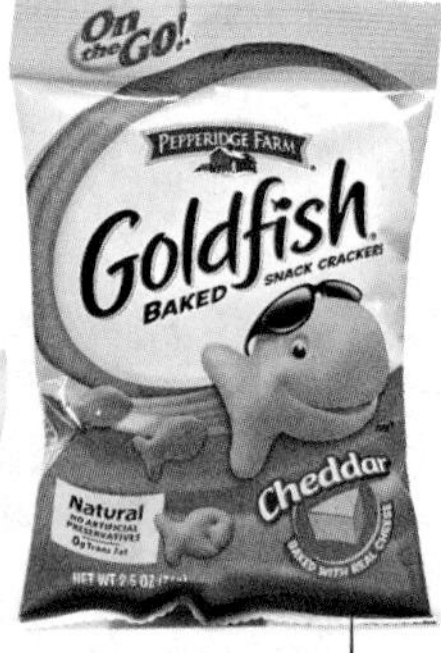

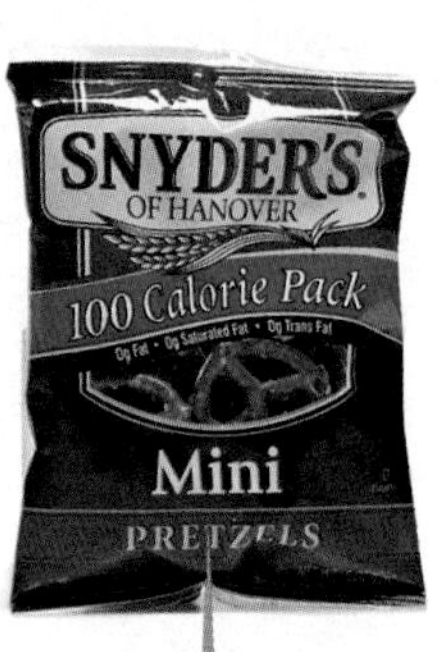

HEATH

Nestlé Crunch

220 calories
11 g fat
(7 g saturated)
24 g sugars

The Crunch bar is less dense than pure milk chocolate, which means less fat and sugar in each bite.

Heath Bar

210 calories
13 g fat
(7 g saturated)
23 g sugars

Toffee is normally incredibly rich and calorie-dense, but Heath pulls off the unexpected by keeping this bar close to 200 calories.

Mini Chips Ahoy!
(1 bag)

140 calories
7 g fat
(2 g saturated)
8 g sugars

Hardly a nutritious snack, but its modest size makes certain that you won't overindulge.

Kraft Bagelful Cinnamon

200 calories
4 g fat
(2.5 g saturated)
190 mg sodium
8 g sugars

Not one of Kraft's bagel-and-cream-cheese fusions has more than 200 calories.

Pepperidge Farm Goldfish Cheddar Crackers
(55 pieces)

140 calories
5 g fat
(1 g saturated)
250 mg sodium

A swap everyone should make.

Snyder's of Hanover Mini Pretzels
(0.9 oz package)

100 calories
1 g fat
(0.5 g saturated)
220 mg sodium

Virtually fat-free, pretzels make for smarter snacking than chips.

Not That!

America's most popular candy is also one of its worst, with more sugar than you'd get in two bowls of Captain Crunch cereal.

Snickers
280 calories
14 g fat (5 g saturated)
30 g sugars

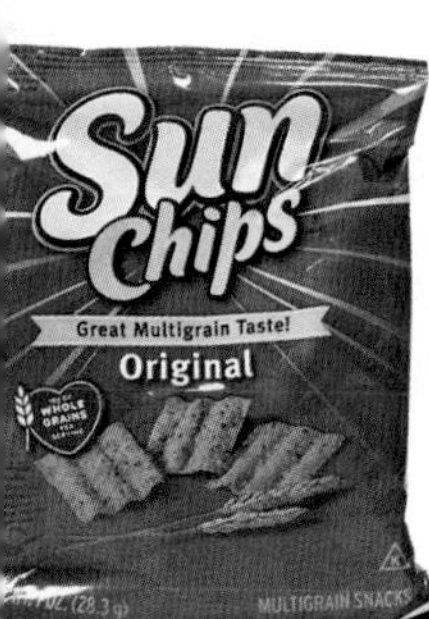

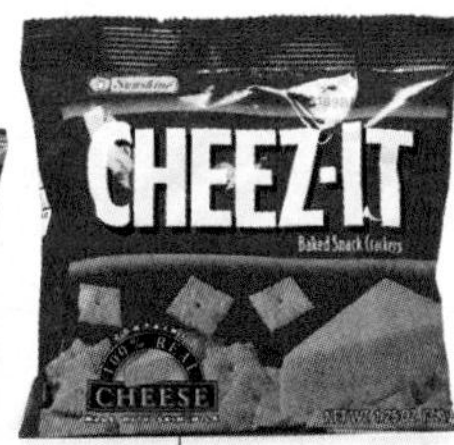

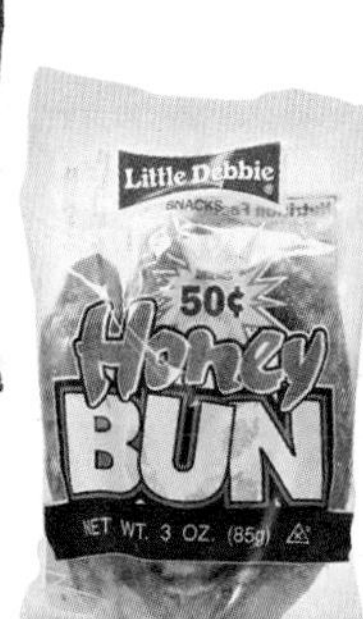

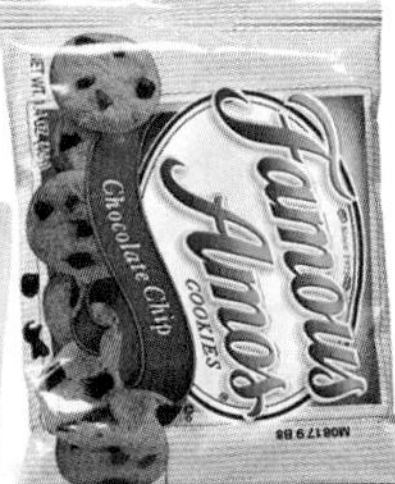

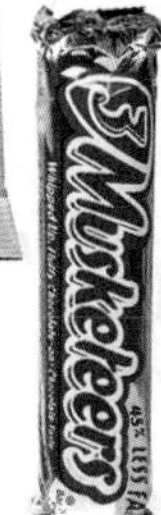

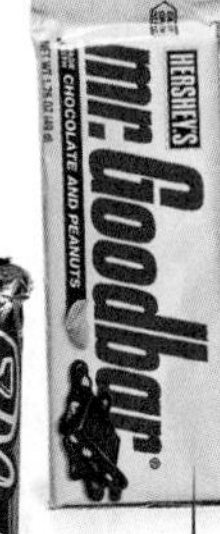

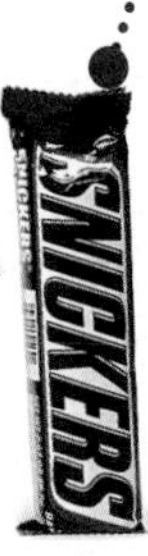

SunChips Original
(1 oz package)
140 calories
6 g fat
(1 g saturated)
120 mg sodium

Marginally better than regular chips, but still far from a healthy snack.

Cheez-It Original Crackers
(1 package)
180 calories
9 g fat
(2 g saturated)
290 mg sodium

About 40 calories worse than your average bag of chips.

Little Debbie Honey Bun
360 calories
20 g fat
(10 g saturated)
19 g sugars

Sticky buns and rolls are among the most calore-dense, fat-laden foods on the planet.

Famous Amos Chocolate Chip Cookies
(1 bag)
240 calories
10 g fat
(4 g saturated)
13 g sugars

The bigger bag will cost you more than a hundred extra calories.

3 Musketeers
260 calories
8 g fat
(5 g saturated)
40 g sugars

It's not the fat that does this bar in; it's the sugar. Forty grams is more than you'd find in three Breyers Oreo Ice Cream sandwiches.

Mr. Goodbar
250 calories
17 g fat
(7 g saturated)
22 g sugars

The only way to make this a truly good bar would be to increase the ratio of peanuts to milk chocolate.

Eat This, Not That! FOR KIDS

6

Being a great parent has always been a challenge.

Think of Adam and Eve, figuring out the whole parenting thing without a guidebook. (Eve: "Should we be concerned about Cain picking on his brother?" Adam: "Nah, they're fine. Hand me an apple.") Or how about Oedipus, who killed his dad, married his mom, and brought disaster to their kingdom? (And you thought your kids feeding Fido their green beans was a big deal.)

But while headaches, backaches, and wallet aches have always been part of the penalty we pay for having children we love, it seems as though parenting has gotten even more complicated in recent years. Technology deserves a lot of the blame: Facebook, texting, and a dozen other wizardly wonders have given our progeny plenty of ways to get around the rules. But the technology that's complicating our lives as parents is a different kind of science entirely.

FOOD SCIENCE.

See, the foods our kids are eating today are very different from the foods we ate as children. The foods on offer in today's supermarkets and on restaurant kids' menus come not from the great green earth, but from the minds of marketers. They're assembled not in warm, welcoming kitchens, but in cold, bright science labs, and their nutritional labels read like the contents of a chemistry set.

Consider, if you will, the humble Cheerio. A little round O of goodness, the Cheerio that you and I grew up with contains only ground oats, a little sugar, some starch, some salt, and two preservatives—one of which is good old vitamin E. Pretty simple.

Until it got complicated. Because now we have not only Cheerios, but also Berry Burst Cheerios, MultiGrain Cheerios, Apple Cinnamon Cheerios, Honey Nut Cheerios, and something called Yogurt Burst Cheerios. Which of these variations are good for your kids? Which are not?

It's hard to tell. Is the "fractionated palm kernel oil" in the Yogurt Burst Cheerios something you should feed your kids? What about the dextrose, the maltodextrin, the corn syrup, the brown sugar syrup, and oh yes, the actual sugar (which is listed twice!)? In fact, this breakfast concoction is a great example of how today's food marketers are taking healthy foods and making them unhealthy by messing around with a complicated combination of confusing chemicals.

The result of all this fiddling about with our food supply is easy to see all around us: Kids are getting fatter. And with that fat comes more than just pleated pants and jokes about

What Our Kids Need Each Day

	1–3 YEARS	4–8 YEARS	9–13 YEARS	14–18 YEARS
CALORIES	1,000–1,400	1,400–1,600	1,800–2,200 (B)	2,200–2,400 (B)
			1,600–2,200 (G)	2,000 (G)
FAT (g)	33–54	39–62	62–85	61–95 (B) 55–78 (G)
SATURATED FAT (g)	<12–16	<16–18	<20–24 (B) <18–22 (G)	<24–27 (B) <22 (G)
SODIUM (mg)	1,000–1,500	1,200–1,900	1,500–2,200	1,500–2,300
CARBS (g)	130	130	130	130
FIBER (g)	19	25	31 (B) 26 (G)	38 (B) 26 (G)
PROTEIN (g)	13	19	31 (B) 26 (G)	52 (B) 46 (G)

being junk-food junkies. Being overweight as a child is a serious health problem. Consider this:

Ten years ago, type-2 diabetes was known as "adult-onset diabetes" because it took several decades of overeating to get your body to the point where it was at risk. But we have so hyperinflated the calories in our foods that even children—children as young as 4!—are now developing this disease. And it's not a pretty disease: Among its complications are blindness, heart attack, stroke, and sexual dysfunction. And the Centers for Disease Control and Prevention (CDC) recently predicted that one in three children born in the year 2000 will develop diabetes at some point in his or her lifetime.

Yet much of the food on offer as "for kids" in America's restaurants and supermarkets is a practical invitation to diabetes and other health complications—from heart disease to cancer to high blood pressure to asthma—later in life.

That's why we've included this chapter. We've analyzed the offerings of all the major restaurant chains and uncovered the real truth about what America is feeding its children. And the great news is this: You can have a major impact on your children's health and future, simply by making a few smart choices.

The power is in your hands.

Eat This Pyramid, Not That One

The USDA has its pyramid, of course, but the iconic image young students learn so well in school leaves a lot to be desired in terms of specifics. According to the vagaries of the image, a serving of white rice and quinoa both count the same toward the recommended six daily servings, despite the fact that one is packed with fiber, healthy fat, and essential amino acids (quinoa) and the other is a nutritional black hole (rice).

It's time for parental discretion. One-quarter of all vegetables consumed by kids are French fries, and according to a government study of 4,000 kids between the ages of 2 and 19, the overwhelming bulk of their nutrients comes from fruit juice and sugary cereals. While those might have a place in the USDA's pyramid, they have no place in ours. It's still important for your kids to go about constructing their pyramids each day—you just need to be sure they have the right building blocks.

FATS AND OILS (USE SPARINGLY)

Eat This
Healthy fats: Olive oil; canola oil; monounsaturated fats from nuts, avocado, and salmon

Not That!
Unhealthy fats: Stick margarine, lard, palm oil, anything with partially hydrogenated oil

DAIRY (2 OR 3 1-CUP SERVINGS)

Eat This
2 percent milk, string cheese, cottage cheese, plain yogurt sweetened with fresh fruit

Not That!
Chocolate milk, ice cream, hot cheese dip, yogurt with fruit on the bottom

MEAT, POULTRY, FISH, EGGS, AND BEANS (2 OR 3 2-OUNCE SERVINGS)

Eat This
Grilled chicken breast; roast pork tenderloin; sirloin steak; scrambled, boiled, or poached eggs; stewed black beans; almonds; unsweetened peanut butter

Not That!
Chicken fingers, crispy chicken sandwiches, cheeseburgers, strip or rib-eye steak, peanut butter with added sugars

VEGETABLES (5 ½-CUP SERVINGS)

Eat This
Sautéed spinach, steamed broccoli, romaine or mixed green salads, roasted mushrooms, grilled pepper and onion skewers, baby carrots, tomato sauce, salsa, homemade guacamole

Not That!
French fries, potato chips, onion rings, vegetables dipped in ranch dressing

FRUIT (3 ½-CUP SERVINGS)

Eat This
Sliced apples or pears; berries; grapes; stone fruit like peaches, plums, and apricots; 100 percent fruit smoothies

Not That!
More than one 8-ounce glass of juice a day; more than a few tablespoons of dried fruit a day; smoothies made with sherbet, frozen yogurt, or added sugar

GRAINS (6 1-OUNCE SERVINGS)

Eat This
Brown rice, whole grain bread, quinoa, whole grain pasta, oatmeal

Not That!
White rice, white bread, pasta, muffins, tortillas, pancakes, waffles, heavily sweetened cereal

6 Rules of Good Nutrition

GREAT FOR YOUR KIDS, AND GREAT FOR YOU

Rule #1
NEVER SKIP BREAKFAST. EVER.

Yes, mornings are crazy. But they're also our best hope at regaining our nutritional sanity. A 2005 study synthesized the results of 47 other studies that examined the impact of starting the day with a healthy breakfast. Here's what they found.

Children skipped breakfast more than any other meal. Skipping is more prevalent in girls, older children, and adolescents.

People who skip breakfast are more likely to take up smoking or drinking, less likely to exercise, and more likely to follow fad diets or express concerns about body weight. Common reasons cited for skipping were lack of time, lack of hunger, or dieting.

► The day that one national breakfast survey was administered, 8 percent of 1- to 7-year-olds skipped, 12 percent of 8- to 10-year-olds skipped, 20 percent of 11- to 14-year-olds skipped, and 30 percent of 15- to 18-year-olds skipped.

Bad news. Sure, it would seem to make sense that skipping breakfast means eating fewer calories, which means weighing less. But it doesn't work that way. Consider:

People who eat breakfast tend to have higher total calorie intakes throughout the day, but they also get significantly more fiber, calcium, and other micronutrients than skippers do. Breakfast eaters also tended to consume less soda and French fries and more fruits, vegetables, and milk.

Breakfast eaters were approximately 30 percent less likely to be overweight or obese. (Think about that—kids who eat breakfast eat more food, but weigh less!)

Rule #2
SNACK WITH PURPOSE.

There's a big difference between mindless munching and strategic snacking. Snacking with purpose means reinforcing good habits, keeping your metabolic rate high, and filling the gaps between meals with the nutrients your child's body craves.

- In the 20 years leading up to the 21st century (1977 to 1996), salty snack portions increased by 93 calories, and soft drink portions increased by 49 calories. So when you give your kid an individual bag of chips and a soda—the same snack you might have enjoyed when you were 10—he's ingesting 142 more calories than you did. Feeding him that just twice a week means he'll weigh 4 more pounds within a year.

Combat portion distortion by sending your kid off to school with healthy snacks that you'll both feel good about: Triscuits and peanut butter; string cheese; a sandwich bag filled with homemade popcorn; or that classic of kid's snacktime nourishment, ants on a log.

Rule #3

BEWARE OF PORTION DISTORTION.

Snack portions aren't the only things that have increased wildly in size. Since 1977, hamburgers have increased by 97 calories, French fries by 68 calories, and Mexican foods by 133 calories, according to analysis of the Nationwide Food Consumption Survey.

- A study published in the *American Journal of Preventive Medicine* looked at 63,380 individuals' drinking habits over a span of 19 years. The results show that for children ages 2 to 18, portions of sweetened beverages increased from 13.1 ounces in 1977 to 18.9 ounces in 1996.

One easy way to short-circuit this growing trend? ***Buy smaller bowls and cups.*** A recent study at the Children's Nutrition Research Center in Houston, Texas, shows that 5- and 6-year-old children will consume a third more calories when presented with a larger portion. The findings are based on a sample of 53 children who were served either 1- or 2-cup portions of macaroni and cheese.

Rule #4

DRINK RESPONSIBLY.

Too many of us keep in mind the adage "watch what you eat," and we forget another serious threat to our health: We don't watch what we drink. In fact, according to research from the University of North Carolina, Americans now slurp up nearly 25 percent of their calories in liquid form—nearly double the rate we used to drink just 20 years ago. One study found that sweetened beverages constituted more than half (51 percent) of all beverages consumed by fourth- through sixth-grade students. The students who consumed the most sweetened beverages took in approximately 330 extra calories per day, and on average they ate less than half the amount of real fruit than did their peers who drank unsweetened or lightly sweetened beverages.

One important strategy is to keep cold, filtered water in a pitcher in the fridge. You might even want to keep some cut-up limes, oranges, or lemons nearby for kids to flavor their own water with. A UK study showed that in classrooms with limited access to water, only 29 percent of students met their daily needs; free access to water led to higher intake.

Be extra careful about the juice you purchase. Too many "juices" are little more than sugar water masquerading as the real thing. Ocean Spray Cran-Raspberry, for instance, has just 15 percent real fruit juice. The other 85 percent? High-fructose corn syrup and water. Make sure the juice you buy says "100 percent Fruit Juice" on the label, and try to choose one made from a single fruit, not a mix of high-sugar fruits like white grapes, which are commonly used in fruit juice blends. And after you find the perfect juice, limit kids to one 8-ounce glass a day. If they want more, hand them a glass of water and a piece of fruit.

Rule #5

EAT MORE WHOLE FOODS AND FEWER SCIENCE EXPERIMENTS.

Here's a rule of healthy eating that will serve you well when picking out foods for your family: The shorter the ingredients list, the healthier the food. (One of the worst foods we've ever found, the Baskin-Robbins Heath Shake, has 73 ingredients—and, by the way, a whopping 2,310 calories and more than 3 days' worth of saturated fat! What happened to the idea that a milk shake was, um, milk and ice cream? Let's be grateful that Baskin-Robbins finally pulled this monstrosity from their menus.) The FDA maintains a list of more than 3,000 ingredients that are considered safe to eat, but we've found reasons for concern for a number of the additives on that long list, and any one of them could wind up in your next box of mac 'n' cheese.

▶ According to USDA reports, most of the sodium in the American diet comes from packaged and processed foods. Naturally occurring salt accounts for only 12 percent of total intake, while 77 percent is added by food manufacturers.

Rule #6
SET THE TABLE.

Children in families with more structured mealtimes exhibit healthier eating habits. Among middle- and high-school girls, those whose families ate together only once or twice per week were more than twice as likely to exhibit weight control issues, compared with those who ate together three or four times per week.

Of course, the notion of a 6 P.M. dinnertime and then everyone into their pj's is a quaint one, but it's hardly realistic in a society where our kids have such highly scheduled social lives that the delineation between "parent" and "chauffeur" is sometimes difficult to parse. While we can't always bring the family together like Ozzie Nelson's (or, heck, even like Ozzy Osbourne's), we can make some positive steps in that direction. One busy family I know keeps Sunday night dinner sacred—no social plans, no school projects, no extra work brought home from the office. Even keeping the family ritual just once a week gives parents the opportunity to point out what is and isn't healthy at the dinner table.

Another smart move: Get your kids involved in cooking. Make a game of trying to pack the most healthful ingredients into your meals. A Texas study showed that children can be encouraged to eat more fruits and vegetables by giving them goals and allowing them to help with preparation. So buy the kids their own aprons and cutting boards and let them peel carrots, stir sauces, and if at the end of the day they've done their duties as dilligent sous chefs, reward them with that priceless kitchen treasure: a few licks of the cake batter off the back of the beaters.

Eat the Rainbow

Better nutrition starts not with cutting out the bad, but with adding in the good. Fill your children's meals with healthful, high-quality foods, and you'll eventually squeeze out the bad stuff.

Let's not pretend that getting a child to eat what's good for him isn't sometimes a struggle. "A lot of parents tell me, 'My kids don't like healthy foods,'" says David Katz, MD, an associate clinical professor of epidemiology and public health at Yale Medical School. "'Finicky' is not an excuse. You never hear a parent say, 'My child doesn't like to look both ways before he crosses the street.' They tell him to do it. More kids today will die of complications from bad foods they eat than will die from tobacco, drugs, and alcohol."

So how do you teach the basics of nutrition to a 7-year-old? Even we grown-ups have trouble understanding how many calories we're supposed to take in each day, which vitamins and minerals we need more of, and which of the complicated chemical ingredients flooding our food system we need to avoid.

Well, here's a simple trick: Just teach your kids to eat as many different colors as they can. And no, We're not talking about red, green, and purple Skittles. We're talking about eating as much of a mix of fruits and vegetables as possible. That's because the colors represented in foods are indicators of nutritional value—and different colors mean different vitamins and minerals.

Not everything on this list is going to appeal to your child (or to you, for that matter). But there's enough variation here that he or she can squeeze one food from each category into a day's eating. For a fun project, make a multicolor checklist and have your kid check off each color as he or she eats it throughout the day.

Or do what our parents did and sell them on the kid-friendly benefits trapped inside of spinach, carrots, and the like. Each group of produce offers seriously cool "superpowers" that appeal to kids' deepest desires to dominate math quizzes and monkey bars alike. Feel free to sell these as hard as you want. Hey, even if it didn't end up making you as strong as Popeye, you still ate your spinach, right?

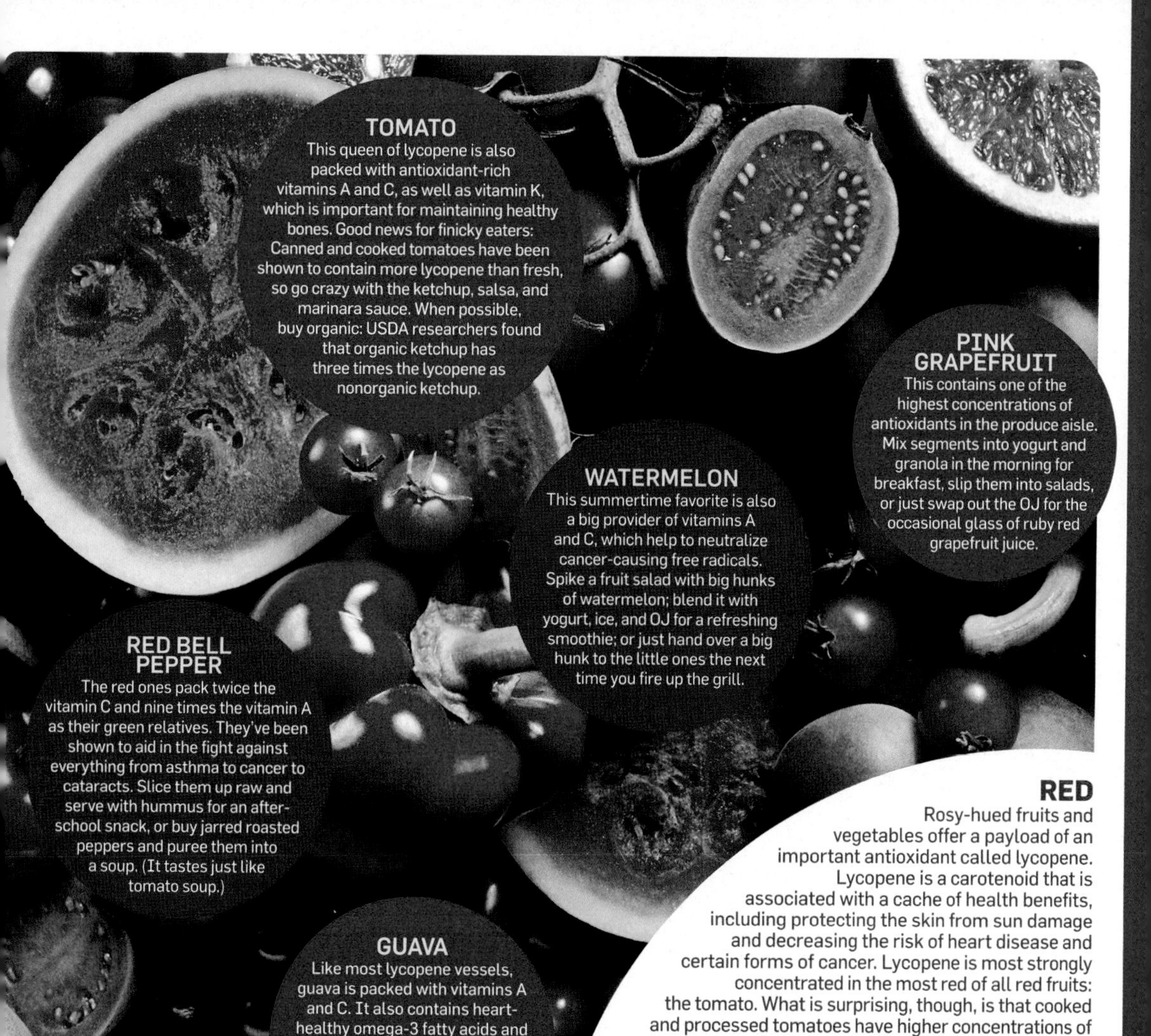

TOMATO

This queen of lycopene is also packed with antioxidant-rich vitamins A and C, as well as vitamin K, which is important for maintaining healthy bones. Good news for finicky eaters: Canned and cooked tomatoes have been shown to contain more lycopene than fresh, so go crazy with the ketchup, salsa, and marinara sauce. When possible, buy organic: USDA researchers found that organic ketchup has three times the lycopene as nonorganic ketchup.

PINK GRAPEFRUIT

This contains one of the highest concentrations of antioxidants in the produce aisle. Mix segments into yogurt and granola in the morning for breakfast, slip them into salads, or just swap out the OJ for the occasional glass of ruby red grapefruit juice.

WATERMELON

This summertime favorite is also a big provider of vitamins A and C, which help to neutralize cancer-causing free radicals. Spike a fruit salad with big hunks of watermelon; blend it with yogurt, ice, and OJ for a refreshing smoothie; or just hand over a big hunk to the little ones the next time you fire up the grill.

RED BELL PEPPER

The red ones pack twice the vitamin C and nine times the vitamin A as their green relatives. They've been shown to aid in the fight against everything from asthma to cancer to cataracts. Slice them up raw and serve with hummus for an after-school snack, or buy jarred roasted peppers and puree them into a soup. (It tastes just like tomato soup.)

GUAVA

Like most lycopene vessels, guava is packed with vitamins A and C. It also contains heart-healthy omega-3 fatty acids and belly-filling fiber. Get your hands on these in the produce aisles of larger supermarkets or Latin grocers, or simply keep a bottle of guava nectar in the fridge.

RED

Rosy-hued fruits and vegetables offer a payload of an important antioxidant called lycopene. Lycopene is a carotenoid that is associated with a cache of health benefits, including protecting the skin from sun damage and decreasing the risk of heart disease and certain forms of cancer. Lycopene is most strongly concentrated in the most red of all red fruits: the tomato. What is surprising, though, is that cooked and processed tomatoes have higher concentrations of lycopene, so don't shy away from the salsa or marinara sauce. **SUPERPOWER:** Red food makes you dash like the Flash! There's a reason he wore red: Lycopene-rich foods have been shown to decrease symptoms of wheezing, asthma, and shortness of breath in people when they exercise.

ORANGE Beta-carotene is the nutrient responsible for fruits and vegetables' dramatic orange color, and although the carotenoid is present in a host of other vegetables (spinach, kale, and broccoli, for instance), the orange ones have the highest concentrations. But the conspicuous hue of this carotenoid does more than just attract your attention; once inside your body, it is converted into vitamin A, a powerful antioxidant that contributes to immune health, improves communication between cells, and helps fight off cell-damaging free radicals. **SUPERPOWER:** Orange foods give you night vision! That's because vitamin A is vital for creating the pigment in the retina responsible for vision in low-light situations. Just think of the benefits: It'll help them beat their friends at hide-and-seek, spy on their brothers or sisters, and spot bogeymen before they can hide under their beds.

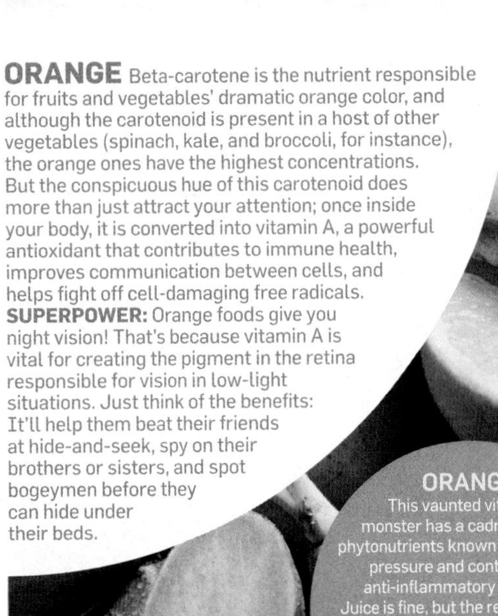

WINTER SQUASH
A true grab bag of nutrients, winter squash is a great source of a dozen different vitamins, including a host of B vitamins, folate, manganese, and fiber. What does that all mean? It means feed it to your kid! And lots of it! The best way is to cut the squash into 1-inch wedges and bake them at 375°F for 40 minutes, until they're soft and caramelized.

ORANGE
This vaunted vitamin C monster has a cadre of critical phytonutrients known to lower blood pressure and contain strong anti-inflammatory properties. Juice is fine, but the real fruit is even better. The secret, though, is that the orange's most powerful healing properties are found in the peel; use a zester to grate the peel over bowls of yogurt, salads, or directly into smoothies.

CANTALOUPE
The surge of vitamin A is important not just for your eyes, but also for healthy lungs, and the megadose of vitamin C helps white blood cells ward off infection. Sliced cantaloupe and yogurt make a killer breakfast, or combine the two in a food processor with a touch of honey and lemon, and puree into a soup. It makes a great low-cal dessert.

SWEET POTATO
The best thing about sweet potatoes, outside of the beta-carotene, is that they're loaded with fiber. That means they have a gentler effect on your kid's blood sugar levels than regular potatoes do. Substitute baked sweet potatoes for baked potatoes, mash them up like you would an Idaho, or make fries out of them by tossing spears with olive oil and roasting in a 400°F oven for 30 minutes.

CARROT
The snack of choice for Bugs Bunny happens to be the richest carotene source of all. Raw baby carrots are perfect for dipping or snacking on, of course, but also try shredding carrots into a salad or marinara for a hint of natural sweetness, or roasting them slowly in the oven with olive oil and salt.

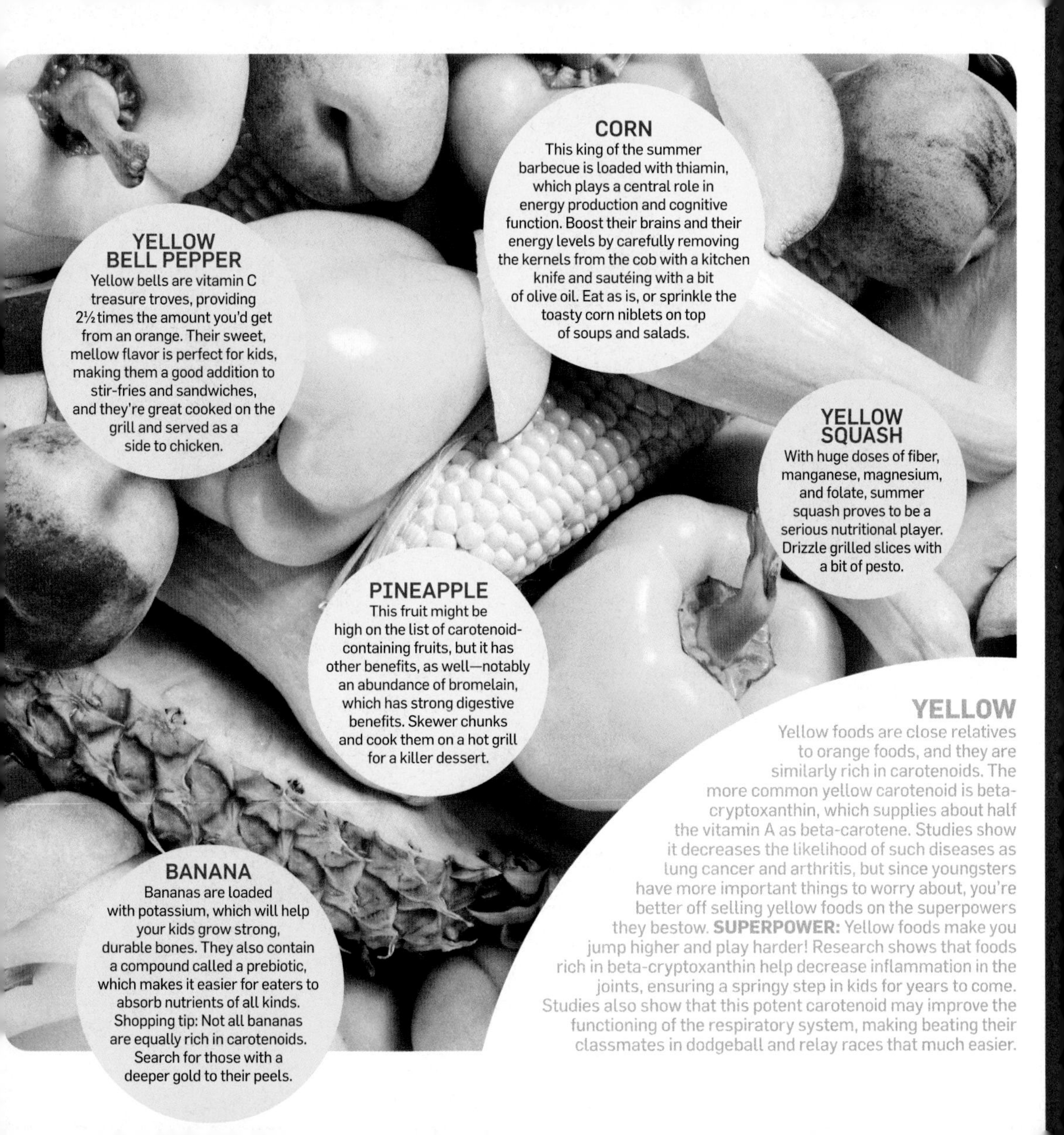

CORN

This king of the summer barbecue is loaded with thiamin, which plays a central role in energy production and cognitive function. Boost their brains and their energy levels by carefully removing the kernels from the cob with a kitchen knife and sautéing with a bit of olive oil. Eat as is, or sprinkle the toasty corn niblets on top of soups and salads.

YELLOW BELL PEPPER

Yellow bells are vitamin C treasure troves, providing 2½ times the amount you'd get from an orange. Their sweet, mellow flavor is perfect for kids, making them a good addition to stir-fries and sandwiches, and they're great cooked on the grill and served as a side to chicken.

YELLOW SQUASH

With huge doses of fiber, manganese, magnesium, and folate, summer squash proves to be a serious nutritional player. Drizzle grilled slices with a bit of pesto.

PINEAPPLE

This fruit might be high on the list of carotenoid-containing fruits, but it has other benefits, as well—notably an abundance of bromelain, which has strong digestive benefits. Skewer chunks and cook them on a hot grill for a killer dessert.

BANANA

Bananas are loaded with potassium, which will help your kids grow strong, durable bones. They also contain a compound called a prebiotic, which makes it easier for eaters to absorb nutrients of all kinds. Shopping tip: Not all bananas are equally rich in carotenoids. Search for those with a deeper gold to their peels.

YELLOW

Yellow foods are close relatives to orange foods, and they are similarly rich in carotenoids. The more common yellow carotenoid is beta-cryptoxanthin, which supplies about half the vitamin A as beta-carotene. Studies show it decreases the likelihood of such diseases as lung cancer and arthritis, but since youngsters have more important things to worry about, you're better off selling yellow foods on the superpowers they bestow. **SUPERPOWER:** Yellow foods make you jump higher and play harder! Research shows that foods rich in beta-cryptoxanthin help decrease inflammation in the joints, ensuring a springy step in kids for years to come. Studies also show that this potent carotenoid may improve the functioning of the respiratory system, making beating their classmates in dodgeball and relay races that much easier.

GREEN Not just potent vitamin vessels capable of strengthening bones, muscles, and brains, green foods are also among the most abundant sources of lutein and zeaxanthin, an antioxidant tag team that, among other things, promotes healthy vision.

SUPERPOWER: Green foods give you sharp vision and superhuman healing abilities! Beyond the peeper protection kids get from lutein and zeaxanthin, green fruits and vegetables get their color from chlorophyll, which studies show plays an important role in stimulating the growth of new tissue and hindering the growth of bacteria. As a topical treatment, it can speed healing time by 25 percent.

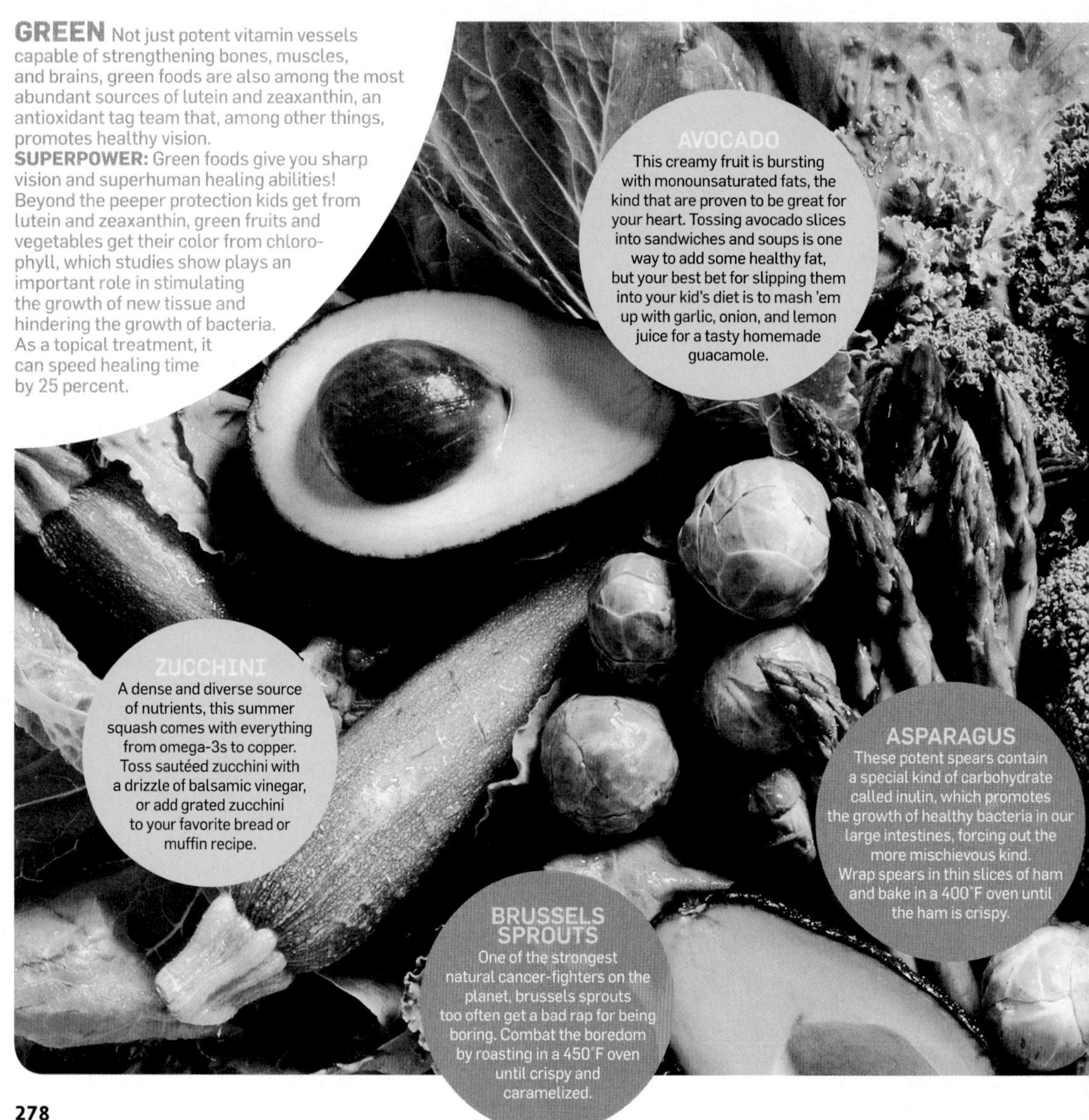

AVOCADO
This creamy fruit is bursting with monounsaturated fats, the kind that are proven to be great for your heart. Tossing avocado slices into sandwiches and soups is one way to add some healthy fat, but your best bet for slipping them into your kid's diet is to mash 'em up with garlic, onion, and lemon juice for a tasty homemade guacamole.

ZUCCHINI
A dense and diverse source of nutrients, this summer squash comes with everything from omega-3s to copper. Toss sautéed zucchini with a drizzle of balsamic vinegar, or add grated zucchini to your favorite bread or muffin recipe.

ASPARAGUS
These potent spears contain a special kind of carbohydrate called inulin, which promotes the growth of healthy bacteria in our large intestines, forcing out the more mischievous kind. Wrap spears in thin slices of ham and bake in a 400°F oven until the ham is crispy.

BRUSSELS SPROUTS
One of the strongest natural cancer-fighters on the planet, brussels sprouts too often get a bad rap for being boring. Combat the boredom by roasting in a 450°F oven until crispy and caramelized.

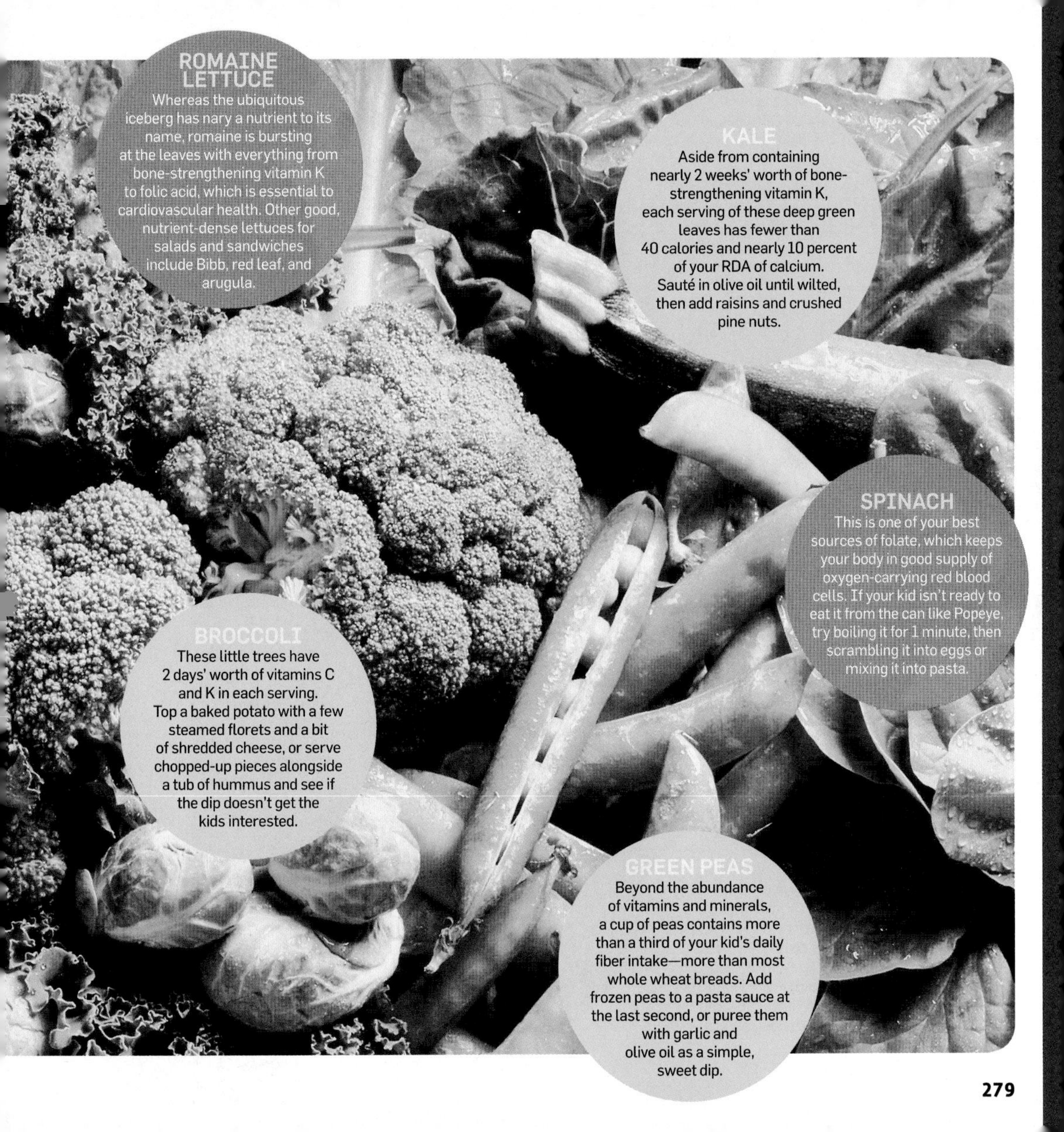
ROMAINE LETTUCE
Whereas the ubiquitous iceberg has nary a nutrient to its name, romaine is bursting at the leaves with everything from bone-strengthening vitamin K to folic acid, which is essential to cardiovascular health. Other good, nutrient-dense lettuces for salads and sandwiches include Bibb, red leaf, and arugula.
KALE
Aside from containing nearly 2 weeks' worth of bone-strengthening vitamin K, each serving of these deep green leaves has fewer than 40 calories and nearly 10 percent of your RDA of calcium. Sauté in olive oil until wilted, then add raisins and crushed pine nuts.
SPINACH
This is one of your best sources of folate, which keeps your body in good supply of oxygen-carrying red blood cells. If your kid isn't ready to eat it from the can like Popeye, try boiling it for 1 minute, then scrambling it into eggs or mixing it into pasta.
BROCCOLI
These little trees have 2 days' worth of vitamins C and K in each serving. Top a baked potato with a few steamed florets and a bit of shredded cheese, or serve chopped-up pieces alongside a tub of hummus and see if the dip doesn't get the kids interested.
GREEN PEAS
Beyond the abundance of vitamins and minerals, a cup of peas contains more than a third of your kid's daily fiber intake—more than most whole wheat breads. Add frozen peas to a pasta sauce at the last second, or puree them with garlic and olive oil as a simple, sweet dip.

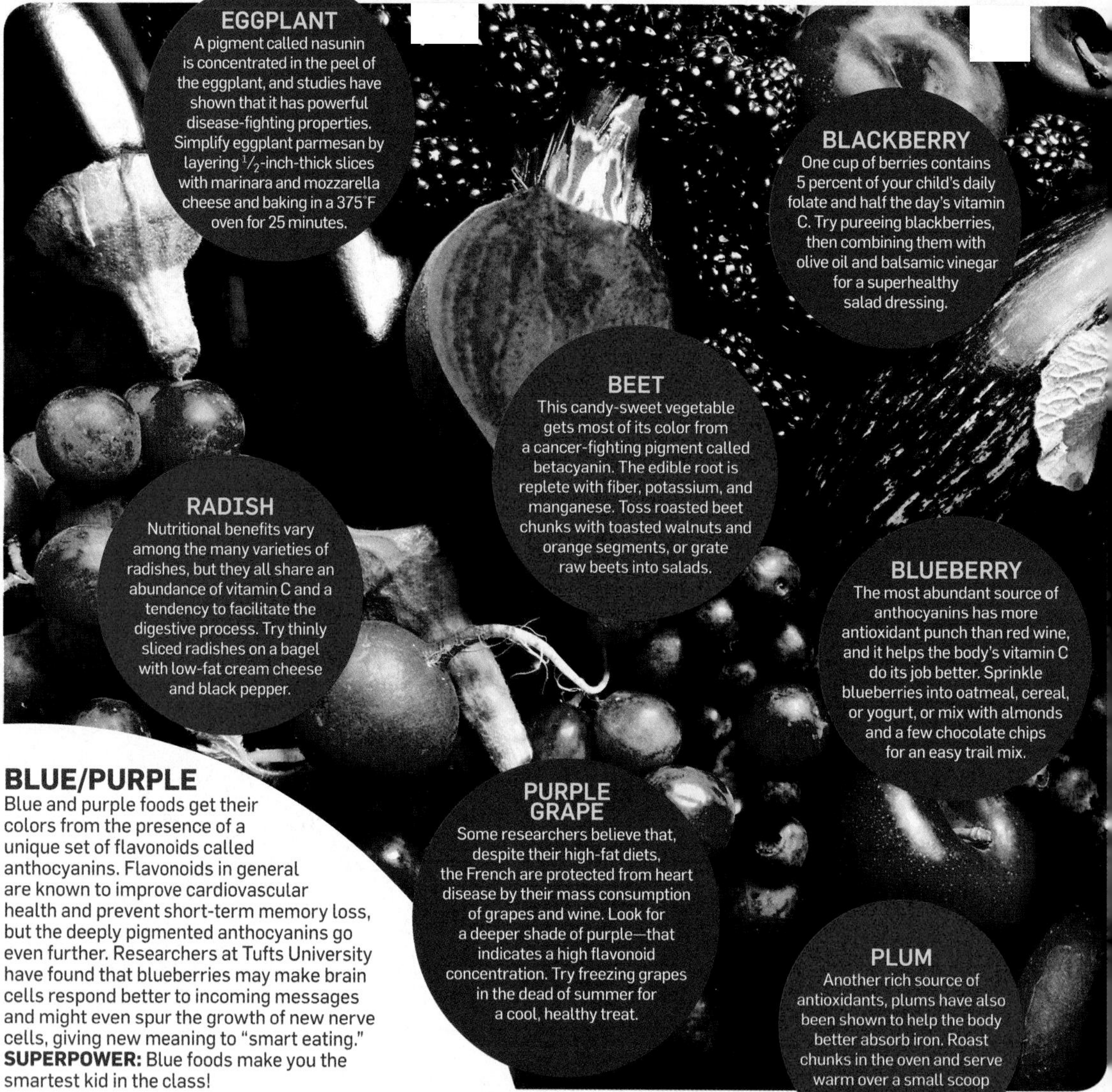

EGGPLANT
A pigment called nasunin is concentrated in the peel of the eggplant, and studies have shown that it has powerful disease-fighting properties. Simplify eggplant parmesan by layering ½-inch-thick slices with marinara and mozzarella cheese and baking in a 375°F oven for 25 minutes.

BLACKBERRY
One cup of berries contains 5 percent of your child's daily folate and half the day's vitamin C. Try pureeing blackberries, then combining them with olive oil and balsamic vinegar for a superhealthy salad dressing.

BEET
This candy-sweet vegetable gets most of its color from a cancer-fighting pigment called betacyanin. The edible root is replete with fiber, potassium, and manganese. Toss roasted beet chunks with toasted walnuts and orange segments, or grate raw beets into salads.

RADISH
Nutritional benefits vary among the many varieties of radishes, but they all share an abundance of vitamin C and a tendency to facilitate the digestive process. Try thinly sliced radishes on a bagel with low-fat cream cheese and black pepper.

BLUEBERRY
The most abundant source of anthocyanins has more antioxidant punch than red wine, and it helps the body's vitamin C do its job better. Sprinkle blueberries into oatmeal, cereal, or yogurt, or mix with almonds and a few chocolate chips for an easy trail mix.

BLUE/PURPLE
Blue and purple foods get their colors from the presence of a unique set of flavonoids called anthocyanins. Flavonoids in general are known to improve cardiovascular health and prevent short-term memory loss, but the deeply pigmented anthocyanins go even further. Researchers at Tufts University have found that blueberries may make brain cells respond better to incoming messages and might even spur the growth of new nerve cells, giving new meaning to "smart eating." **SUPERPOWER:** Blue foods make you the smartest kid in the class!

PURPLE GRAPE
Some researchers believe that, despite their high-fat diets, the French are protected from heart disease by their mass consumption of grapes and wine. Look for a deeper shade of purple—that indicates a high flavonoid concentration. Try freezing grapes in the dead of summer for a cool, healthy treat.

PLUM
Another rich source of antioxidants, plums have also been shown to help the body better absorb iron. Roast chunks in the oven and serve warm over a small scoop of vanilla ice cream.

Kids' Restaurant Report Card

Just as your kids are tested every day on state capitals and basic arithmetic, restaurants need to be closely examined based on the fare they serve to our future doctors, lawyers, and multimedia mavens. After all, the difference between one restaurant's chicken finger meal and another's can be 500 calories and 30 grams of fat or more. And over the course of adolescence, those differences add up in a big way. That's why we've put 21 major chain restaurants—the titans of the food industry—under the spotlight, picking apart the details of their Happy Meals and not-so-happy meals, in order to help you make better decisions about where and what your family should eat next time you venture out in search of sustenance. Do your kids' favorite restaurants make the grade?

APPLEBEE'S

F Applebee's is one of a handful of restaurant-industry titans that refuses to give up the goods on their nutritional information. Until they tell diners what they're putting in their bodies, we'll be forced to fail them.

SURVIVAL STRATEGY

Two Mini Cheeseburgers, fries, and a soft drink add up to a shocking 1,425 calories, making it one of the worst kids' meals in America. The better bet is to pair a hot dog or a grilled chicken sandwich with applesauce and milk, juice, or water.

BASKIN-ROBBINS

C- It's hard to serve just ice cream and still make the grade, but Baskin-Robbins does nothing to help its case. It serves up some of the fattiest scoops in the industry, plus 900-calorie soft serve concoctions, smoothies with more sugar than fruit, and a handful of the worst shakes and sundaes on the planet.

SURVIVAL STRATEGY

Baskin does deserve credit for offering plenty of lighter options, such as sherbets, sorbets, and low-sugar ice creams; each of these lines offers ample opportunity to feel indulgent without really being so.

BURGER KING

C- The standard kids' fare—hamburger, cheeseburger, chicken tenders—is no better or worse here than it is at most fast-food joints. But BK still clings to the use of trans fat, despite the pledge to follow the lead of other chain restaurant and remove it from the menu by the end of 2008.

SURVIVAL STRATEGY

Burger King deserves credit for one of the finest inventions of the 21st century: apple fries, the ultimate healthy decoy for deep-fried potatoes. Pair them with a 4-piece Chicken Tenders and water or milk for an impressive kids' meal.

CHILI'S

C- Chili's gets the award for the longest, most diverse kids' menu we've seen, and many of the items on it represent reasonable nutritional options. Unfortunately, sodium is a major problem. And the adult menu, where older kids might be tempted to wander, is nothing but trouble.

SURVIVAL STRATEGY

Choose wisely, as the difference between good (corn dog) and bad (chicken strips) can be 700 calories once sides are factored in. On the adult menu, the Chicken Fajita Pita is the best choice.

DOMINO'S PIZZA

C+ Domino's suffers the same pitfalls as any other pizza purveyor: too much cheese, bread, and greasy toppings. If you don't know the pitfalls, you might bag your child a pizza with more than 350 calories per slice. To its credit, Domino's does keep the trans fat off the pizza, and it also offers the lowest-calorie thin crust option out there.

SURVIVAL STRATEGY

Stick with the Crunchy Thin Crust pizzas sans sausage and pepperoni. Whenever possible, try to sneak a vegetable or two onto each pie.

DUNKIN' DONUTS

C After years as a major trans-fat transgressor, Dunkin' has cleaned up its act and cut it almost entirely from the menu. They've also shown encouraging signs of health-consciousness with their new lines of flatbread sandwiches. Unfortunately, between deleterious donuts and bloated bagels, the majority of the menu is still pure waistline-expanding rubbish.

SURVIVAL STRATEGY

Go for sandwiches made on English muffins for breakfast and flatbread sandwiches (preferably the Ham and Swiss) at all other times. If the kids really want a doughnut, limit them to one, and make it a raised doughnut instead of a cake doughnut.

IHOP

F IHOP refuses to serve up nutritional information, but thanks to the New York City Board of Health, they were forced to publish calorie counts on their menus in April 2008. The big reveal shocked New York diners: 1,700-calorie cheeseburgers and salads with more than 1,000 calories. For the kids, trouble comes in the form of the 790-calorie Cheese Omelette and the 620-calorie Grilled Cheese Sandwich.

SURVIVAL STRATEGY

Write letters, make phone calls, beg, scream, and plead for IHOP to provide nutritional information on all of their products. While those complaints are being processed, know that the best breakfast option for kids is the Funny Face pancake at 420 calories and the best option the rest of the day is the Crispy Chicken Strips at 510 calories.

KFC

B- For a place with the word "fried" in its acronymic title, KFC manages to downplay the damage of their namesake goods by offering low-calorie Snacker sandwiches and a variety of relatively healthy vegetable sides. The new line of grilled chicken is a good sign that the Colonel is willing to step away from the fryer.

SURVIVAL STRATEGY

Skip over the fried chicken—unless your family likes it skinless, in which case, have at it—and look instead to the Snackers, the Crispy Strips, and the grilled chicken. Don't miss the opportunity to sneak a serving or two of vegetables into your kid's diet, assuming those veggies don't come out of the fryer.

MCDONALD'S

B Though not blessed with an abundance of healthy options for kids, Mickey D's isn't burdened with any major calorie bombs, either. Kid standards like McNuggets and cheeseburgers both come in right around the 300-calorie mark.

SURVIVAL STRATEGY

Apple Dippers and 2 percent milk with a small entrée make for a pretty decent meal. McDonald's quintessential Happy Meal makes this possible—just beware the usual French fries and soda pitfalls.

OLIVE GARDEN

C We're happy to see Olive Garden finally offer up full nutritional info on their menu items. We're not so happy to see, however, that the pasta purveyor is serving up 800-calorie portions of fettuccine Alfredo to young eaters.

SURVIVAL STRATEGY

The kids' menu is short and straightforward, which makes finding the high points and avoiding the caloric potholes that much easier. Skip the Alfredo, the Cheese Pizza, and anything with a 400-calorie serving of fries. The 250-calorie plate of spaghetti and the grilled chicken and pasta both make fine meals.

OUTBACK STEAKHOUSE

F For years we've pestered Outback to provide us with nutritional information. A spokesperson once told us: "Ninety percent of our meals are prepared by hand. Any analysis would be difficult to measure consistently." Yet no fewer than 50 national chain restaurants do just that.

SURVIVAL STRATEGY

The 410-calorie Joey Sirloin, the 390-calorie Grilled Cheese-A-Roo, and the 240-calorie Grilled Chicken on the Barbie all make great meals, as long as you pair them with smart sides (i.e., the baked potato or the veggies).

PAPA JOHN'S

C Pizza joints suffer the curse of bad report cards because of their thick crusts, fat-speckled meats, and blankets of cheese. That said, Papa John's does have a few advantages over the competition: the absence of trans fat, the assortment of nonsoda beverage options, and the first whole wheat crust offered by a big US pizza chain.

SURVIVAL STRATEGY

Order Chicken Strips with Pizza Sauce to blunt the family's collective hunger. Follow with a slice of thin or wheat crust cheese or Spinach Alfredo pizza. Whatever you do, be sure to avoid Papa's pan crust like it's the plague.

PIZZA HUT

D+ Expect no surprises from this quintessential pizza parlor. The chain offers no kid-friendly beverage or side options, and with nothing else to choose from, a couple of breadsticks and a soda tack hundreds of calories onto a pizza dinner. A thin-crust delivery can be a lifesaver in a pinch, but as for truly nourishing options, you won't find many here.

SURVIVAL STRATEGY

First off, nix the pepperoni. If the kids want meat, stick to ham and chicken, but try to add veggies whenever possible. The best possible scenario? Fit 'N Delicious Pizzas. Any of them.

QUIZNOS

C+ Toasty or not, Quiznos offers some of America's worst sandwiches, including the 1,760-calorie large Tuna Melt. Cookies and fatty salads don't make matters any better. What does improve matters is the line of kid-size Sammies—the rare bright spot on an otherwise dark menu.

SURVIVAL STRATEGY

With a handful of Sammies at 200 calories each, they make perfect meals for younger kids. You can double up for the older eaters—even two of the healthier Sammies will be better than many small sandwiches.

RED LOBSTER

B+ Red Lobster boasts one of America's healthiest adult menus, and some of that magic rubs off on their kids' offerings: Broiled fish, crab legs, and even popcorn shrimp all make good picks, as do a few of the eight side options. Still, the ever-appealing chicken fingers and fries together pack 744 calories and more than 2,000 milligrams of sodium —some choppy seas in an otherwise smooth sail.

SURVIVAL STRATEGY

The biggest battle here is fought on the sides front. Broccoli, salad, and a baked potato are all strong options; the fries, Caesar, and Cheddar Bay Biscuit, not so much. Match one of the former options with grilled chicken or any of the seafood choices for a great meal.

RUBY TUESDAY

D One of the worst kids' menus we've seen, with only a single dish containing fewer than 400 calories: the 217-calorie chicken breast. Beyond that safe zone lies a dangerous milieu of high-cal pastas, fat-strewn fried fare, and "mini" burgers with more calories than Wendy's infamous Baconator.

SURVIVAL STRATEGY

Pair the Chicken Breast or the Chop Steak with a fresh vegetable side and there is hope for a happy, healthy dinner. If not, your kid could very well end up consuming half her day's calories in one sitting.

STARBUCKS

C- As any caffeine-addicted parent knows, there are few options for kids at a coffee shop. Starbucks is no exception. Whether due to an excess of sugar or a surge of caffeine (or both), nearly every drink here will have your kid treating your furniture like a trampoline. The food isn't much better, though Starbucks has started to show real signs of improvement in the edibles department.

SURVIVAL STRATEGY

Try giving your kid one of the fiber-rich, fruit-based Vivanno smoothies—he'll think he's getting a reward for good behavior. As for food, skip the baked goods in favor of Perfect Oatmeal or a hot breakfast wrap.

SUBWAY

A- A menu based on lean protein and vegetables is always going to score well in our book. With more than half a dozen kid-friendly sandwiches less than 300 calories, plus a slew of soups and healthy sides to boot, Subway can satisfy even the pickiest eater without breaking the caloric bank. But despite what Jared may want you to believe, Subway is not nutritionally infallible: Most of those rosy calorie counts posted on the menu boards include neither cheese nor mayo (add 160 calories per 6-inch sub), and some of the toasted subs, like the Meatball Marinara, contain hefty doses of calories, saturated fat, and sodium.

SURVIVAL STRATEGY

Cornell researchers have discovered a "health halo" at Subway—this refers to the tendency to reward yourself or your kid with chips, cookies, and large soft drinks because your entrée is healthy. Avoid the halo, and all will be well.

T.G.I. FRIDAY'S

F We applaud Friday's efforts to offer smaller portion sizes for high-calorie dishes, but we don't approve of their reluctance to provide hard nutritional data on any of their dishes. Between the array of deep-fried starters and mammoth sandwiches, it's clear they have something to hide.

SURVIVAL STRATEGY

Our research has found that nearly every kids' menu option flirts with the 1,000-calorie barrier. The best option, surprisingly enough, is the Mac & Cheese. Still, your child would be better off ordering the 480-calorie Dragonfire Chicken or the 400-calorie Shrimp Key West from the adult menu.

TACO BELL

C Diners live and die by the mix-and-match opportunities Taco Bell presents, where any two items can either be a reasonable 400-calorie meal or a 900-calorie saturated fat and sodium fest.

SURVIVAL STRATEGY

Cut out the big-ticket items like Mexican Pizzas and Nachos, and direct your kid's attention to the crunchy tacos, bean burritos, and anything on the Fresco menu.

WENDY'S

A- Wendy's official kids' menu may be a tiny concession to little eaters, but it is free of the belly-busters that hamper most menus. Plus, the rest of the menu offers ample options for a growing kid; a cup of chili and a baked potato, chicken salad, or even a burger with a cup of mandarin oranges all qualify as nutritionally commendable meals.

SURVIVAL STRATEGY

The Super Value Menu is full of solid choices, as long as you avoid the 480-calorie add-on of fries and a regular soft drink.

Burger King

Eat This

Chicken Tender

(6 piece) with Barbecue Dipping Sauce and Apple Fries with Caramel Sauce

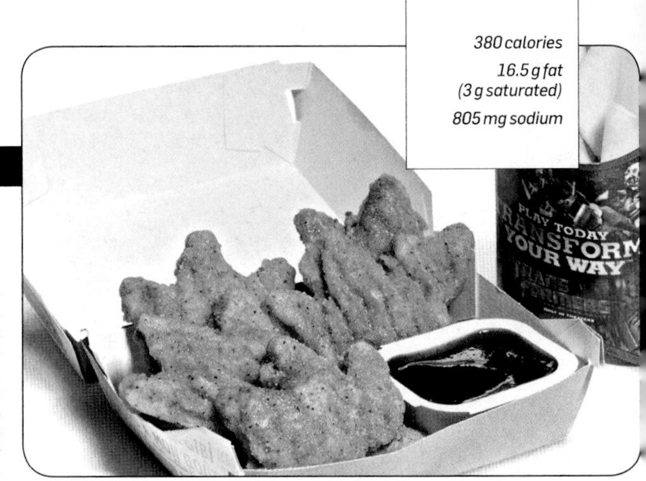

380 calories
16.5 g fat (3 g saturated)
805 mg sodium

At just 63 calories a piece, these rank among the best nuggets/tenders/fingers in the fast-food world. Add to that the genius product that is Apple Fries and you have a pretty sound kid's meal.

Dunkin' Donuts

Eat This

Glazed Chocolate Cake Munchkins

(4)

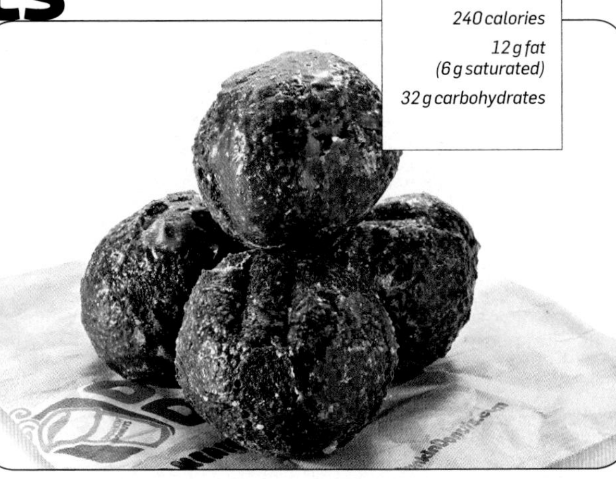

240 calories
12 g fat (6 g saturated)
32 g carbohydrates

No, this is not a typo. A pile of chocolate doughnut holes is better for you than a bagel with light cream cheese in almost every major nutritional category. Still, don't let your kids make a habit of it, since they are really just a glorified dessert.

680 calories

33 g fat (10.5 g saturated, 0.5 g trans)

1,360 mg sodium

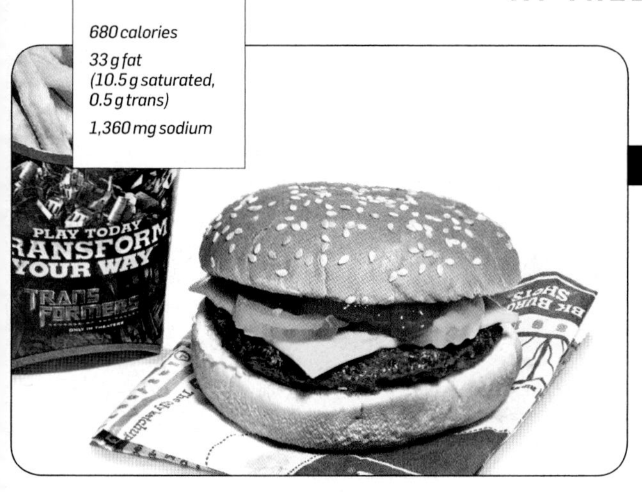

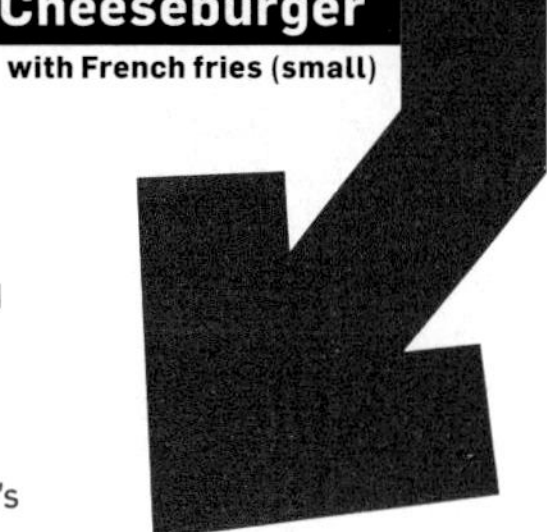

Not That!

Cheeseburger

with French fries (small)

The cheeseburger, with 340 calories and 7 grams of saturated fat, gets trounced by the tenders, while the small French fries double the meal's caloric load without adding any real nutrition to the equation.

---

430 calories

11 g fat (5.5 g saturated)

76 g carbohydrates

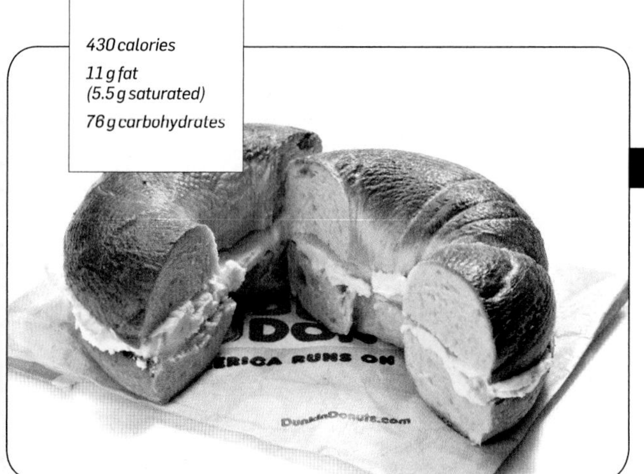

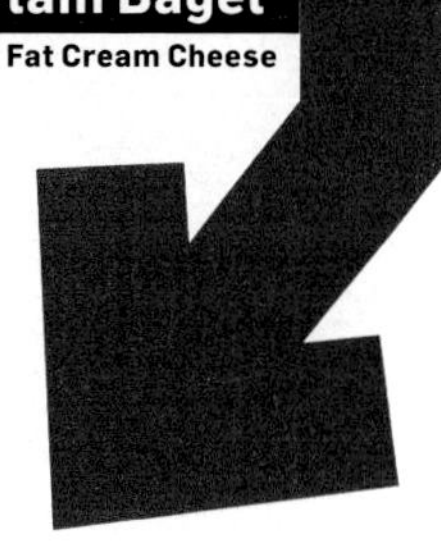

Not That!

Plain Bagel

with Reduced Fat Cream Cheese

The reduced fat cream cheese will save you 50 calories over the regular stuff, but it won't cut any of the refined carbs—and those are to blame for the high calorie count and the denigrated reputation of the bagel in this book series.

KFC

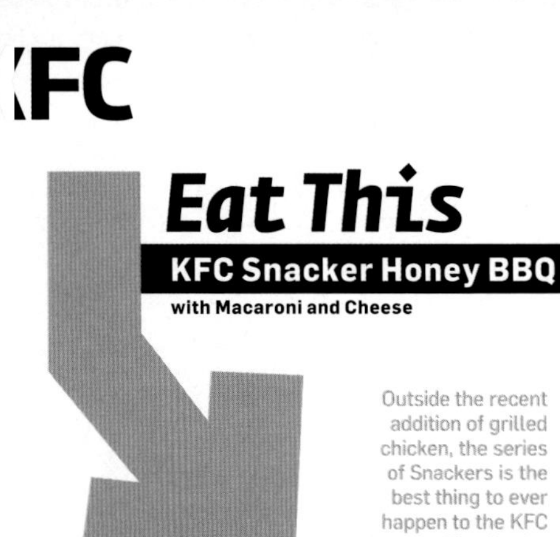

Eat This

KFC Snacker Honey BBQ

with Macaroni and Cheese

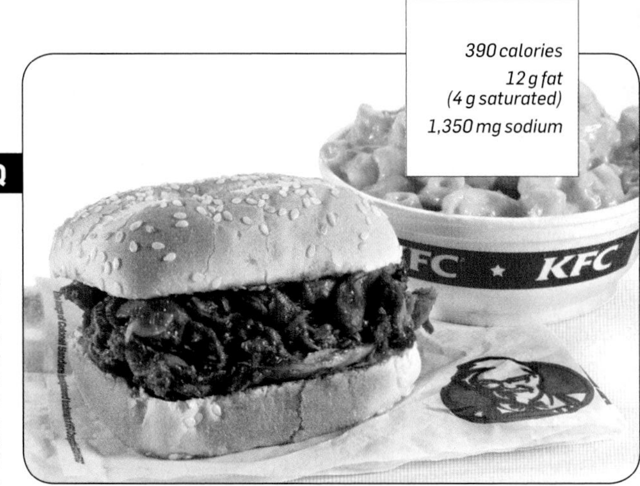

390 calories
12 g fat
(4 g saturated)
1,350 mg sodium

Outside the recent addition of grilled chicken, the series of Snackers is the best thing to ever happen to the KFC menu. They're the perfect size for a kid, and the Honey BBQ (the best of them all) has just 210 calories.

McDonald's

Eat This

Happy Meal:

Chicken McNuggets (4 piece), Apple Dippers with Caramel Sauce, and 1% Low-Fat White Milk Jug

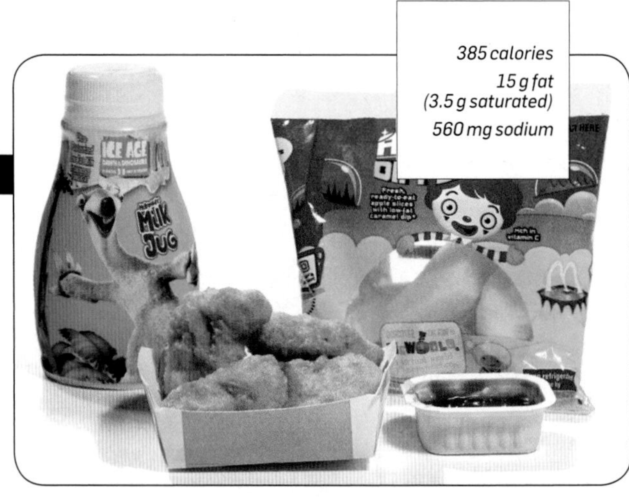

385 calories
15 g fat
(3.5 g saturated)
560 mg sodium

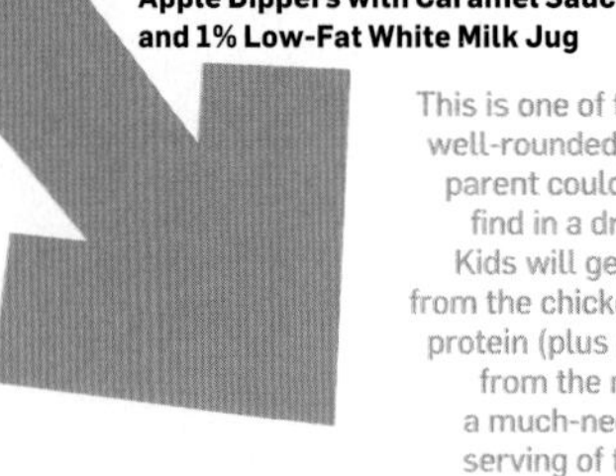

This is one of the most well-rounded meals a parent could hope to find in a drive-thru. Kids will get protein from the chicken, more protein (plus calcium) from the milk, and a much-needed full serving of fruit with the beloved dippers.

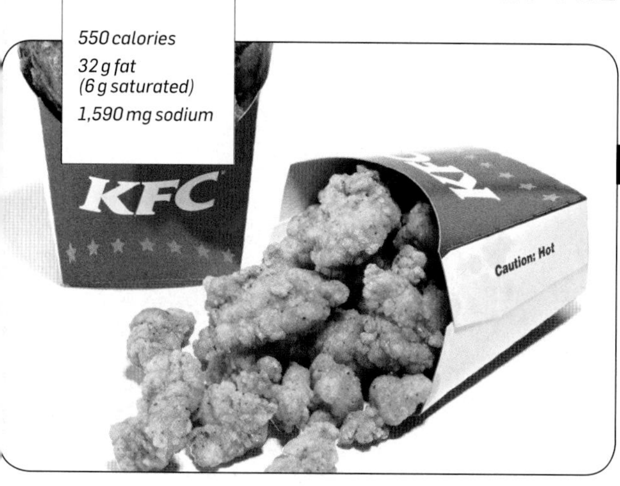

550 calories

32 g fat (6 g saturated)

1,590 mg sodium

Not That!

Kids Popcorn Chicken

with Potato Wedges

If your kid really wants fried chicken at KFC, let her order the Crispy Strips. Two substantial fingers run 250 calories. As for potato products, swap in the mashed taters with gravy for the wedges and save 130 calories.

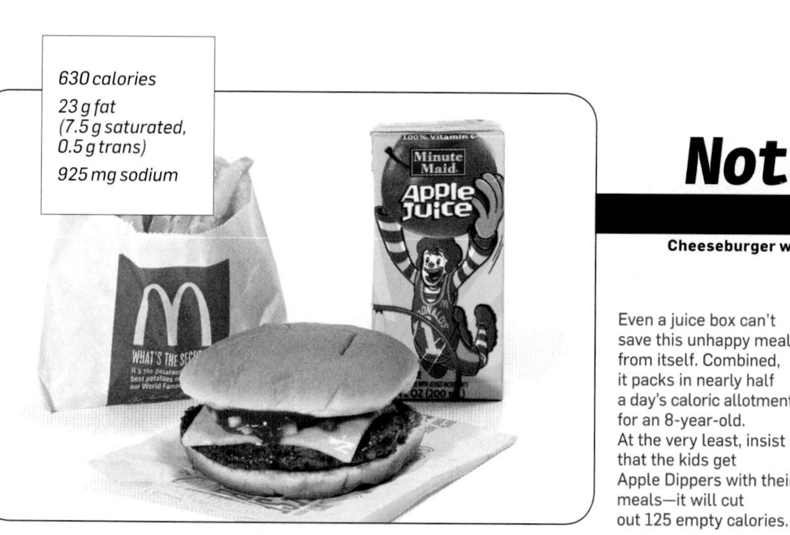

630 calories

23 g fat (7.5 g saturated, 0.5 g trans)

925 mg sodium

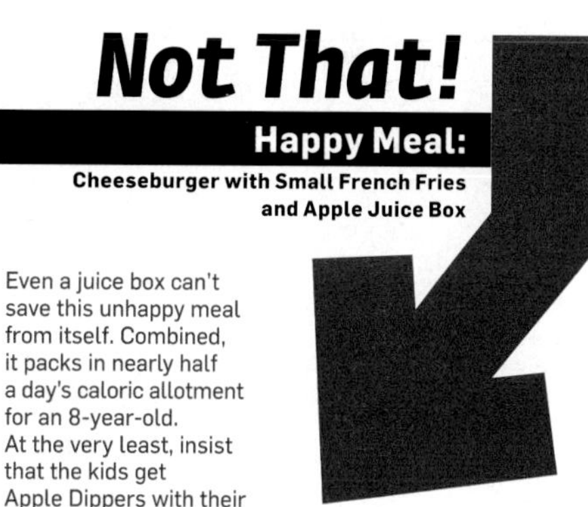

Not That!

Happy Meal:

Cheeseburger with Small French Fries and Apple Juice Box

Even a juice box can't save this unhappy meal from itself. Combined, it packs in nearly half a day's caloric allotment for an 8-year-old. At the very least, insist that the kids get Apple Dippers with their meals—it will cut out 125 empty calories.

Subway

Eat This

Turkey Breast and Swiss Cheese

(6", with lettuce, tomatoes, and onions)

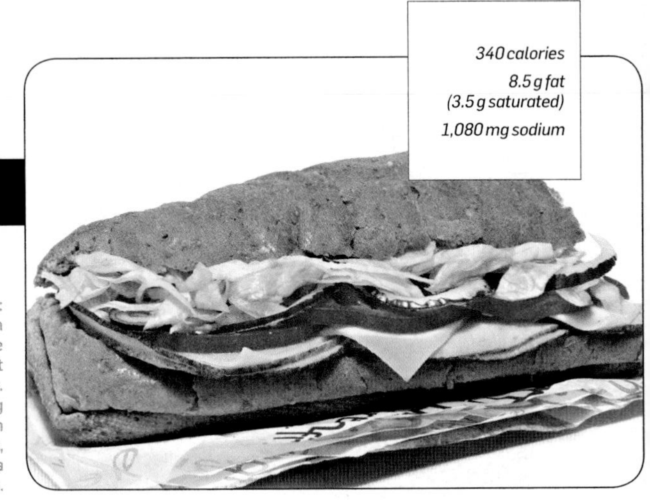

340 calories
8.5 g fat
(3.5 g saturated)
1,080 mg sodium

Turkey and swiss: a classic combination that proves to be the blueprint for a great kids' meal at Subway. It has everything your kid needs: lean protein, fresh produce, calcium, and a bit of cheesy incentive.

Taco Bell

Eat This

Crunchy Fresco Tacos

(2)

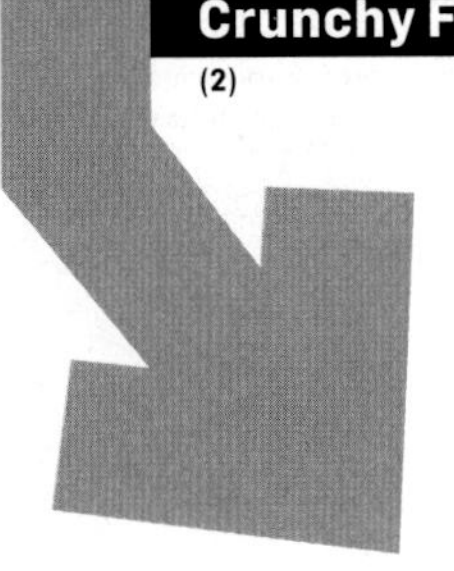

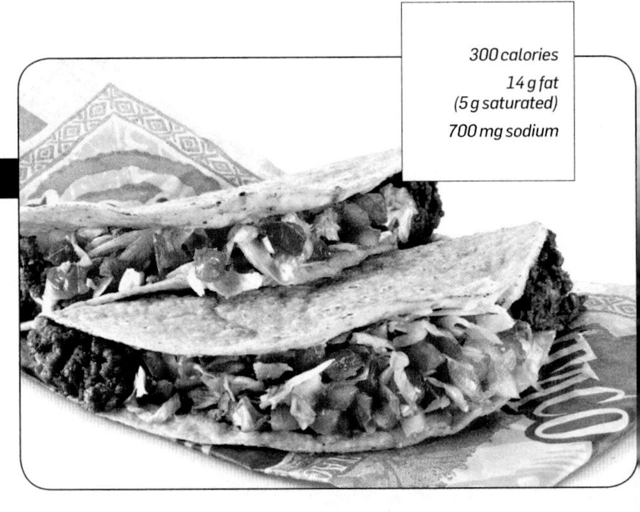

300 calories
14 g fat
(5 g saturated)
700 mg sodium

Kids love crunchy stuff and parents love fresh produce, and these tacos satisfy both affections. If you can get your kids to take Fresco treatment, then Taco Bell ranks among the best eateries for the younger set.

680 calories
22 g fat
(9 g saturated)
1,070 mg sodium

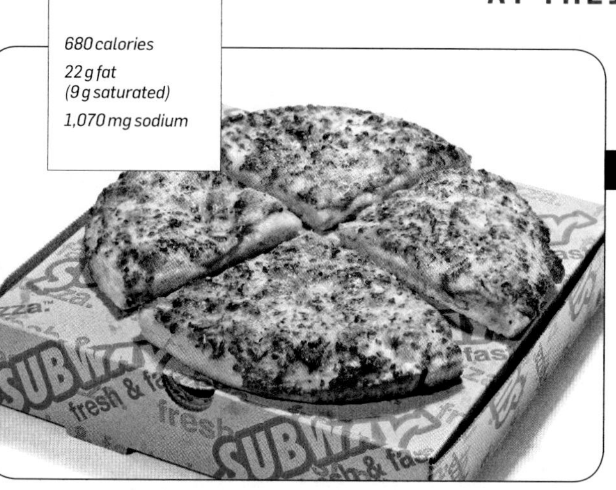

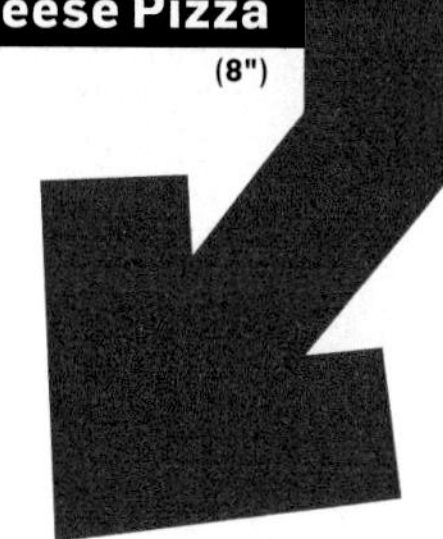

Not That!

Individual Cheese Pizza

(8")

Let's hope this new addition to the Subway menu becomes discontinued soon. In the meantime, don't let your kids fall for the allure of pizza in a sub shop. This pie packs more calories and fat than most footlong sandwiches.

470 calories
26 g fat
(11 g saturated, 0.5 g trans)
1,170 mg sodium

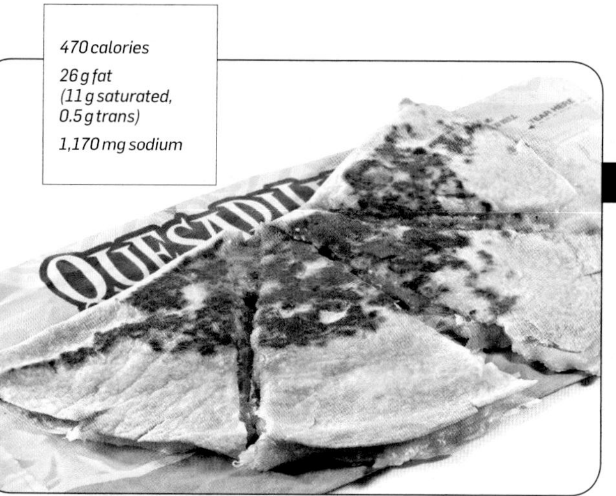

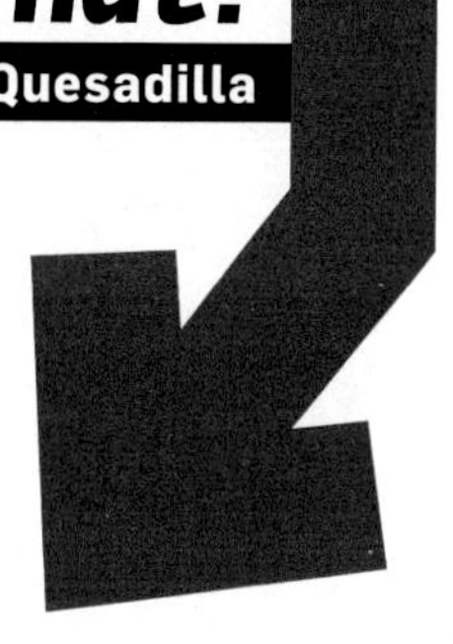

Not That!

Cheese Quesadilla

The quesadilla is Mexico's answer to the grilled cheese sandwich, and this one at the Bell delivers more than half a day's worth of saturated fat and sodium between the toasty tortillas.

Eat This, Not That!

ON A BUDGET

7

Waiting for some good news that finally scratches off the tarry black outlook of the economy and reveals a shiny silver lining beneath? We've got it for you.

The last 12 months have been a challenge—both in the United States and around the world—thanks to what appears to be a small group of balding men in suits and ties with private jets and mysterious jobs and the magic power to make everyone else's money instantly disappear.

How do they do that?

Well, we're still working on an answer to that one. We're not quite sure what happened to the other half of our 401(k), except that it had something to do with things called credit-default swaps, subprime loans, and the Glass-Steagall Act, which only the very smart guys who lost all the money in the first place supposedly comprehend. (And we thought understanding "high-fructose corn syrup" was a challenge.) But we do know that when the economy gets tough, the tough do one smart thing: They cook at home.

And there's the silver lining.

You see, the power to control your weight and your health comes down to the power to control the foods you feed into your body.

Once you hop into the car and head to your local eatery—whether it's the eggs-and-bacon diner you've been going to for 20 years or the hot new hipster joint that sells "microbrews" instead of beer—you've given up control over what's in your food and handed that control over to a bunch of folks who have less invested in your health and well-being than you do.

Sure, you can special order, you can parse the menu for the best choices, and you can quiz the waiter about what, exactly, is in the blue plate special. But you don't really know what's happening back there behind the kitchen doors, where the sizzling sound could be caused by freshly picked vegetables caressing heart-healthy canola oil or by frozen nuggets taking a bath in the deep fryer.

So cooking at home is not only a smart way to cut down on waste but also a smart way to stop adding to your waist.

That said, the grocery bill is always an ugly thing to look at. And over the last 2 years, prices of foods like vegetables, meat, fruit, and other high-nutrition, low-calorie treats have skyrocketed. A combination of unstable oil prices, bad weather, and a growing world population has made eating healthy more expensive.

But eating in an unhealthy way? Oh, that's still plenty cheap. In fact, junk food prices have actually decreased slightly over the past few years, which is why in many stores you can buy a couple of Twinkies for less than the cost of a single apple. Researchers at the University of Washington recently estimated the cost of a diet based on high-calorie foods versus one based on healthy, low-calorie foods. The high-calorie diet you could eat for $3.52 a day. The low-cal diet? A whopping $36.32 per diem.

Now, that sounds pretty bad. But remember, people in the United States still spend a smaller percentage of their incomes on food than almost any other people on earth—just under 10 percent. And shopping at the grocery store—and making our own food at home—gives us a tremendous budgetary advantage. (Want to make an easy $800? Brew your own coffee each day instead of stopping for a latte on your way to work.)

The key to trimming your belly while trimming your bills is to make your kitchen the center of your home and use it to its full advantage. And we show you how to do exactly that in our Save-

Money Shopping Guide in this chapter.

Of course, you're not going to be eating at home every night. Or every morning. Or even most afternoons. And the local diner, fast-food joint, or fancy sit-down restaurant still has its magical allure even when you know you should just pack a PB&J and head out.

Restaurants know this, of course, and they also know that your dollars are tight and the competition for them is rabid. Since McDonald's introduced their dollar menu in the early 2000s, cheap restaurant food has gotten even cheaper. But remember what we said at the top of this chapter: When you eat out, you give up control of what's in your food. So being extra smart about how you approach the menu will make all the difference in keeping your wallet padded—and not the rest of you.

In this chapter, we've taken a hard look at some of the "cheap eats" out there and figured out which of them are good investments and which are just throwing your money away. Put your money in the safe deposit box, turn the lock, and read on.

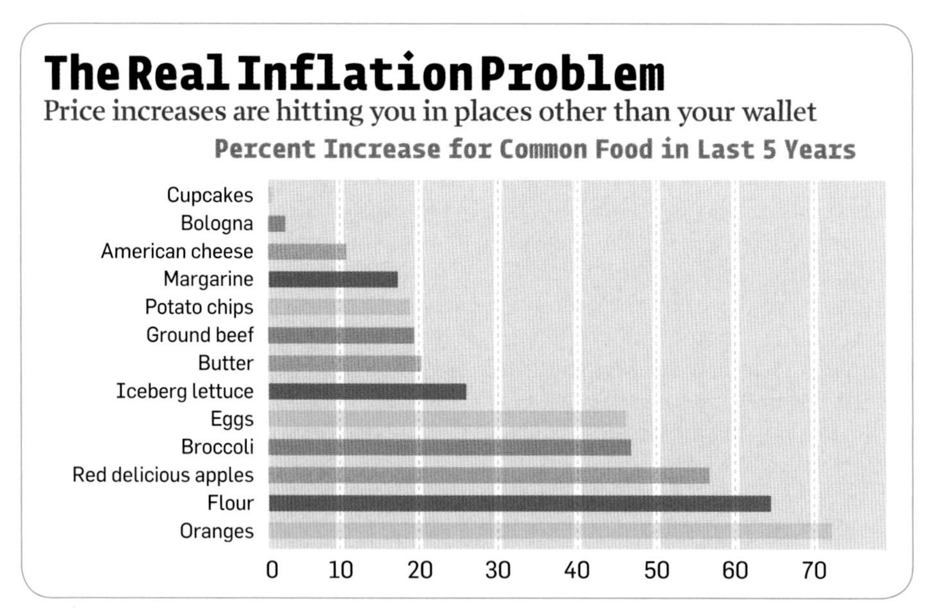

Your Save-Money Shopping Guide

Cut out the empty calories and maximize the quality of your supermarket score with these six rules of savvy shopping.

- **Avoid quickies.** A study published by the Marketing Science Institute found that shoppers who made "quick trips" to the store purchased an average of 54 percent more merchandise than they planned. Instead, be thoughtful in your planning—keep a magnet-based notepad on your fridge and make notes throughout the week about what you need. (And avoiding extra trips will cut down on your gasoline costs as well.)

- **Write the perfect shopping list.** Before you head out, organize your list of needs by grocery-store section: produce, dairy, meat, cleaning products, cosmetics, etc. (Rewrite the list if you need to.) Then bring a pencil and, as you add each item to your cart, tick it off from your list. No loitering, no wandering aimlessly through the store. Try to make each visit a minute or two shorter than the last—you'll find that the more time you save, the more money and calories you save too!

- **Check yourself out.** Maybe those creepy mechanical voices weird you out, or maybe you just like waiting in long lines to chat with retirees. But waiting in line for a checkout person is an invitation to caloric chaos. A study by IHL Group found that when shoppers used the self-checkout line, impulse purchases dropped by more than 16 percent for men—and more than 32 percent for women. (That's good news for your body as well. Eighty percent of candy and 61 percent of salty snacks are bought on impulse.)

- **Make Wednesday grocery night.** According to *Progressive Grocer*, only 11 percent of shoppers go to the store on Wednesdays, and only 4 percent of customers shop on any day after 9 P.M. If your store's open late, it might be the best way to avoid the crowds—

and to avoid the impulse spending that accompanies being stuck in the checkout line.

• **Watch your weight.** Okay, so one brand of crackers costs $4 and the other $4.50. But before you assume which is cheaper, take a closer look at the net weight. You'll often find the more expensive box contains more actual food—and as such, the food is really cheaper. Net weight is also a great way of making sure you're not paying for a lot of packaging, only to get home and discover most of what's inside the box is air.

• **Eat before you shop.** A 2008 study in the *Journal of Consumer Research* found that consumers are likely to spend more if their appetite is revving full throttle before making a purchase. (And it's not just food you'll spend more on. In the study, women who were given a whiff of a chocolate-scented candle were four times as likely to want to shop for a new sweater than those who weren't. Damn you, Auntie Anne's!)

Five Can't-Beat Cheap Eats

Stretch your dollar and shrink your waistline with these prudent picks

FROZEN CHICKEN BREASTS: Lean protein for about half the price of fresh chicken. In our taste tests, where we seasoned and grilled chicken breasts, we found it impossible to tell the difference between fresh and frozen.

CANOLA OIL: Save the pricey olive oil for dressing salads or drizzling over grilled fish. Canola's neutral flavor is great for cooking, and it happens to have a better ratio of monounsaturated to saturated fat than the vaunted extra virgin. Olive oil can cost as much as a dollar per ounce, while canola oil costs about $0.25.

DRY LENTILS: For about the price of a bottle of water, you can boil up a massive pot of soup- and salad-ready lentils. A 1-pound bag has 11 grams of fiber and 10 grams of protein in each of its 13 servings.

SALSA: It's twice as versatile as ketchup. Look to the bottom shelf for store-brand bulk containers and you'll find a half-gallon for less than 6 bucks, a month's supply for about the price of a Chipotle Burrito.

POPCORN: Paper-bag popcorns run about $3.50 for 9 ounces, versus $1.25 a pound for straight kernels. Why pay a premium for grease? Make popcorn the old fashioned way: straight from the jar. Just fill the bottom of a large saucepan with kernels and a touch of oil and cover. After it's popped, season it with herbs, citrus, or chili powder.

Cook Off the Pounds!

Cut calories and save cash with these 10 decadent dishes

The best way to take control of your diet as well as your food finances is to grab a chef's knife and a sauté pan and start cooking. According to studies, people consume 50 percent more calories, fat, and sodium when they eat out than when they cook at home. Add the fact that you're likely to save some serious coin with a bit of savvy shopping and you have a potent case for the power of a little down-home cooking.

In hopes of inspiring you to turn up the heat in your kitchen, we've taken 10 of America's most popular dishes and remade them, with quality nutrition, prudent spending, and maximum gustatory pleasure all considered in equal measure. As you'll see with the calorie comparisons we provide, these also happen to be 10 dishes the restaurant industry has egregiously hijacked and corrupted. To help you take back the food you love most, we built each recipe around some of the finest products in the supermarket, which will allow you to enjoy top-notch eating on a shoestring.

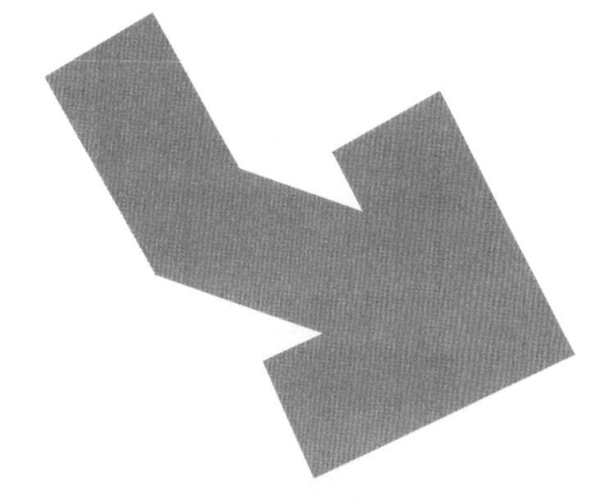

Blueberry Pancakes

Eat This

YOU'LL NEED:

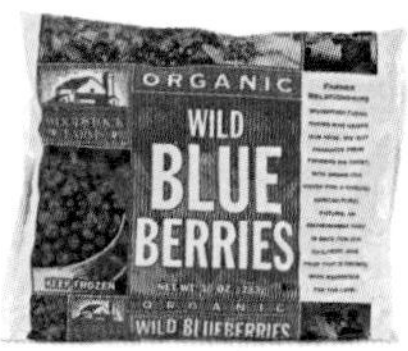

2 cups frozen wild blueberries

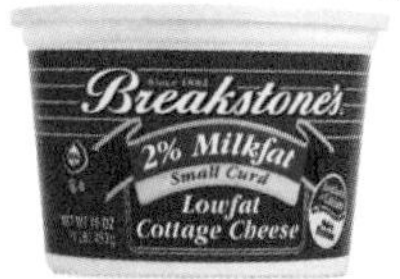

1 cup low-fat cottage cheese or ricotta

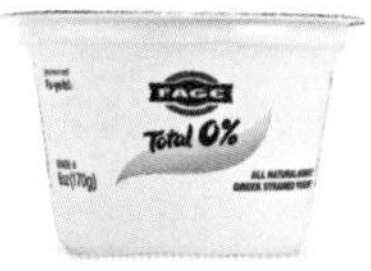

1 cup Fage 0% yogurt

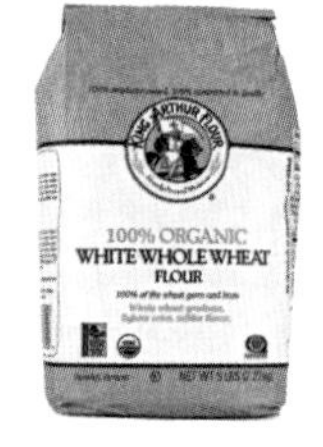

1 cup King Arthur White Whole Wheat Flour

YOU'LL ALSO NEED:

½ cup water
¼ cup sugar
3 eggs
Juice of 1 lemon
½ tsp baking soda
Pinch of salt

The use of yogurt and cheese to make these pancakes does two things: It brings extra protein to the breakfast table, and it helps produce the lightest, moistest pancake you've ever had. And once you try this simple blueberry compote, you'll never go back to lackluster syrup again.

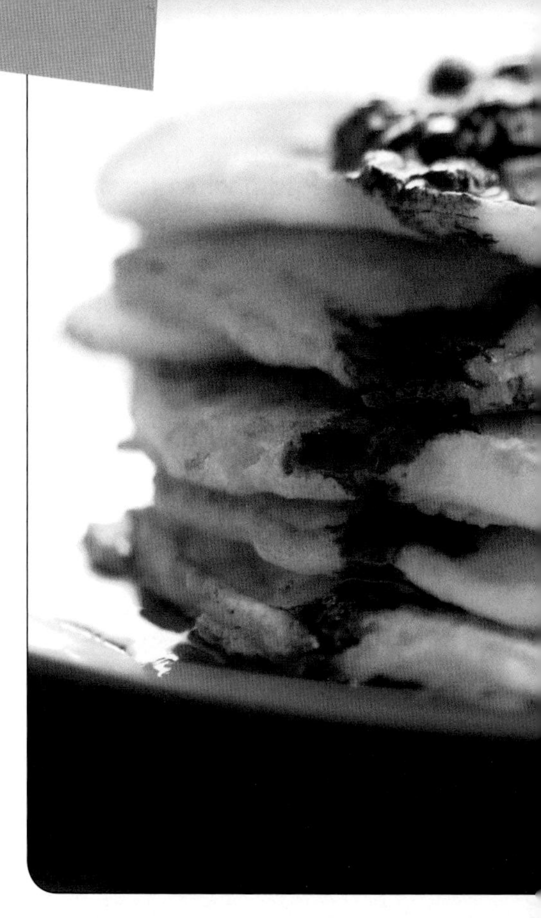

310 calories
8 g fat
(3.5 g saturated)
500 mg sodium

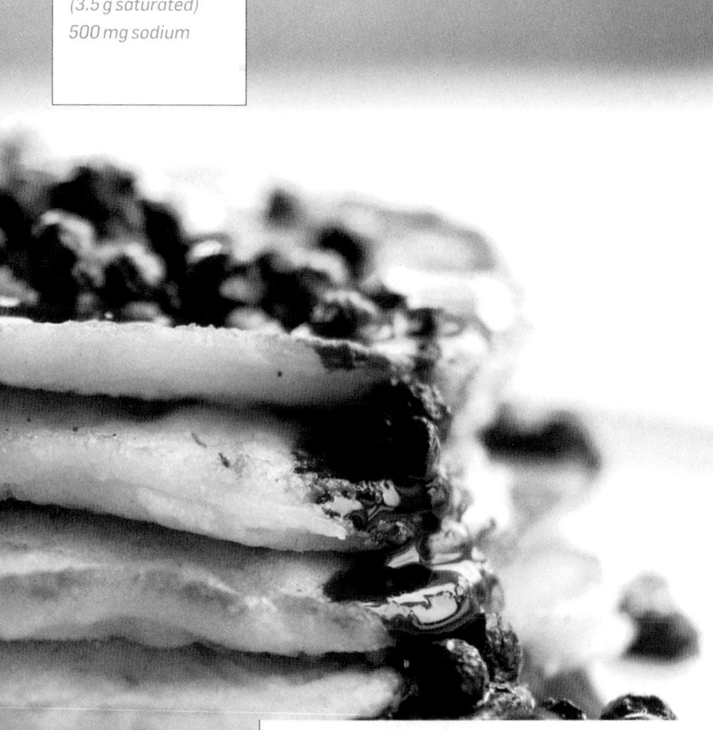

Not That!

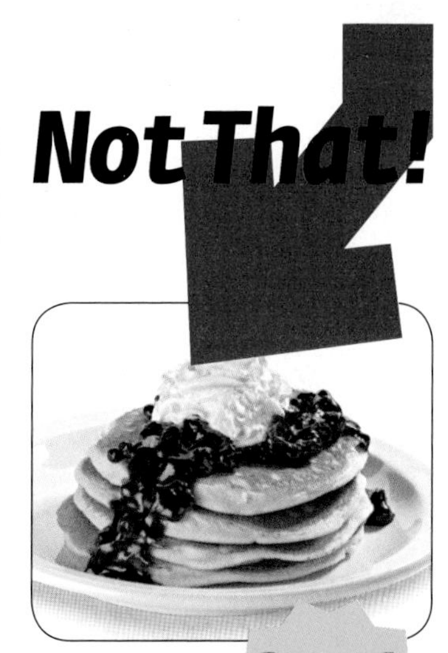

IHOP Blueberry Pancakes

710 calories

(IHOP does not provide anything other than calorie counts for its menu items.)

Cost: $7.99

Save!
Cost: $5.76
Calories: 400

How to Make It:

Mix the blueberries, water, and sugar in a saucepan. Cook over low heat, stirring often, for 10 minutes or until the blueberries begin to break apart.

Whisk together the yogurt, cottage cheese, eggs, and lemon juice in a bowl. Mix the flour, baking soda, and salt in another bowl. Add the flour to the yogurt mixture and stir just until blended.

Heat a large skillet over medium-low heat. Coat with nonstick spray and add batter in large spoonfuls (about 1/4 cup). Flip the pancakes when the tops begin to bubble, 3 to 5 minutes, and cook the second side until browned. Serve with the warm blueberries.

Makes 4 servings / Cost per serving: $2.23

Breakfast Burrito

Eat This

YOU'LL NEED:

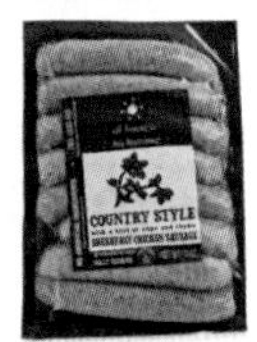

2 cooked chicken sausage links, diced

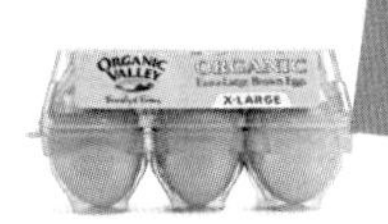

6 large eggs, lightly beaten

+

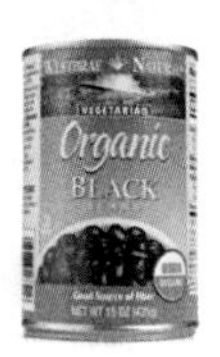

1 cup black beans, rinsed, drained, and heated

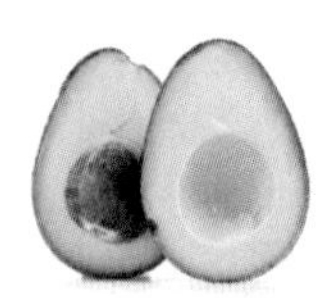

1 avocado, pitted, peeled, and sliced

+

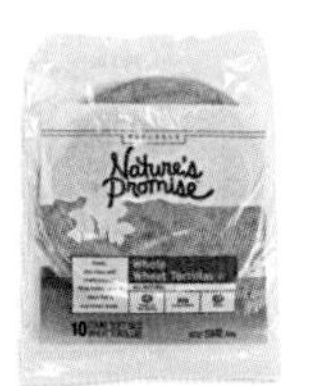

4 medium (10") whole wheat tortillas

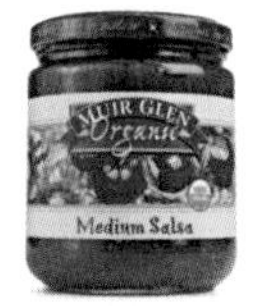

Salsa, to taste

YOU'LL ALSO NEED:

½ Tbsp olive oil

1 red onion, diced

Salt and pepper

Chopped cilantro

½ cup low-fat shredded Cheddar or Jack cheese

Pickled jalapeños (optional)

Take an oversize tortilla and stuff it full of sausage and cheese and you're bound for a rude awakening. By swapping worthless white tortillas for whole wheat, fatty pork sausage for the lean chicken variety, and adding fiber-rich beans and fresh avocado, we've slashed the calories in half while increasing overall nutrition (and deliciousness).

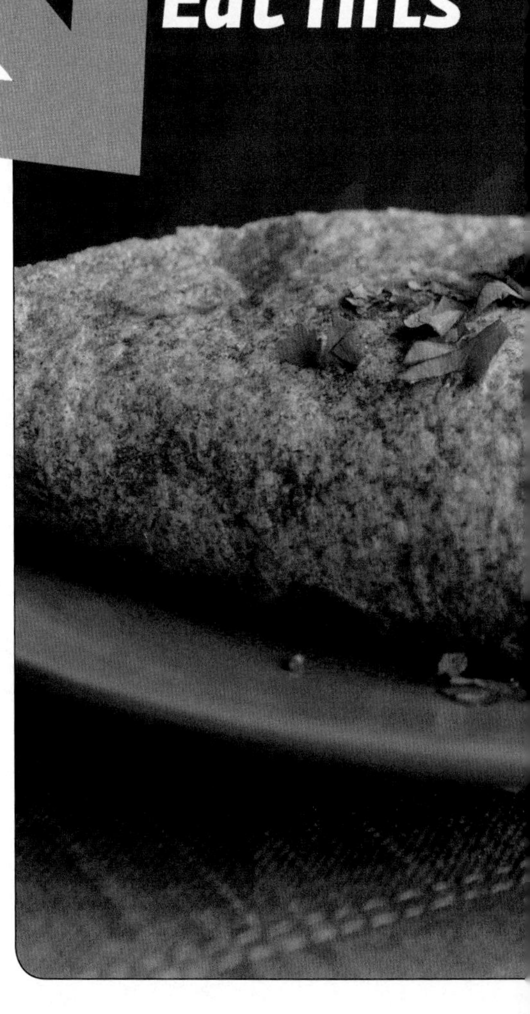

415 calories
17 g fat
(5 g saturated)
625 mg sodium

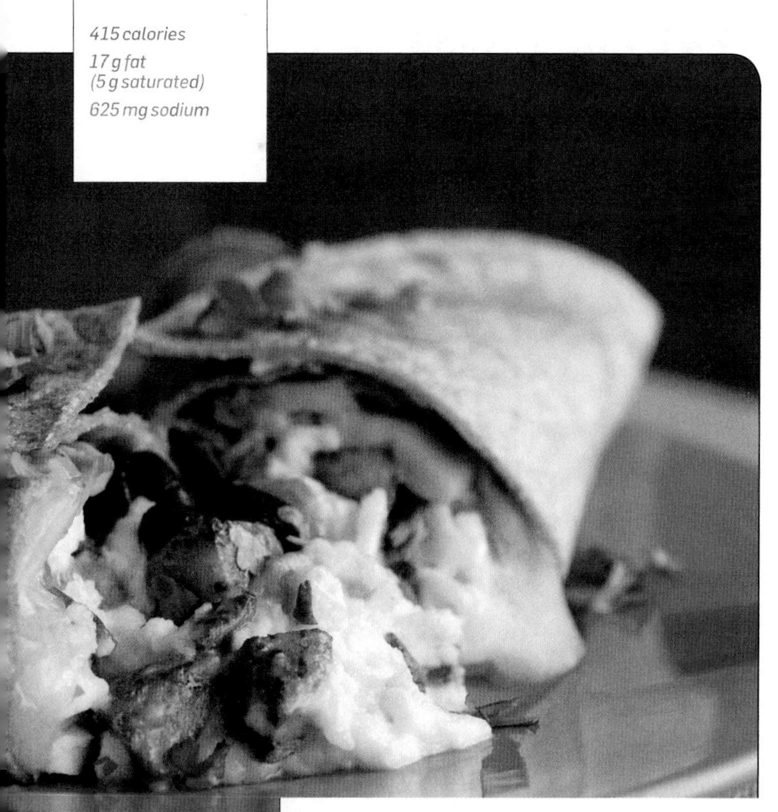

Not That!

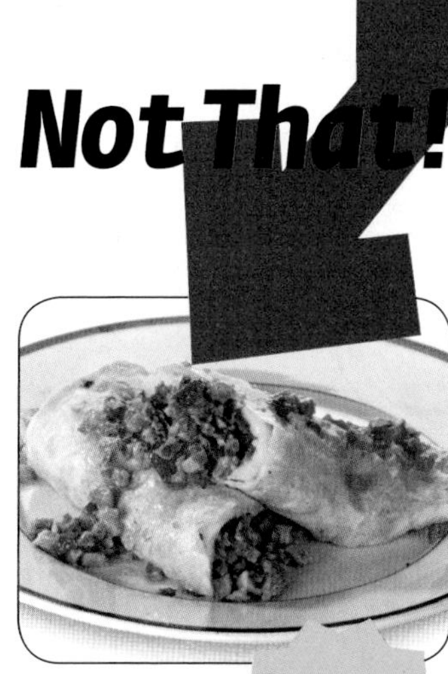

Bob Evans Meat Lover's BoBurrito

799 calories
49 g fat
(19 g saturated)
2,427 mg sodium
Cost: $5.99

Save!
Cost:$3.57
Calories:384
Fat:32g

How to Make It:

Heat the oil in a large skillet over medium heat. Add the sausage and onion; cook for 5 minutes or until lightly browned. Turn the heat to low.

Pour the eggs into the skillet. Cook slowly, constantly stirring with a wooden spoon until the eggs are firm but still moist. Remove from the heat, season with salt and pepper, and stir in cilantro.

Wrap the tortillas in a damp, clean kitchen towel and heat in the microwave for 45 seconds. (Or, if time allows, heat them individually in a dry pan until warm and lightly toasted.) Divide the eggs, beans, cheese, and avocado among the tortillas. Top each burrito with salsa, more cilantro, and jalapeños (if using).

Makes 4 servings / Cost per serving: $2.42

Artichoke Dip

Eat This

YOU'LL NEED:

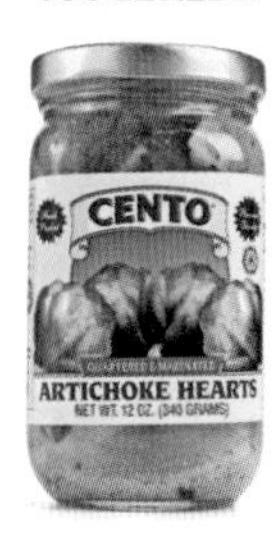

1 (12 oz) jar artichoke hearts in water, drained and chopped

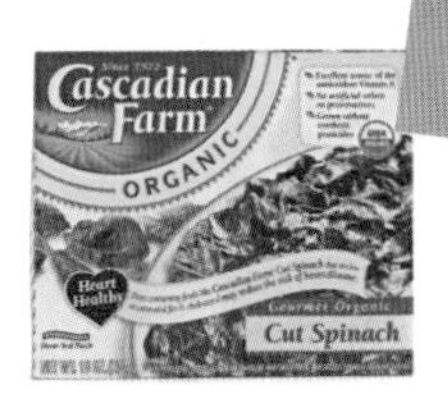

1 (16 oz) box chopped frozen spinach, thawed

+

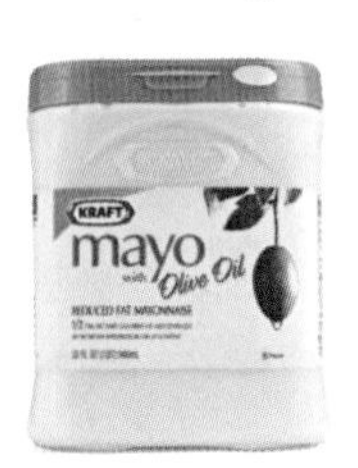

2 Tbsp olive-oil based mayonnaise (made by both Kraft and Hellman's)

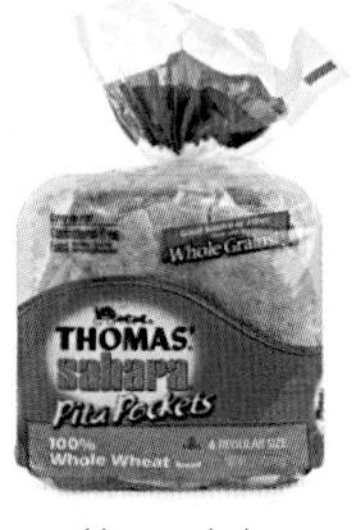

4 large whole wheat pitas

+

YOU'LL ALSO NEED:

½ Tbsp butter

1 onion, finely chopped

3 cloves garlic, finely chopped

1 small can roasted green chiles, drained and chopped

2 Tbsp whipped light cream cheese

Juice of 1 lemon

Salt and fresh cracked pepper, to taste

This classic dip is normally hijacked by a roguish team of full-fat mayo and cream cheese; somewhere, hidden within, lies a token amount of spinach and artichoke. Here, we turn that ratio on its head, plus use a flavorful olive-oil based mayo to cut calories and boost nutrition. Chiles bring some extra heat to the equation, while toasted wheat pitas work as super scoopers. Overall, this reimagined appetizer packs an amazing 14 grams of fiber.

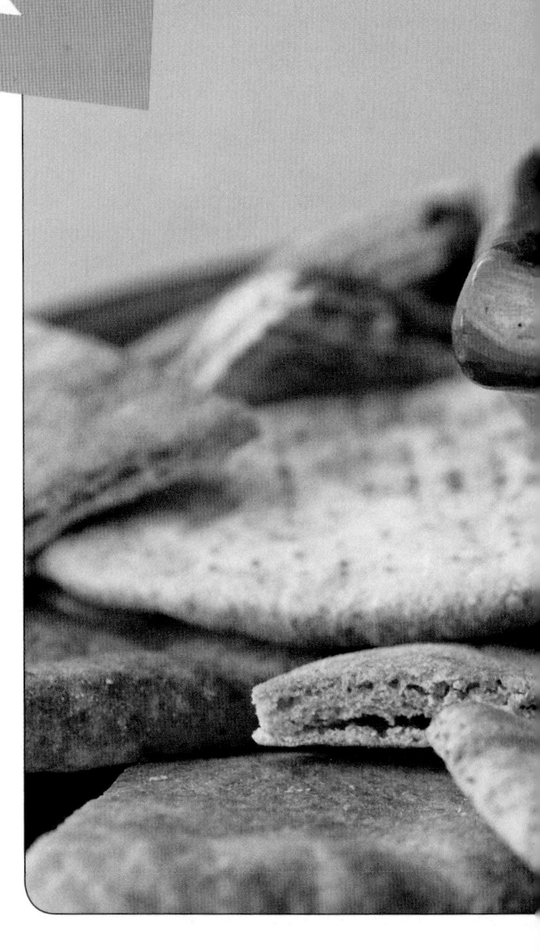

270 calories
10 g fat
(2.5 g saturated)
520 mg sodium

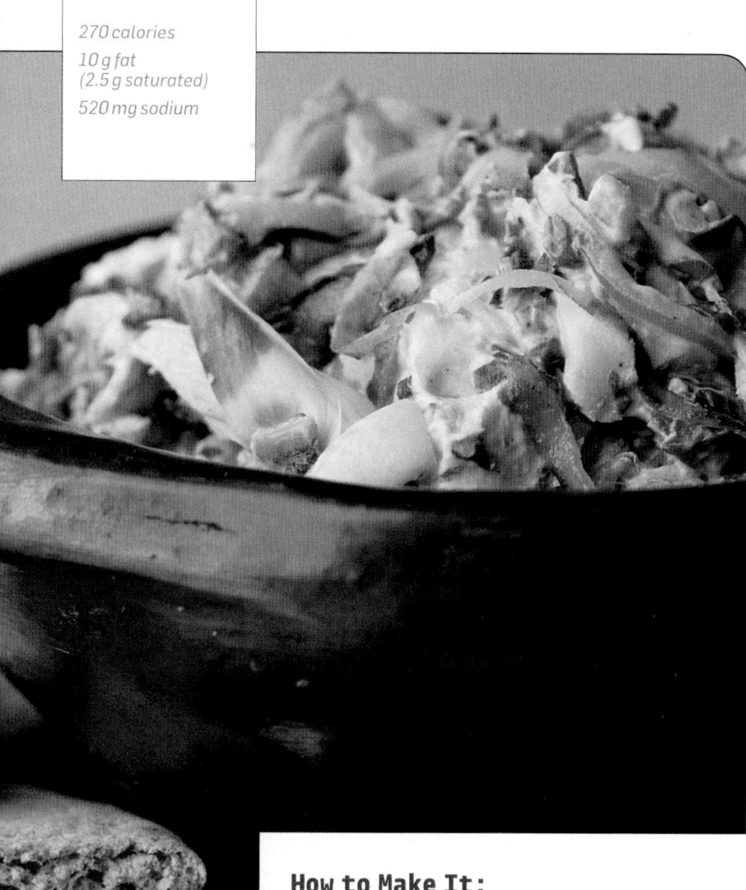

Not That!

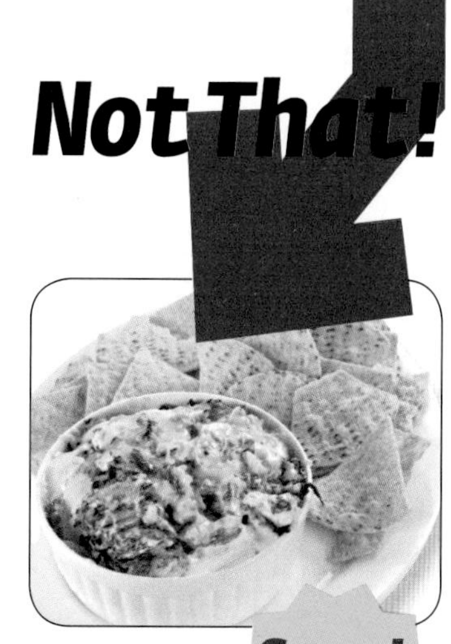

Chili's Hot Spinach & Artichoke Dip with Chips

930 calories
77 g fat
(34 g saturated)
3,130 mg sodium
Cost: $7.99

Save!
Cost: $5.92
Calories: 660
Fat: 67 g

How to Make It:

Cut the pitas into 6 to 8 wedges each and separate the layers. Spread on 2 baking sheets and bake at 400°F for 5 minutes or until crisp.

Heat the butter in a large skillet over medium heat. Add the onion and garlic and cook for 5 minutes or until softened. Add the artichokes, spinach, chiles, mayonnaise, cream cheese, and lemon juice. Cook, stirring often, for 5 minutes or until hot. Season with salt and pepper.

Serve with the pita wedges.

Makes 4 servings / Cost per serving: $2.07

Chicken Parmesan

Eat This

YOU'LL NEED:

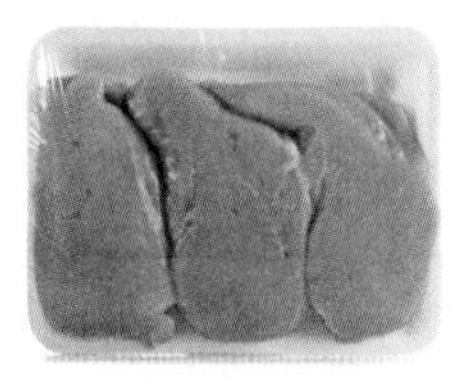

4 small boneless skinless chicken breasts (4 to 6 oz each)

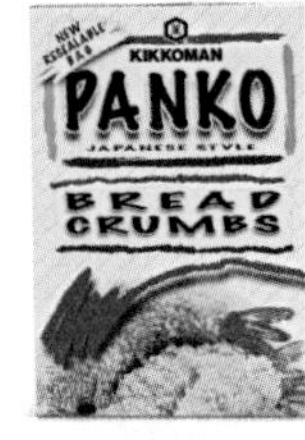

1 cup bread crumbs, preferably panko

+

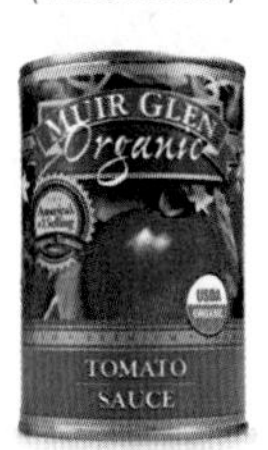

1 cup your favorite tomato sauce (we love anything from Muir Glen)

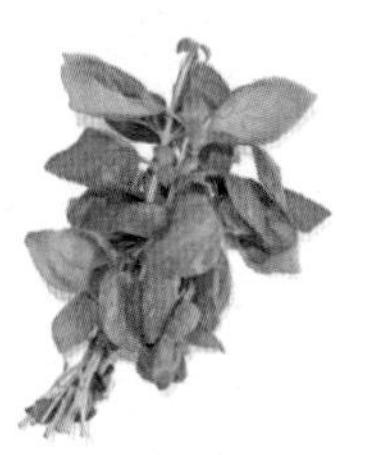

Fresh basil leaves (optional)

+

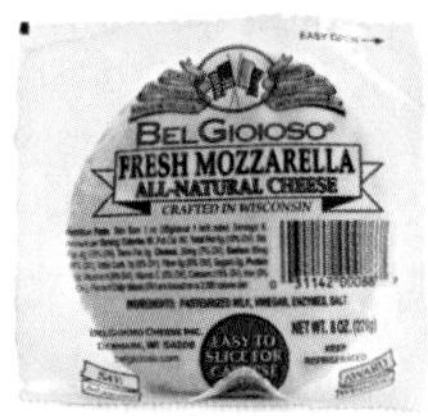

4 oz fresh mozzarella cheese, sliced thinly (shredded low-moisture mozzarella also works fine)

YOU'LL ALSO NEED:

½ tsp salt

½ tsp black pepper

2 egg whites, lightly beaten

2 Tbsp grated Parmesan cheese

½ Tbsp dried Italian seasoning

1 Tbsp extra-virgin olive oil

This Italian-American staple normally suffers from a glut of oil, an excess of cheese, and a huge bed of carb-heavy spaghetti as the base. We shallow-fry a modest portion of chicken to minimize oil soakage, then use fresh mozz (which is lower in calories and fat) to top it off. For sides, trade the spaghetti bed for garlicky sautéed spinach.

340 calories

11 g fat
(4 g saturated)

670 mg sodium

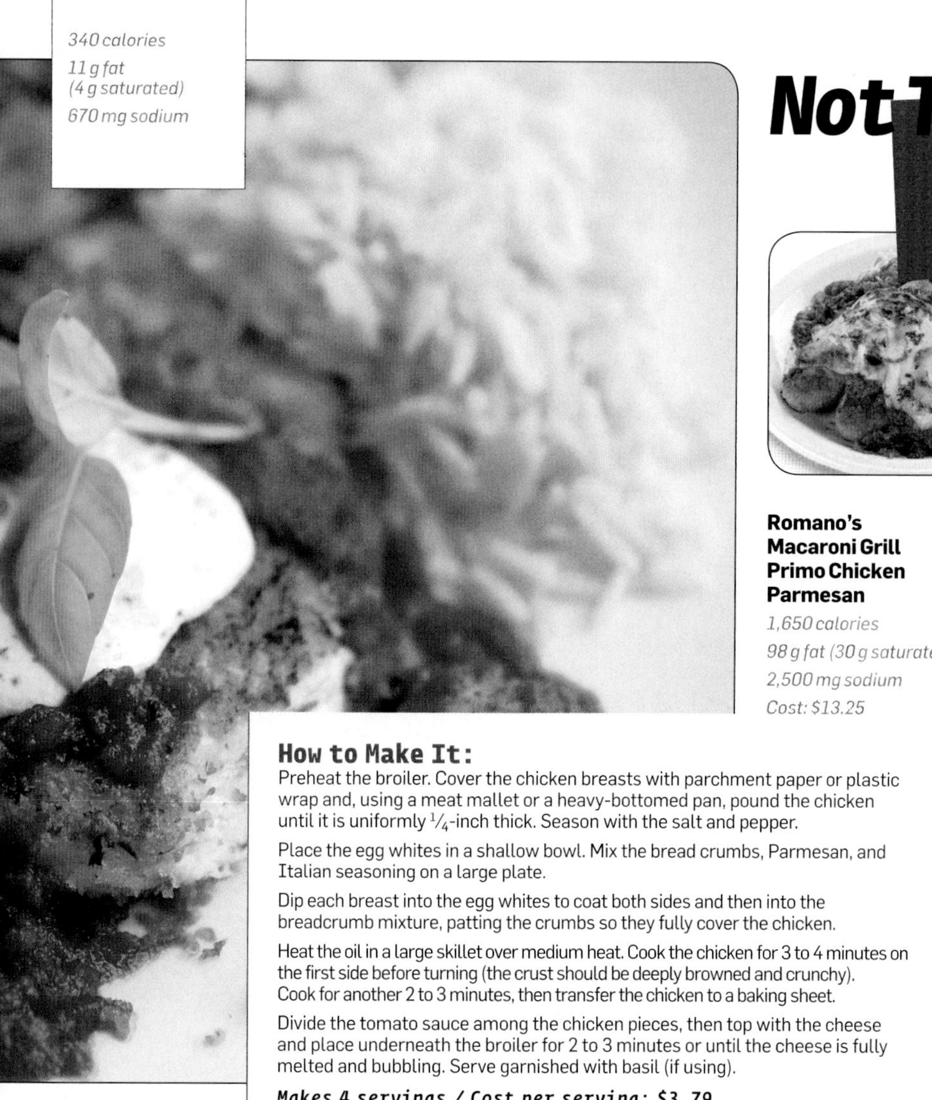

Not That!

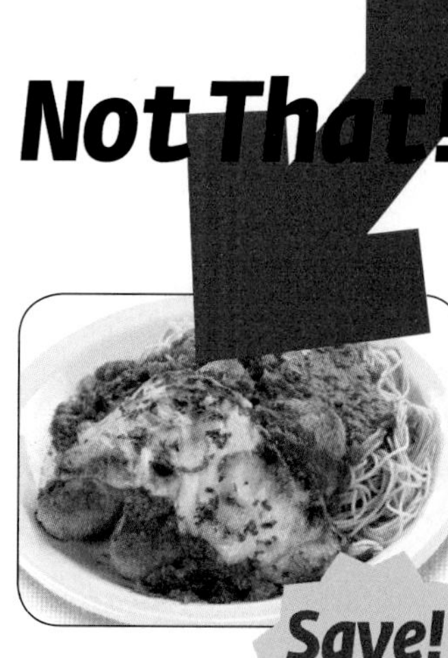

Save!
Cost: $9.46
Calories: 1,310
Fat: 87g

Romano's Macaroni Grill Primo Chicken Parmesan

1,650 calories

98 g fat (30 g saturated)

2,500 mg sodium

Cost: $13.25

How to Make It:

Preheat the broiler. Cover the chicken breasts with parchment paper or plastic wrap and, using a meat mallet or a heavy-bottomed pan, pound the chicken until it is uniformly $\frac{1}{4}$-inch thick. Season with the salt and pepper.

Place the egg whites in a shallow bowl. Mix the bread crumbs, Parmesan, and Italian seasoning on a large plate.

Dip each breast into the egg whites to coat both sides and then into the breadcrumb mixture, patting the crumbs so they fully cover the chicken.

Heat the oil in a large skillet over medium heat. Cook the chicken for 3 to 4 minutes on the first side before turning (the crust should be deeply browned and crunchy). Cook for another 2 to 3 minutes, then transfer the chicken to a baking sheet.

Divide the tomato sauce among the chicken pieces, then top with the cheese and place underneath the broiler for 2 to 3 minutes or until the cheese is fully melted and bubbling. Serve garnished with basil (if using).

Makes 4 servings / Cost per serving: $3.79

Pepper Sirloin

Eat This

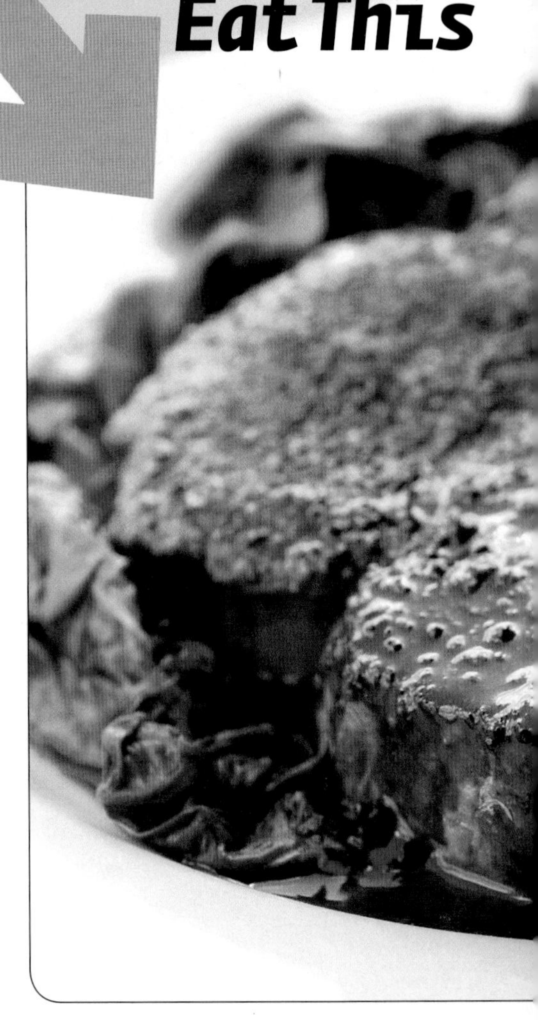

YOU'LL NEED:

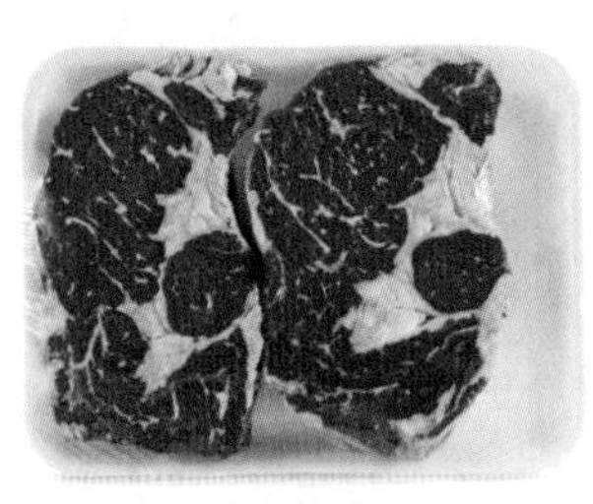

2 sirloin steaks
(6 to 8 oz each),
trimmed of excess fat

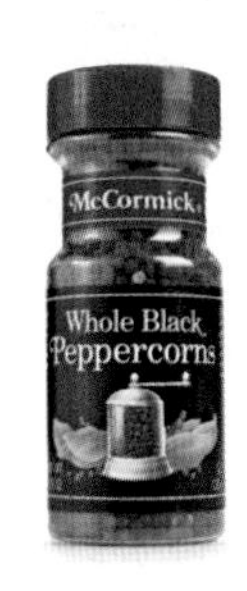

1 Tbsp coarsely
cracked peppercorns

+

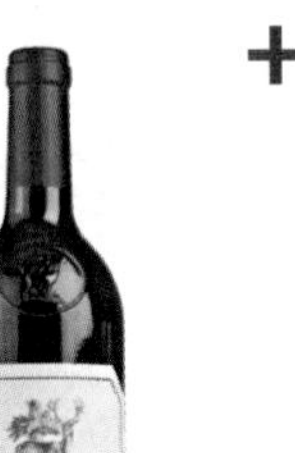

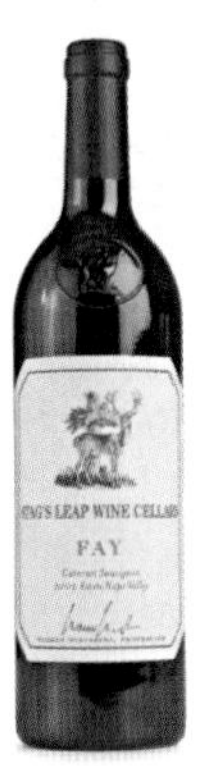

½ cup red wine, preferably
Cabernet Sauvignon
or Pinot Noir

YOU'LL ALSO NEED:

Kosher salt

½ Tbsp olive oil

½ cup low-sodium
beef broth

1 Tbsp butter

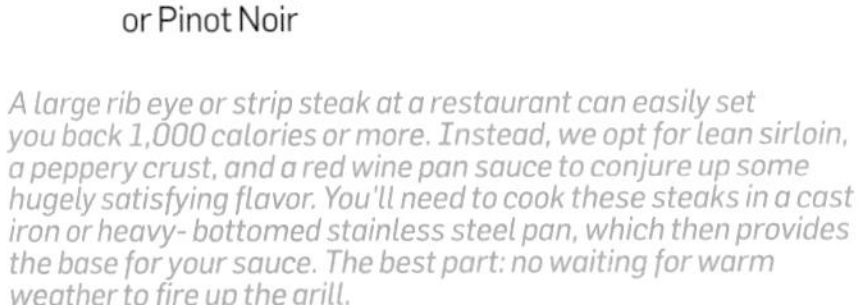

A large rib eye or strip steak at a restaurant can easily set you back 1,000 calories or more. Instead, we opt for lean sirloin, a peppery crust, and a red wine pan sauce to conjure up some hugely satisfying flavor. You'll need to cook these steaks in a cast iron or heavy- bottomed stainless steel pan, which then provides the base for your sauce. The best part: no waiting for warm weather to fire up the grill.

410 calories
19 g fat
(8 g saturated)
470 mg sodium

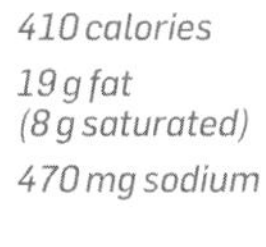

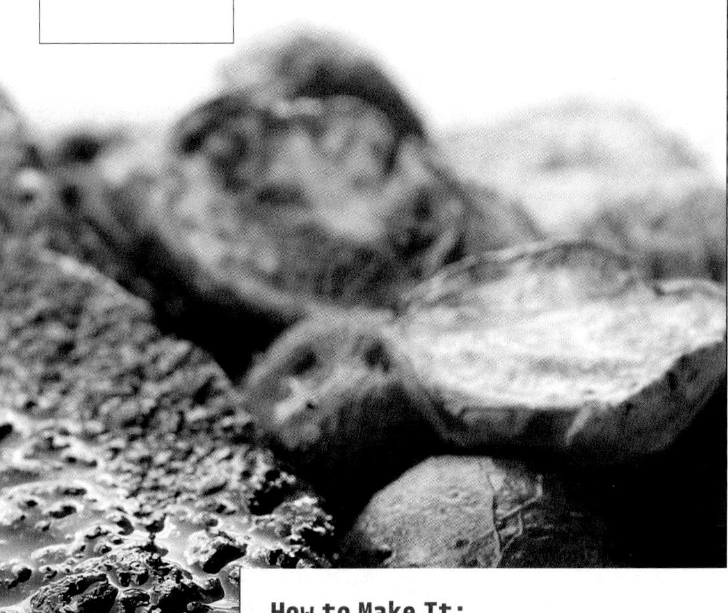

Not That!

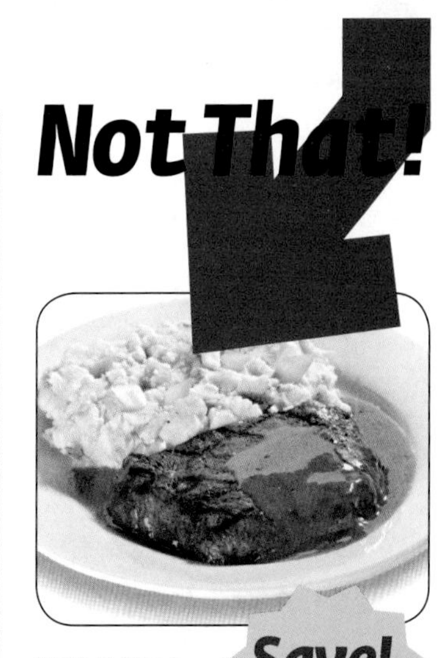

T.G.I. Friday's New York Strip Steak with Burgundy Sauce

1,530 calories

Cost: $17.00

Save!
Cost: $11.24
Calories: 1,120

How to Make It:

Remove the steaks from the fridge 30 minutes before cooking. Season each with a few pinches of salt and half of the pepper, using your palms to press the peppercorns into the meat.

Heat a large skillet over high heat. Add the oil; when it smokes lightly, add the steaks. (The pan should be very hot, so the steaks should sizzle vigorously when they hit the surface.) Cook, untouched, until a deep crust develops on the underside, about 4 minutes. Flip and cook for another 3 to 4 minutes for medium-rare. Transfer the steaks to a plate and set aside to rest.

Add the wine and broth to the skillet and use a wooden spoon to scrape up any bits of meat stuck to the bottom of the pan. Continue to cook over medium-high heat until the liquid is reduced and thick enough to coat the back of a spoon, about 5 minutes. Remove from the heat and swirl in the butter. Serve the steaks with the sauce drizzled over the top and a side of oven-roasted red potatoes.

Makes 2 servings / Cost per serving: $5.76

Cobb Salad

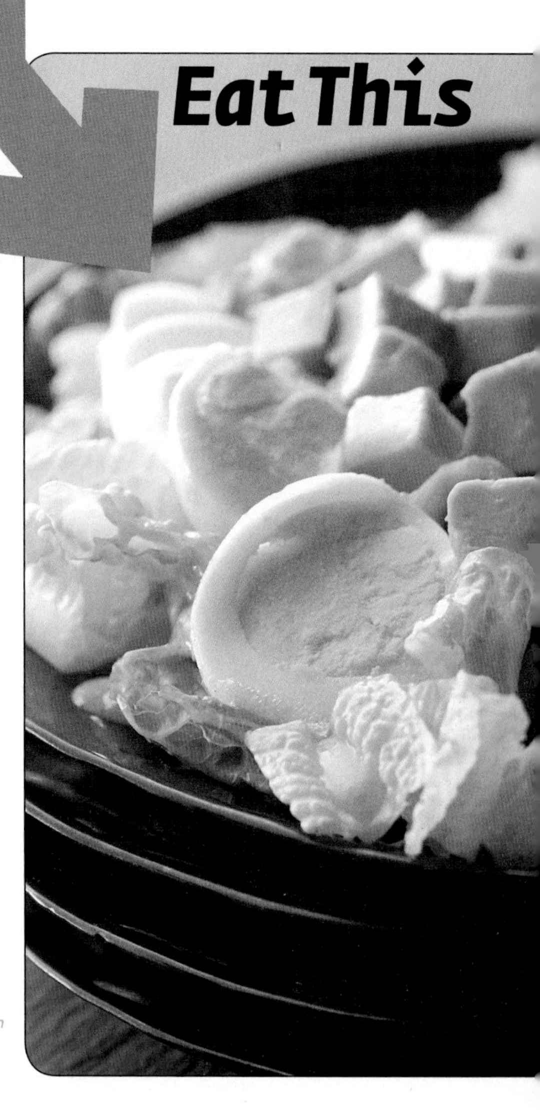

YOU'LL NEED:

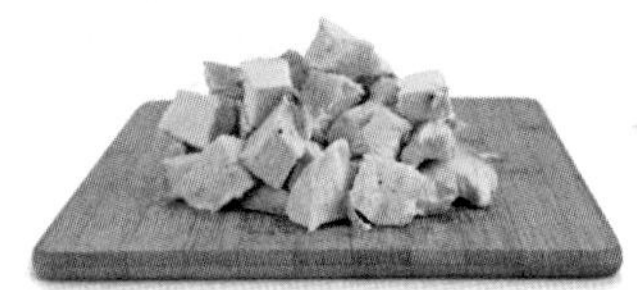

2 cups chopped cooked chicken (store-bought rotisserie chickens work great)

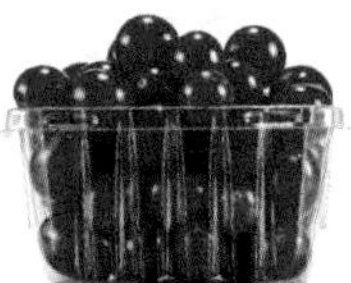

1 pint cherry tomatoes

+

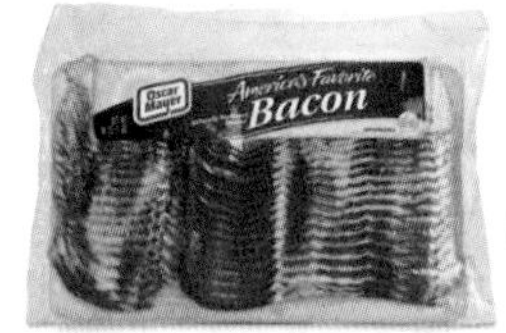

4 strips bacon, cooked and crumbled

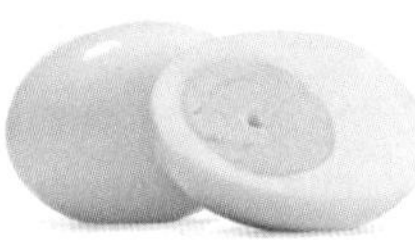

2 hard-boiled eggs, sliced

+

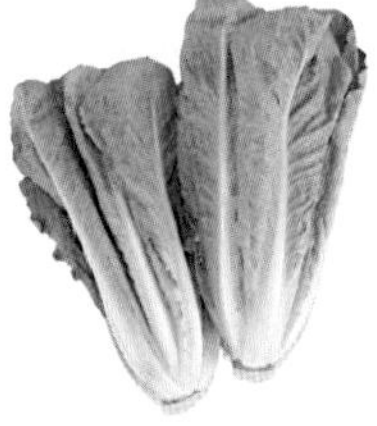

2 heads Bibb or 1 large head romaine lettuce, torn into bite-size pieces

YOU'LL ALSO NEED:

¼ cup extra-virgin olive oil
Juice of 1 lemon
1 tsp Dijon mustard
Salt and pepper
1 avocado, pitted, peeled, and cut into ¼-inch pieces
¼ cup crumbled blue cheese

Considering what most restaurants do to even the simplest salads, this multi-component California classic is truly dangerous in the hands of corporate chefs across America. Use leftover grilled chicken or a shredded store-bought rotisserie bird, use the cheese and the bacon sparingly, and make the dressing yourself—it takes 2 minutes and can save you up to 200 calories a serving.

420 calories
28 g fat
(6 g saturated)
430 mg sodium

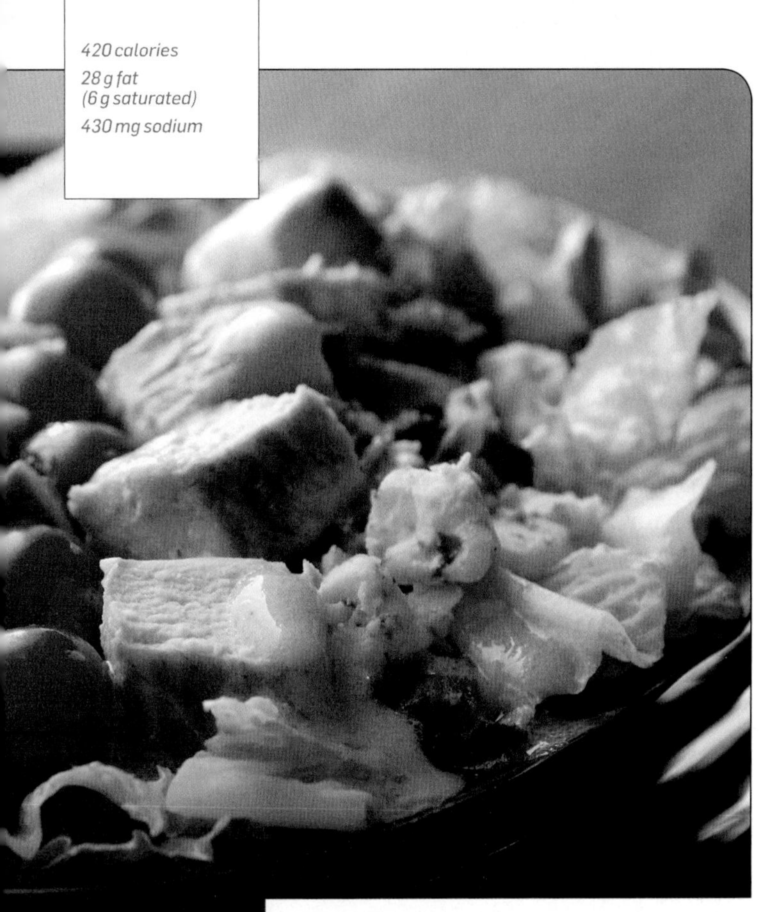

Not That!

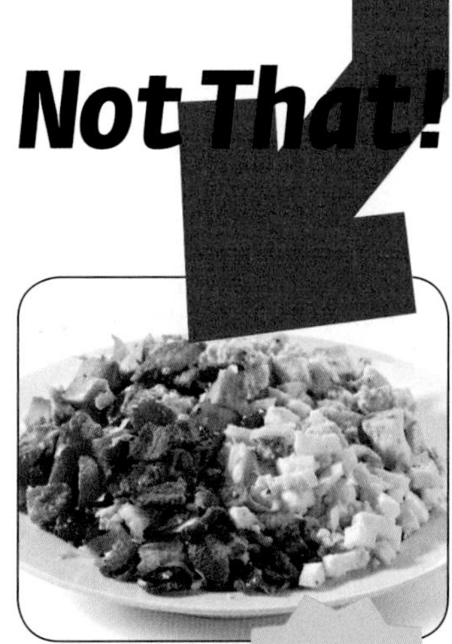

California Pizza Kitchen CPK Cobb Salad

1,138 calories

Cost: $13.25

Save!
Cost: $9.28
Calories: 718

How to Make It:

Whisk together the oil, lemon juice, and mustard. Season with salt and pepper. Place the lettuce in a large bowl and pour three-quarters of the dressing over it; toss until lightly coated. Divide the lettuce among chilled plates.

Top with the chicken, avocado, tomatoes, bacon, eggs, and cheese. Drizzle with the remaining dressing and serve.

Makes 4 servings / Cost per serving: $3.97

Loaded Pizza

Eat This

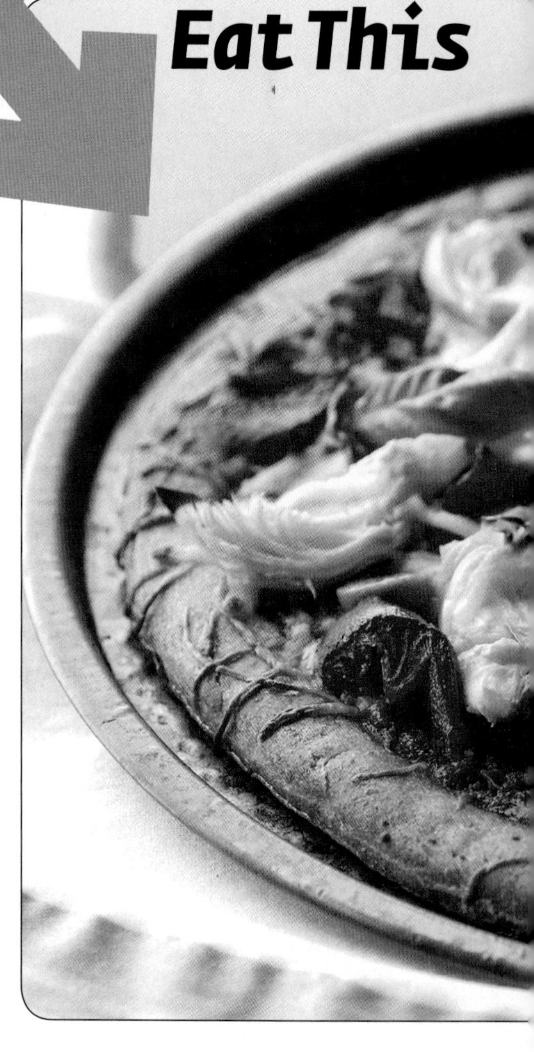

YOU'LL NEED:

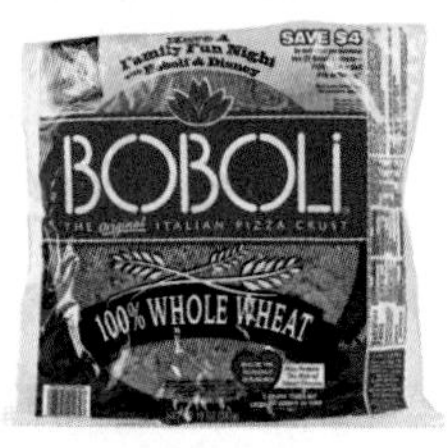

12" Boboli 100% Whole Wheat Thin Crust

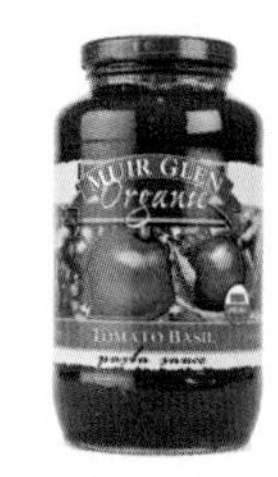

1 cup Muir Glen Tomato Basil Pasta Sauce

+

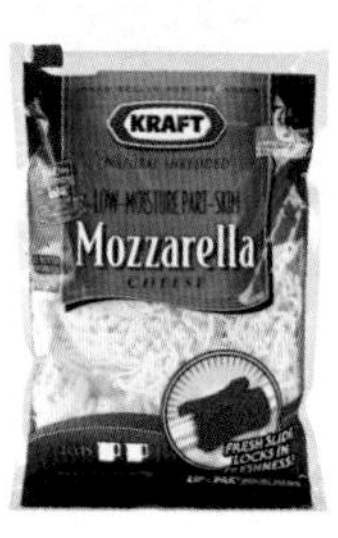

2 cups Kraft Natural Low-Moisture Part-Skim Mozzarella Shreds

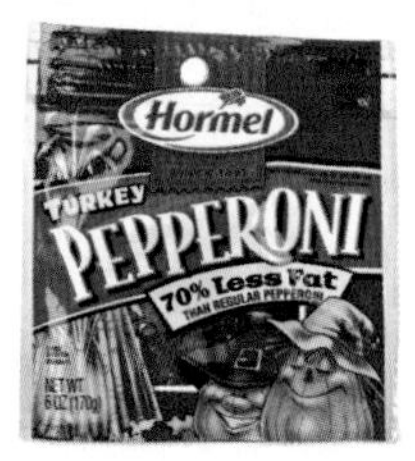

15 slices Turkey Pepperoni

+

YOU'LL ALSO NEED:

½ cup onion, sliced

½ cup roasted red peppers

½ cup chopped green olives

2 garlic cloves, minced

½ tsp red pepper flakes

1 (6-oz) jar artichoke hearts, drained

1 cup fresh basil leaves (optional)

Ordering a supreme pizza for delivery is an open invitation for caloric calamity. Best case scenario, you're looking at 250 calories a slice; worst case, 500 or more. Here, we use Boboli's new whole wheat thin crust shell as a low-cal, fiber-rich base. We then load the pizza with a team of nutritional all-stars (red peppers, artichokes, fresh basil) and a good amount of turkey pepperoni. Torn deli ham or Canadian bacon would also work great here.

300 calories
14 g fat
(6 g saturated)
780 mg sodium

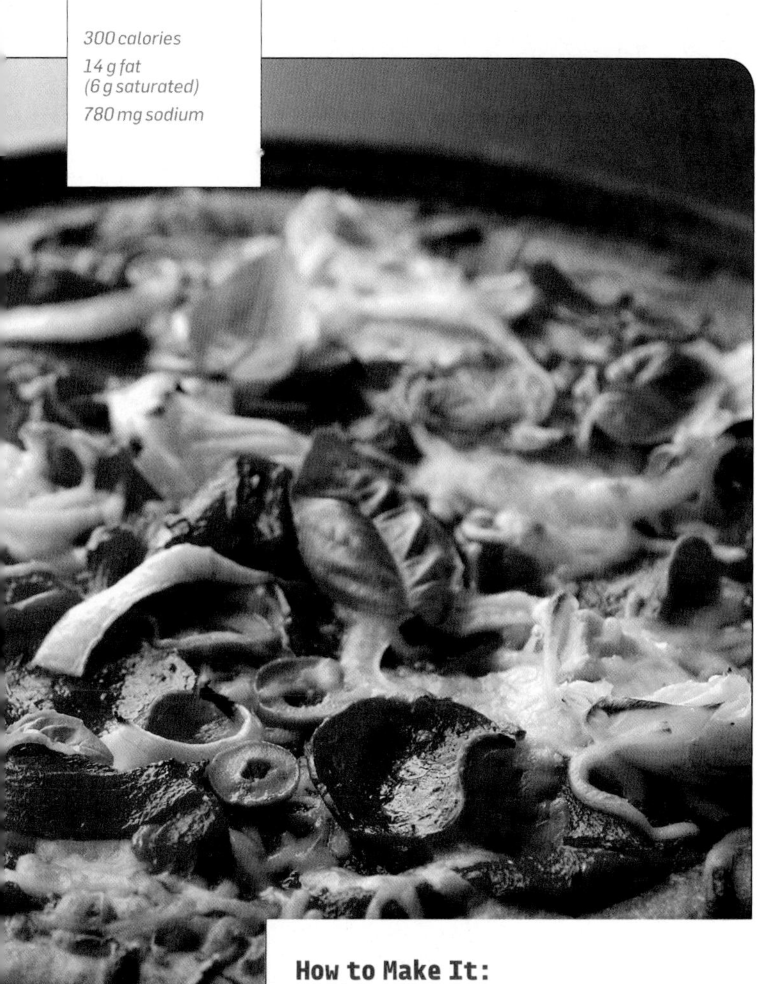

Not That!

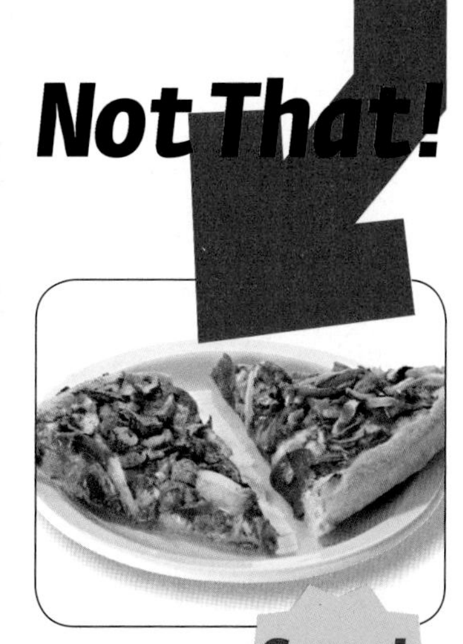

Pizza Hut Supreme Pan Pizza (2 slices)

800 calories
40 g fat
(16 g saturated)
1,780 mg sodium
Cost: $4.55

Save!
Cost: $1.48
Calories: 500
Fat: 26g

How to Make It:

Preheat the oven to 400°F. Cover the crust with sauce and then cheese. Sprinkle with the pepperoni, onion, peppers, olives, garlic, pepper flakes, and artichokes. Bake for 12 to 15 minutes, until the cheese is melted and bubbling. Top with the basil and serve immediately.

Makes 4 servings / Cost per serving: $3.07

Grilled Fish Tacos

Eat This

YOU'LL NEED:

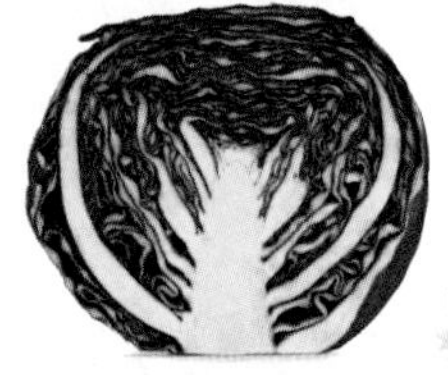

1 cup finely shredded red cabbage

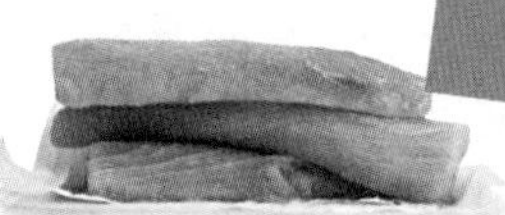

1 mahimahi fillet (12 oz)

+

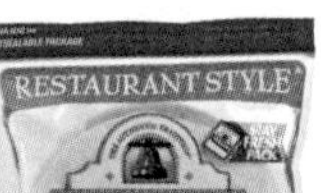

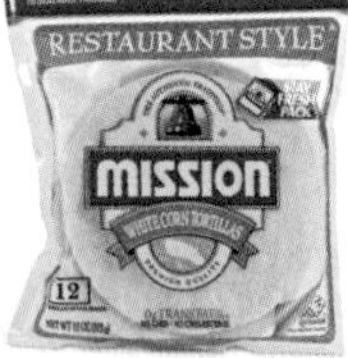

4 small corn tortillas

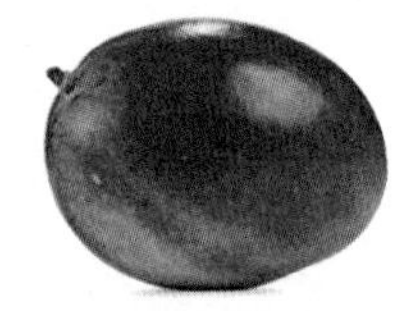

1 mango, peeled, pitted, and cubed

+

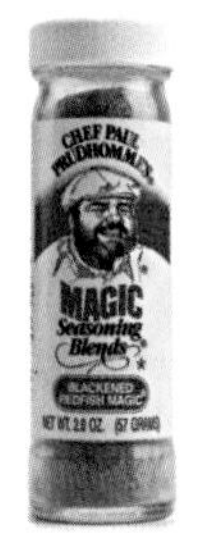

½ Tbsp blackening spice

YOU'LL ALSO NEED:

1 avocado, pitted, peeled, and cubed

½ red onion, finely chopped

2 limes

Chopped cilantro

Salt and pepper

Canola oil

Who doesn't love fish tacos? South of the border, the fish is always battered and fried and served with an aggressive dousing of mayonnaise. We wanted to ditch the frying oil and mayo but maintain the flavor, so instead we subbed a spicy blackening seasoning and a nutrient-rich mango-avocado salsa, which cuts the heat and pairs perfectly with the fish. This salsa would make shoe leather taste good.

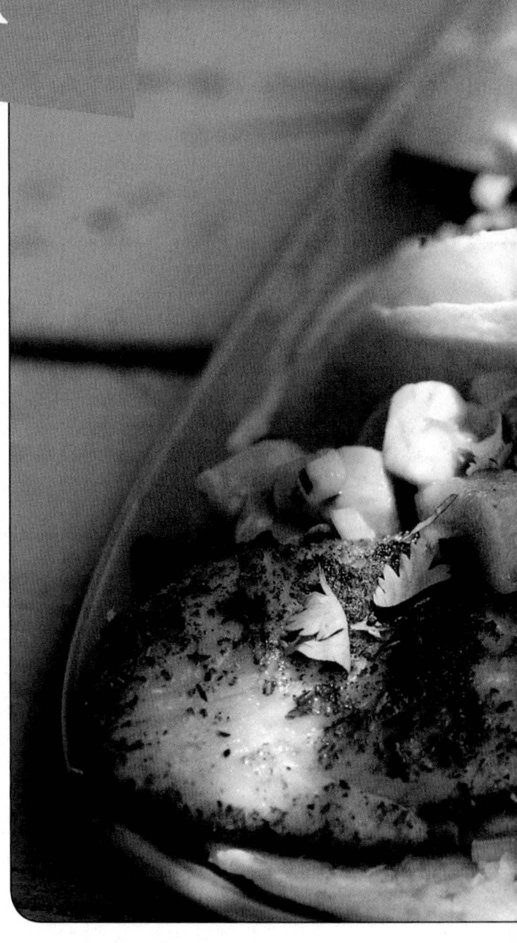

470 calories
15 g fat
(2 g saturated)
240 mg sodium

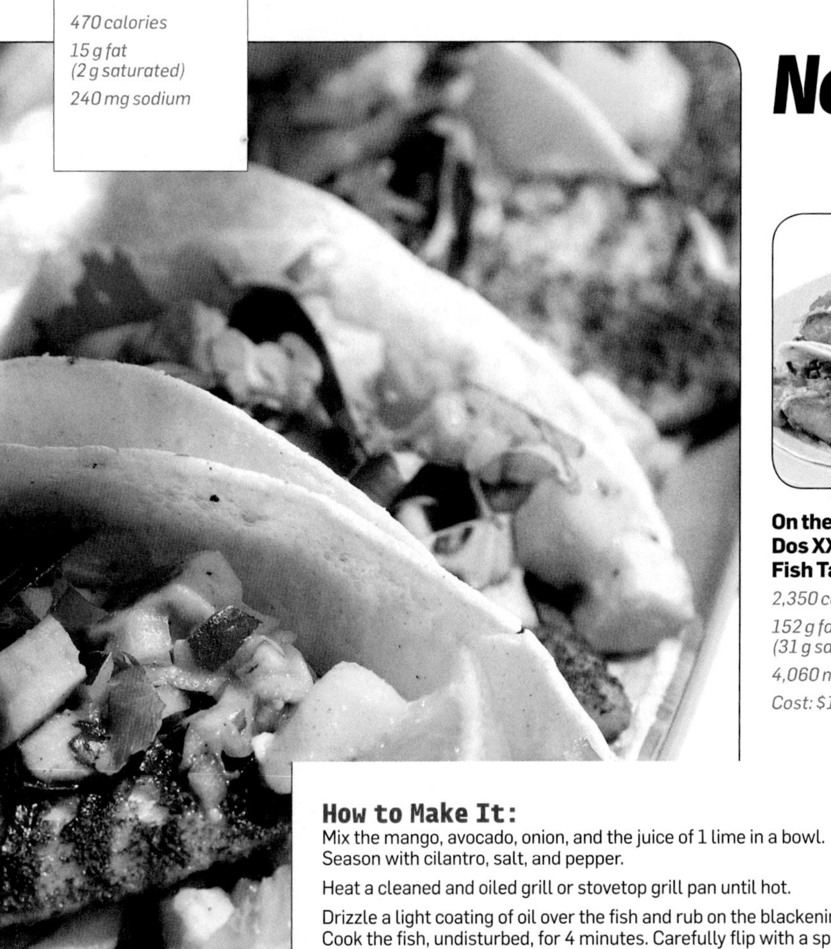

Not That!

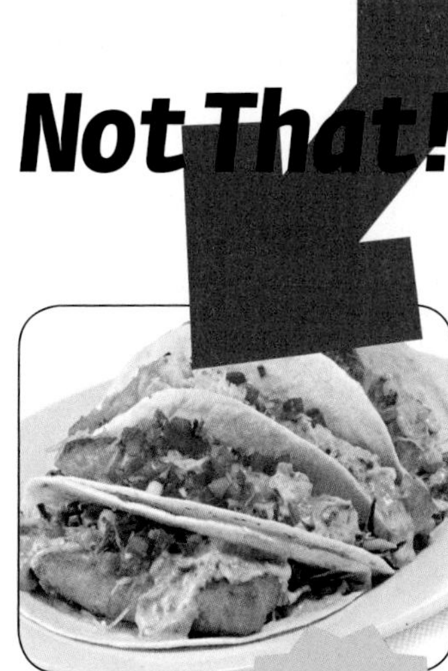

On the Border Dos XX Fish Tacos

2,350 calories
152 g fat
(31 g saturated)
4,060 mg sodium
Cost: $13.95

Save!
Cost: $10.04
Calories: 1,880
Fat: 137 g

How to Make It:

Mix the mango, avocado, onion, and the juice of 1 lime in a bowl. Season with cilantro, salt, and pepper.

Heat a cleaned and oiled grill or stovetop grill pan until hot.

Drizzle a light coating of oil over the fish and rub on the blackening spice. Cook the fish, undisturbed, for 4 minutes. Carefully flip with a spatula and cook for another 4 minutes. Remove. Warm the tortillas on the grill for 1 to 2 minutes or wrap in damp paper towels and microwave for 1 minute.

Break the fish into chunks and divide among the warm tortillas. Top with cabbage and the mango mixture. Serve with lime wedges.

Makes 2 servings / Cost per serving: $3.91

Fettuccine Alfredo

Eat This

YOU'LL NEED:

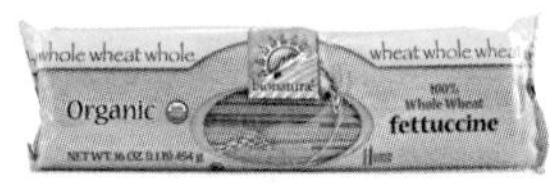

12 oz whole wheat fettuccine (we like Ronzoni Healthy Harvest)

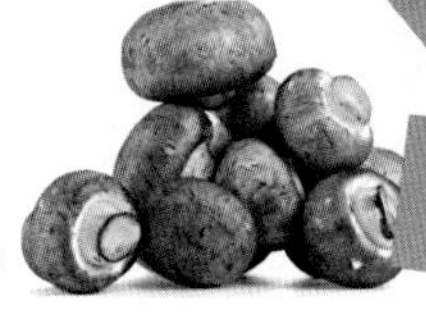

8 oz cremini mushrooms, sliced

+

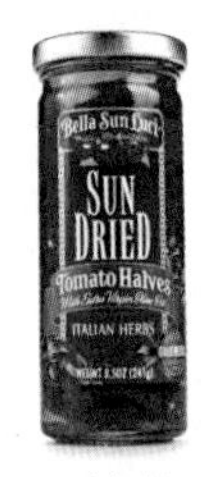

¼ cup sun-dried tomatoes, chopped

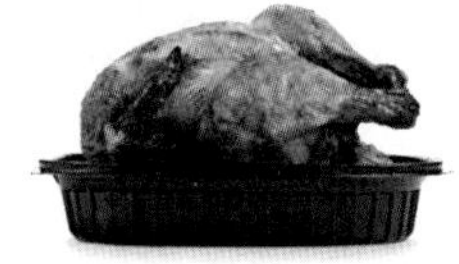

8 oz cooked chicken breast, thinly sliced (store-bought rotisserie chickens work well)

+

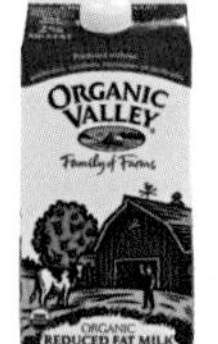

2 cups 2% milk

YOU'LL ALSO NEED:

2 Tbsp unsalted butter
3 Tbsp all-purpose flour
2 garlic cloves, chopped
2 Tbsp grated Parmesan cheese
Salt and pepper
½ Tbsp olive oil
2 cups broccoli florets cut into bite-size pieces

The recipe for Alfredo is this: cream, butter, and cheese. We ditched the cream and made a basic bechamel sauce with flour, milk, butter, and Parmesan. We solved the other major shortcoming of pasta Alfredo (that is, a dearth of any true nutrition) and improved the dish substantially by adding chicken, broccoli, mushrooms, and, for good measure, sun-dried tomatoes. You'll never go back to the old version.

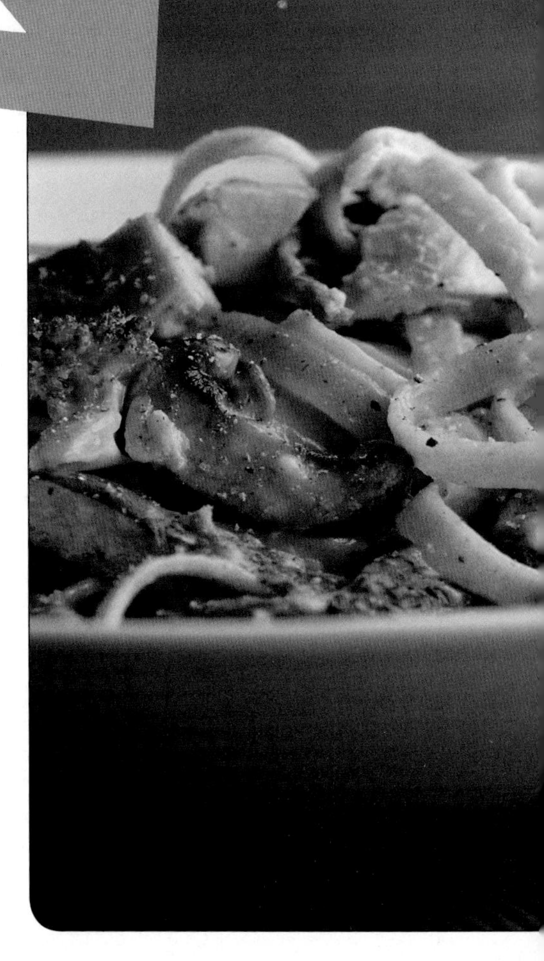

540 calories
14 g fat
(6 g saturated)
520 mg sodium

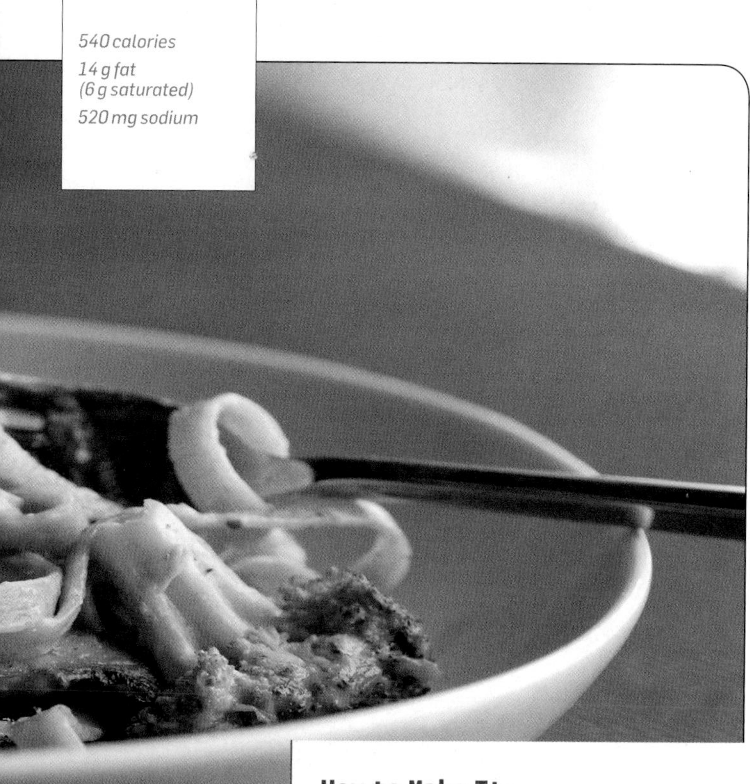

Not That!

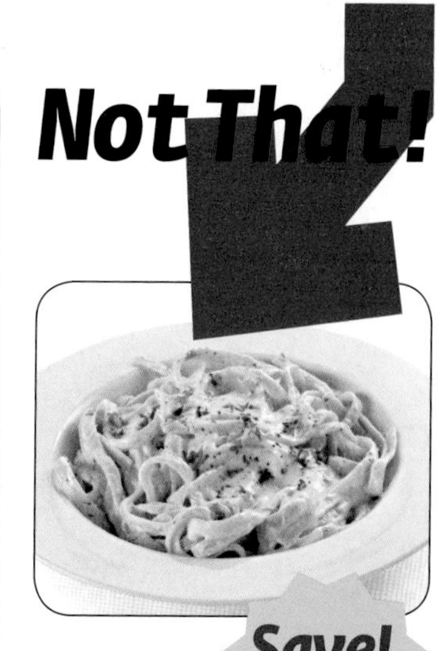

Olive Garden Fettuccine Alfredo

1,220 calories
75 g fat
(47 g saturated)
1,350 mg sodium
Cost: $12.00

Save!
Cost: $8.37
Calories: 680
Fat: 61 g

How to Make It:

Melt the butter in a saucepan over medium-low heat. Whisk in the flour. Cook, stirring, until lightly golden. Slowly whisk in the milk to prevent any lumps from forming. Add the garlic and simmer, whisking often, for 10 to 15 minutes or until thickened. Stir in the Parmesan and season with salt and pepper. Set aside.

Heat the oil in a large skillet over medium-high heat. Add the broccoli and cook for 3 to 4 minutes. Add the mushrooms and tomatoes. Cook for 5 minutes or until the vegetables have lightly caramelized. Stir in the chicken. Season with salt and pepper.

Meanwhile, cook the pasta according to the package directions. Drain, reserving 1 cup of the cooking water. Return the pasta to the pot, add the sauce, and the chicken mixture and toss to coat. If the sauce is too thick, add some of the pasta water until you reach the desired consistency. Serve immediately.

Makes 4 servings / Cost per serving: $3.63

The Ultimate Burger

Eat This

YOU'LL NEED:

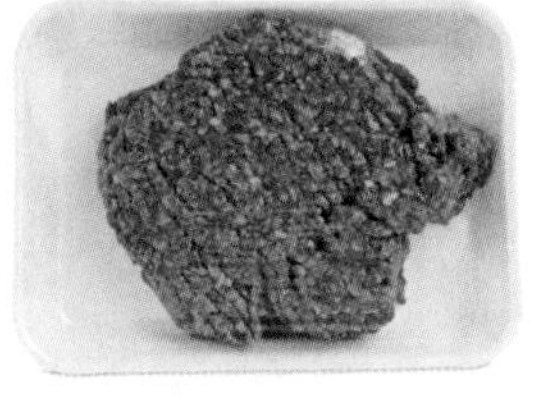

10 oz ground brisket

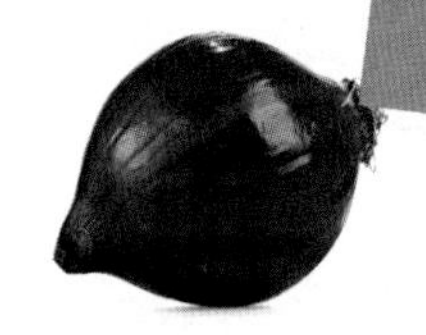

1 red onion, sliced

+

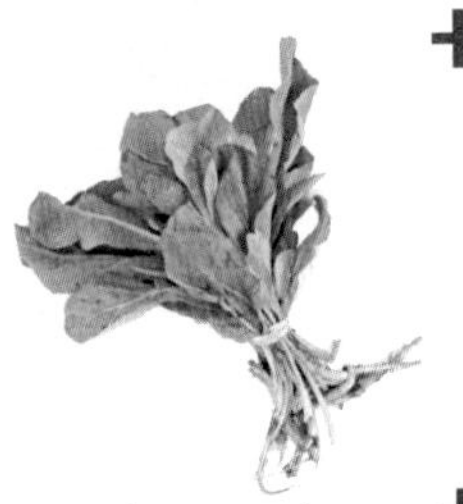

2 cups arugula

+

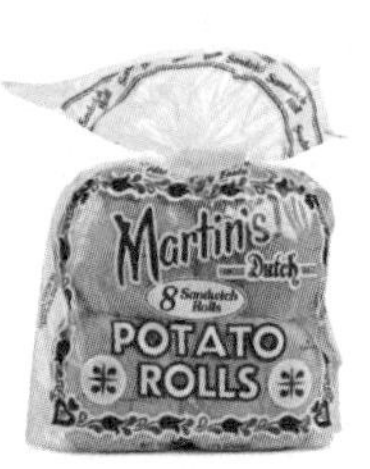

4 Martin's Potato Rolls, toasted

It is nearly impossible to find a burger at a sitdown restaurant with fewer than 1,000 calories. Blame the high-fat meat and heavy condiments. Here, we start with ground brisket, which is relatively lean but packed with perfect burger flavor. The butcher at your local market should be happy to grind up a hunk for you. We solve the condiment crisis by slowly caramelizing a full red onion until it's sweet and moist. Combine that with the great beef and peppery arugula for a first-class burger experience. If you must add cheese, a bit of crumbled blue goes well here.

YOU'LL ALSO NEED:

1 Tbsp butter

1 tsp each salt and fresh cracked pepper

10 oz ground sirloin

320 calories

12 g fat
(6 g saturated)

710 mg sodium

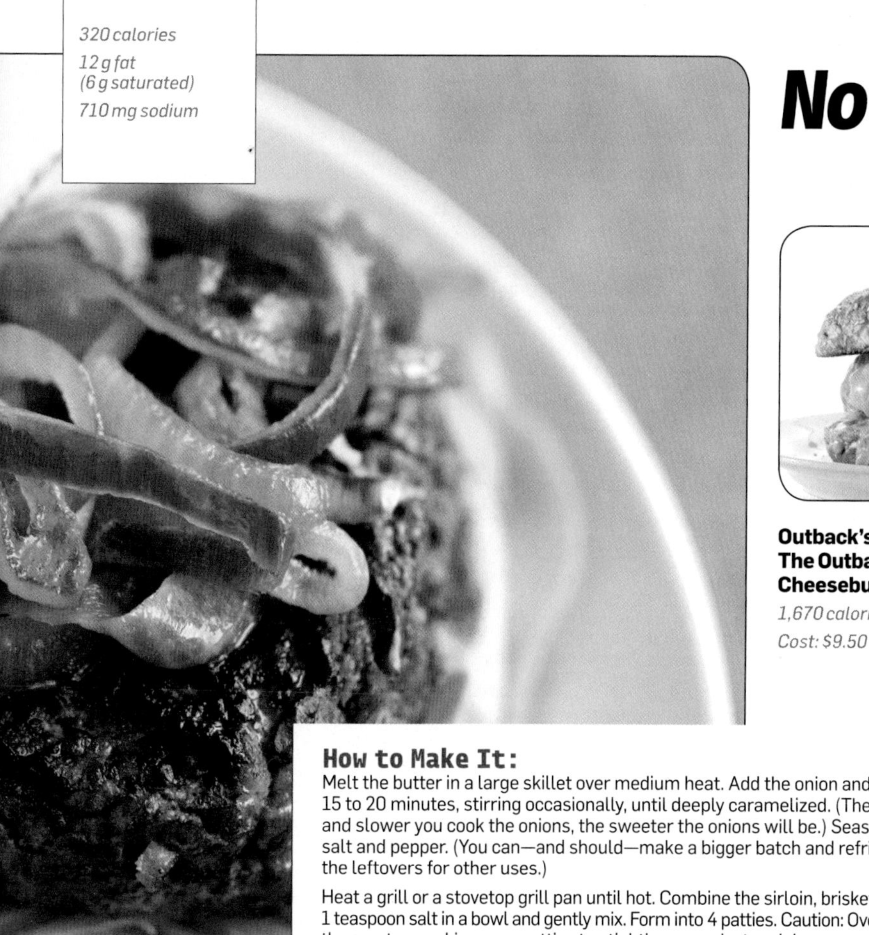

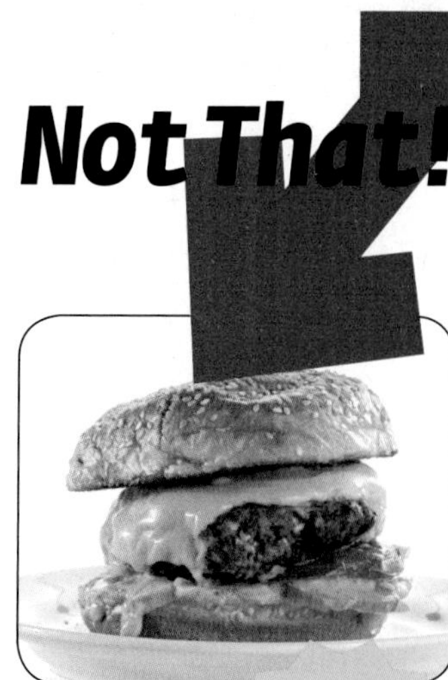

Not That!

Outback's The Outbacker Cheeseburger

1,670 calories

Cost: $9.50

Save!

Cost: $6.52

Calories: 1,350

How to Make It:

Melt the butter in a large skillet over medium heat. Add the onion and cook for 15 to 20 minutes, stirring occasionally, until deeply caramelized. (The longer and slower you cook the onions, the sweeter the onions will be.) Season with salt and pepper. (You can—and should—make a bigger batch and refrigerate the leftovers for other uses.)

Heat a grill or a stovetop grill pan until hot. Combine the sirloin, brisket, and 1 teaspoon salt in a bowl and gently mix. Form into 4 patties. Caution: Overworking the meat or packing your patties too tightly can make tough burgers.

Cook the burgers for 2 to 3 minutes and flip. Cook on the other side for another 2 to 3 minutes, until nicely charred on the outside but still medium-rare to medium within. (The center of the patty should be firm but easily yielding—like a Nerf football.) After you remove the burgers, toast the buns briefly.

Divide the arugula among the buns and top with the burgers and onions.

Makes 4 servings / Cost per serving: $2.98

Index

Boldface page references indicate photographs. Underscored references indicate boxed text.